Diagnostic, Prognostic and Predictive Biological Markers in Bladder Cancer —Illumination of a Vision 2.0

Diagnostic, Prognostic and Predictive Biological Markers in Bladder Cancer —Illumination of a Vision 2.0

Editors

Thorsten Ecke
Thomas Otto

MDPI • Basel • Beijing • Wuhan • Barcelona • Belgrade • Manchester • Tokyo • Cluj • Tianjin

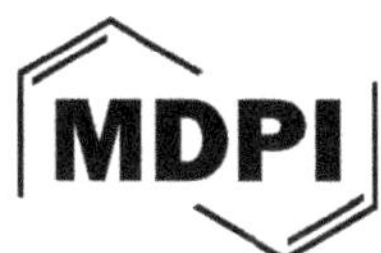

Editors
Thorsten Ecke
HELIOS Hospital Bad Saarow
Germany

Thomas Otto
Rheinland Klinikum Neuss
Germany

Editorial Office
MDPI
St. Alban-Anlage 66
4052 Basel, Switzerland

This is a reprint of articles from the Special Issue published online in the open access journal *International Journal of Molecular Sciences* (ISSN 1422-0067) (available at: https://www.mdpi.com/journal/ijms/special_issues/bladder_cancer_2019).

For citation purposes, cite each article independently as indicated on the article page online and as indicated below:

LastName, A.A.; LastName, B.B.; LastName, C.C. Article Title. *Journal Name* **Year**, *Article Number, Page Range.*

ISBN 978-3-03943-685-9 (Hbk)
ISBN 978-3-03943-686-6 (PDF)

Cover image courtesy of Aleksandra and Alicja Ecke.

Contents

About the Editors

Thorsten Ecke gained his medical degree from Humboldt University, Berlin—Charité (Germany) in 2000 after medical studies in Berlin and Turku (Finland). In 2005, he qualified in urology. In 2012, he became Head of the Prostate Center at Helios Hospital Bad Saarow (Germany). Since 2013 he has been teaching as an Associate Professor at Universitätmedizin Berlin Charité (Germany). He is the author and co-author of more than 80 articles. His areas of clinical and scientific expertise include uro-oncology, tumor markers, urinary-based markers, molecular biology, men's health, and the development of new diagnostic tools.

Thomas Otto gained his medical degree from the University of Essen (Germany) in 1983, and went on to work in the Department of General and Vascular Surgery at the Evangelisches Krankenhaus Mulheim/Ruhr. Between 1987 and 2004, he worked at the University of Essen in the Department of Urology, in addition to undertaking postdoctoral research in the Department of Cell Biology and Molecular Oncology. In 1996, he became an Associate Professor, and in 2001 a Professor of Urology. In 1993, Professor Dr. Otto qualified in urology, and qualified in urological surgery in 2004. In 2004, Professor Dr. Otto became the Head of the Department of Urology at the Städtische Kliniken Lukaskrankenhaus in Neuss. Since 2005, he has also been Head of the Institute of Tissue Engineering at the Städtische Kliniken Lukaskrankenhaus. He is the author and co-author of more than 400 articles. Professor Dr. Otto's areas of clinical expertise include oncology, pediatric urology, urinary incontinence, men's health, and tissue engineering. He is an expert in GMP (good manufacturing practice) and European pharmaceutical law. He has received several awards, including the German Association of Urology's Maximilian Nitze Award, the C.E. Alken Award, the European Association for Urology's (EAU) Scientific Newsflash Award, and the UNESCO Award in Bioethics.

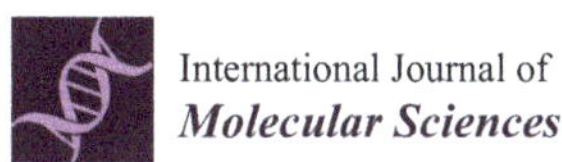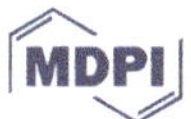

International Journal of
Molecular Sciences

Editorial

Illumination of a Vision 2020—Urinary Based Biomarkers for Bladder Cancer on the Way to Clinical Decisions—Dream or Nightmare?

Thorsten H. Ecke [1,*] and Thomas Otto [2,3,*]

[1] Department of Urology, HELIOS Hospital Bad Saarow, D-15526 Bad Saarow, Germany
[2] Department of Urology, Lukaskrankenhaus Neuss, D-41464 Neuss, Germany
[3] University Hospital Essen, D-45147 Essen, Germany
* Correspondence: thorsten.ecke@helios-kliniken.de (T.H.E.); totto@lukasneuss.de (T.O.)

Received: 13 January 2020; Accepted: 28 February 2020; Published: 2 March 2020

Bladder cancer is one of the most frequent malignancies worldwide [1]. For decades, it has been known that bladder cancer is heterogenous and therefore new markers are still needed for many different questions concerning diagnosis and therapy. Tumor grade and stage alone are not accurate in predicting the biological behavior and thus guiding the choice of treatment, especially in high risk cases [2–4].

Keeping the immense costs for bladder cancer patients from diagnosis to death with a calculation between US\$96,000 and \$187,000 in 2001 in mind, cheaper tests than cytology and tests preventing expensive and painful cystoscopies could help in reducing costs in the healthcare system [5,6]. However, additional information on risk profiles as well as personalized therapies are needed to reduce costs.

Up to date, no bladder cancer markers have been recommended in international guidelines, though cytology is still recommended in diagnostics [7]. Nevertheless, there are three interesting urinary-based fast tests that detect proteins on the market: UBC®, *rapid* test, BTA stat, and NMP22 [8–10]. All of these markers can show more or less high sensitivities in total or in some subgroups of bladder cancer, but none of them can be included into a routine or recommended in international guidelines. The lack of such meta-analysis lies in the problem that such studies are difficult to compare as test systems change during the years and studies differ significantly between each other regarding aim, material, and comparison. Therefore, the need of a study comparing these fast tests in comparison to the old gold standard cytology following the Paris system is needed [11]. On the other hand, in multicenter studies with a high volume of samples, the UBC® *rapid* test is close to the sensitivity of cytology, especially for high grade tumors [12]. It seems that urinary based fast tests that detect proteins could be the way to replace cytology, which is still a subjective method [13].

Referring again to the European Association of Urology (EAU) guidelines, we can observe that positive results of cytology as well as UroVysion (FISH), NMP22, FGFR3/TERT, and microsatellite analysis in patients with negative cystoscopy and upper tract work-up may identify patients who more likely to experience disease and possible progression [7]. Most molecular tests are very expensive and difficult to analyze, but even in that field of diagnostics, there have been attempts to produce commercially available tests with high sensitivity and specificity at lower costs than in previous years. Mutations of TERT and FGFR3 can easily be detected by Uromonitor, a urinary based fast test that showed high sensitivities and specificities in an actual study [14].

Clinical evidence and molecular studies suggest that there are two pathways in human bladder carcinogenesis: the pTa pathway and the CIS (carcinoma in situ) pathway [15]. In most cases, pTa tumors are low-grade, even high-grade in a few cases, and they often recur, but rarely progress to lamina propria-invasive (pT1) and muscle-invasive tumors (pT2-T4), whereas CIS are high-grade by definition and are thought to be the most common precursor of invasive tumors. A urinary-based assay that can diagnose bladder cancer confined by the urothelium/CIS could fulfil the criterion to differ between both. This model has also been confirmed by other publications in the past [16–18].

There is a clinical need for markers to determinate the recurrence and progression of bladder cancer; these markers will contribute to establishing better treatments for the individual patient. Molecular staging of urological tumors will allow for the selection of cases that will require systemic and/or target treatment [19,20].

Clinical needs in uro-oncology are related to diagnosis, prognosis, and treatment. Uro-oncology is diverse, since genitourinary tumors differ histologically in their origin and various clinical behavior [21].

In the past, more and more genetic and epigenetic markers could show its predictive and/or prognostic value regarding overall survival and even cancer specific survival. As an example of how a tumor marker can predict therapeutic success, the results of the phase 2 KEYNOTE-052 (NCT02335424) study showed how a marker could influence therapeutic decisions on one hand, and that negative marker results were also not a certain predictor of therapeutic success [22]. PD-L1 positive is defined as a combined positive score (CPS) $\geq$10. In patients with CPS <10 (n = 251), the overall response rate (ORR) was 20%, while in patients with CPS $\geq$10 (n = 110), the ORR was 47%. This shows that even patients with negative CPS could have the benefit of pembrolizumab in this case.

This Special Issue has been introduced with the aim of offering the possibility of publishing new research results in the field of bladder cancer basic research. While editing this Special Issue, we have learned that enormous enthusiasm is necessary move forward in bladder cancer research. In our eyes, bladder cancer is, on one hand, a very heterogenous malignancy, which is why it so difficult to focus on a single bladder cancer marker in diagnostic and follow-up. Due to the mass of all these markers, it is impossible to report them all. This Special Issue tries to highlight the role of bladder cancer markers in diagnosis and the most important biomarkers studied and recently reported. Due to the determination of recurrence and progression, markers will contribute to establishing better treatments for the individual patient. Molecular staging of urological tumors will allow for cases to be selected that will require systemic treatment. However, as above-mentioned at the moment, it is not clear if clinical decisions based on tumor markers are still a dream, or perhaps a real nightmare. However, is still necessary and more important than before to integrate the same objectives under basic and clinical research.

The editors thank all submitting authors for their efforts and time spent for each manuscript. The lead editor would like to thank all editors for the time spent in reviewing, assigning reviews, and commenting on the submitted manuscripts. As an editorial team, we hope that this Special Issue will prove useful in research work regarding bladder cancer in the future. Hopefully, many researchers will use any kind of art to improve their professional success to ameliorate diagnostics and therapy in bladder cancer!

References

1. Ferlay, J.; Steliarova-Foucher, E.; Lortet-Tieulent, J.; Rosso, S.; Coebergh, J.W.; Comber, H.; Forman, D.; Bray, F. Cancer incidence and mortality patterns in Europe: Estimates for 40 countries in 2012. *Eur. J. Cancer* **2013**, *49*, 1374–1403. [CrossRef] [PubMed]
2. Theodorescu, D.; Wittke, S.; Ross, M.M.; Walden, M.; Conaway, M.; Just, I.; Mischak, H.; Frierson, H.F. Discovery and validation of new protein biomarkers for urothelial cancer: A prospective analysis. *Lancet Oncol.* **2006**, *7*, 230–240. [CrossRef]
3. Sanchez-Carbayo, M.; Cordon-Cardo, C. Molecular alterations associated with bladder cancer progression. *Semin. Oncol.* **2007**, *34*, 75–84. [CrossRef] [PubMed]
4. Mhawech-Fauceglia, P.; Cheney, R.T.; Schwaller, J. Genetic alterations in urothelial bladder carcinoma: An updated review. *Cancer* **2006**, *106*, 1205–1216. [CrossRef] [PubMed]
5. Botteman, M.F.; Pashos, C.L.; Redaelli, A.; Laskin, B.; Hauser, R. The health economics of bladder cancer: A comprehensive review of the published literature. *Pharmacoeconomics* **2003**, *21*, 1315–1330. [CrossRef] [PubMed]

6.   Mitra, N.; Indurkhya, A. A propensity score approach to estimating the cost-effectiveness of medical therapies from observational data. *Health Econ.* **2005**, *14*, 805–815. [CrossRef] [PubMed]

7.   Babjuk, M.; Bohle, A.; Burger, M.; Capoun, O.; Cohen, D.; Compérat, E.M.; Hernández, V.; Kaasinen, E.; Palou, J.; Rouprêt, M.; et al. EAU Guidelines on Non-Muscle-invasive Urothelial Carcinoma of the Bladder: Update 2016. *Eur. Urol.* **2017**, *71*, 447–461. [CrossRef]

8.   Lu, P.; Cui, J.; Chen, K.; Lu, Q.; Zhang, J.; Tao, J.; Han, Z.; Zhang, W.; Song, R.; Gu, M. Diagnostic accuracy of the UBC((R)) Rapid Test for bladder cancer: A meta-analysis. *Oncol. Lett.* **2018**, *16*, 3770–3778. [CrossRef]

9.   Guo, A.; Wang, X.; Gao, L.; Shi, J.; Sun, C.; Wan, Z. Bladder tumour antigen (BTA stat) test compared to urine cytology in the diagnosis of bladder cancer: A meta-analysis. *Can. Urol. Assoc. J.* **2014**, *8*, E347–E352. [CrossRef]

10.   Wang, Z.; Que, H.; Suo, C.; Han, Z.; Tao, J.; Huang, Z.; Ju, X.; Tan, R.; Gu, M. Evaluation of the NMP22 BladderChek test for detecting bladder cancer: A systematic review and meta-analysis. *Oncotarget* **2017**, *8*, 100648–100656. [CrossRef]

11.   Barkan, G.A.; Wojcik, E.M.; Nayar, R.; Savic-Prince, S.; Quek, M.L.; Kurtycz, D.F.I.; Rosenthal, D.L. The Paris System for Reporting Urinary Cytology: The quest to develop a standardized terminology. *J. Am. Soc. Cytopathol.* **2016**, *5*, 177–188. [CrossRef] [PubMed]

12.   Ecke, T.H.; Weiss, S.; Stephan, C.; Hallmann, S.; Arndt, C.; Barski, D.; Otto, T.; Gerullis, H. UBC((R)) Rapid Test-A Urinary Point-of-Care (POC) Assay for Diagnosis of Bladder Cancer with a focus on Non-Muscle Invasive High-Grade Tumors: Results of a Multicenter-Study. *Int. J. Mol. Sci.* **2018**, *19*, 3841. [CrossRef] [PubMed]

13.   Schmitz-Drager, B.J.; Todenhofer, T.; van Rhijn, B.; Pesch, B.; Hudson, M.A.; Chandra, A.; Ingersoll, M.A.; Kassouf, W.; Palou, J.; Taylor, J. Considerations on the use of urine markers in the management of patients with low-/intermediate-risk non-muscle invasive bladder cancer. *Urol. Oncol.* **2014**, *32*, 1061–1068. [CrossRef] [PubMed]

14.   Batista, R.; Vinagre, J.; Prazeres, H.; Sampaio, C.; Peralta, P.; Conceição, P.; Sismeiro, A.; Leão, R.; Gomes, A.; Furriel, F.; et al. Validation of a Novel, Sensitive, and Specific Urine-Based Test for Recurrence Surveillance of Patients With Non-Muscle-Invasive Bladder Cancer in a Comprehensive Multicenter Study. *Front. Genet.* **2019**, *10*, 1237. [CrossRef]

15.   Spruck, C.H., 3rd; Ohneseit, P.F.; Gonzalez-Zulueta, M.; Esrig, D.; Miyao, N.; Tsai, Y.C.; Lerner, S.P.; Schmütte, C.; Yang, A.S.; Cote, R.; et al. Two molecular pathways to transitional cell carcinoma of the bladder. *Cancer Res.* **1994**, *54*, 784–788.

16.   Van Rhijn, B.W.; van der Kwast, T.H.; Vis, A.N.; Kirkels, W.J.; Boevé, E.R.; Jöbsis, A.C.; Zwarthoff, E.C. FGFR3 and P53 characterize alternative genetic pathways in the pathogenesis of urothelial cell carcinoma. *Cancer Res.* **2004**, *64*, 1911–1914. [CrossRef]

17.   Bakkar, A.A.; Wallerand, H.; Radvanyi, F.; Lahaye, J.B.; Pissard, S.; Lecerf, L.; Kouyoumdjian, J.C.; Abbou, C.C.; Pairon, J.C.; Jaurand, M.C.; et al. FGFR3 and TP53 gene mutations define two distinct pathways in urothelial cell carcinoma of the bladder. *Cancer Res.* **2003**, *63*, 8108–8112.

18.   Hernandez, S.; Lopez-Knowles, E.; Lloreta, J.; Kogevinas, M.; Jaramillo, R.; Amorós, A.; Tardón, A.; García-Closas, R.; Serra, C.; Carrato, A.; et al. FGFR3 and Tp53 mutations in T1G3 transitional bladder carcinomas: Independent distribution and lack of association with prognosis. *Clin. Cancer Res.* **2005**, *11*, 5444–5450. [CrossRef]

19.   Lopez-Beltran, A.; Montironi, R. Non-invasive urothelial neoplasms: According to the most recent WHO classification. *Eur. Urol.* **2004**, *46*, 170–176. [CrossRef]

20.   Montironi, R.; Lopez-Beltran, A. The 2004 WHO classification of bladder tumors: A summary and commentary. *Int. J. Surg. Pathol.* **2005**, *13*, 143–153. [CrossRef]

21.   Agarwal, P.K.; Black, P.C.; Kamat, A.M. Considerations on the use of diagnostic markers in management of patients with bladder cancer. *World J. Urol.* **2008**, *26*, 39–44. [CrossRef] [PubMed]

22.   Suzman, D.L.; Agrawal, S.; Ning, Y.M.; Maher, V.E.; Fernandes, L.L.; Karuri, S.; Tang, S.; Sridhara, R.; Schroeder, J.; Goldberg, K.B.; et al. FDA Approval Summary: Atezolizumab or Pembrolizumab for the Treatment of Patients with Advanced Urothelial Carcinoma Ineligible for Cisplatin-Containing Chemotherapy. *Oncologist* **2019**, *24*, 563–569. [CrossRef] [PubMed]

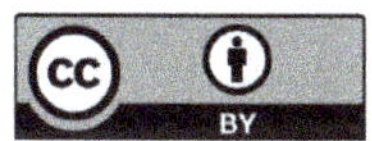

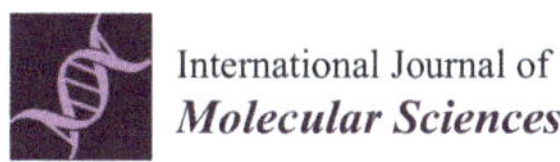
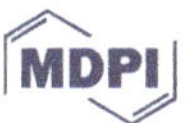

International Journal of
Molecular Sciences

Article

Prognostic Role of Survivin and Macrophage Infiltration Quantified on Protein and mRNA Level in Molecular Subtypes Determined by RT-qPCR of *KRT5*, *KRT20*, and *ERBB2* in Muscle-Invasive Bladder Cancer Treated by Adjuvant Chemotherapy

Thorsten H. Ecke [1,2,*], Adisch Kiani [3], Thorsten Schlomm [3], Frank Friedersdorff [3], Anja Rabien [3,4], Klaus Jung [3,4], Ergin Kilic [5], Peter Boström [6], Minna Tervahartiala [7], Pekka Taimen [8], Jan Gleichenhagen [9], Georg Johnen [9], Thomas Brüning [9], Stefan Koch [2,10], Jenny Roggisch [10] and Ralph M. Wirtz [11]

[1] Department of Urology, HELIOS Hospital Bad Saarow, DE-15526 Bad Sarrow, Germany

[2] Brandenburg Medical School, DE-14770 Brandenburg, Germany; stefan.koch@helios-gesundheit.de

[3] Department of Urology, Charité—Universitätsmedizin, Corporate Member of Freie Universität Berlin, Humboldt-Universität zu Berlin, and Berlin Institute of Health, DE-10098 Berlin, Germany; adisch.kiani@charite.de (A.K.); thorsten.schlomm@charite.de (T.S.); frank.friedersdorff@charite.de (F.F.); Anja.Rabien@charite.de (A.R.); klaus.jung@charite.de (K.J.)

[4] Berlin Institute for Urological Research, DE-10098 Berlin, Germany

[5] Institute of Pathology, DE-51375 Leverkusen, Germany; e.kilic@pathologie-leverkusen.de

[6] Department of Urology, Turku University Hospital, FI-20521 Turku, Finland; peter.j.bostrom@gmail.com

[7] MediCity Research Laboratory, Department of Medical Microbiology and Immunology, University of Turku, FI-20520 Turku, Finland; mmbost@utu.fi

[8] Institute of Pathology, Turku University Hospital, FI-20521 Turku, Finland; pepeta@utu.fi

[9] Institute for Prevention and Occupational Medicine of the German Social Accident Insurance (IPA), Institute of the Ruhr University Bochum, DE-44789 Bochum, Germany; Gleichenhagen@ipa-dguv.de (J.G.); johnen@ipa-dguv.de (G.J.); bruening@ipa-dguv.de (T.B.)

[10] Institute of Pathology, HELIOS Hospital Bad Saarow, DE-15526 Bad Sarrow, Germany; jenny.roggisch@helios-gesundheit.de

[11] STRATIFYER Molecular Pathology GmbH, DE-50935 Cologne, Germany; ralph.wirtz@stratifyer.de

* Correspondence: thorsten.ecke@helios-gesundheit.de; Tel.: +49-33631-72267; Fax: +49-33631-73136

Received: 29 July 2020; Accepted: 30 September 2020; Published: 8 October 2020

Abstract: Objectives: Bladder cancer is a heterogeneous malignancy. Therefore, it is difficult to find single predictive markers. Moreover, most studies focus on either the immunohistochemical or molecular assessment of tumor tissues by next-generation sequencing (NGS) or PCR, while a combination of immunohistochemistry (IHC) and PCR for tumor marker assessment might have the strongest impact to predict outcome and select optimal therapies in real-world application. We investigated the role of proliferation survivin/*BIRC5* and macrophage infiltration (CD68, MAC387, CLEVER-1) on the basis of molecular subtypes of bladder cancer (KRT5, KRT20, ERBB2) to predict outcomes of adjuvant treated muscle-invasive bladder cancer patients with regard to progression-free survival (PFS) and disease-specific survival (DSS). Materials and Methods: We used tissue microarrays (TMA) from n = 50 patients (38 males, 12 female) with muscle-invasive bladder cancer. All patients had been treated with radical cystectomy followed by adjuvant triple chemotherapy. Median follow-up time was 60.5 months. CD68, CLEVER-1, MAC387, and survivin protein were detected by immunostaining and subsequent visual inspection. *BIRC5*, *KRT5*, *KRT20*, *ERBB2*, and *CD68* mRNAs were detected by standardized RT-qPCR after tissue dot RNA extraction using a novel stamp technology. All these markers were evaluated in three different centers of excellence. Results: Nuclear staining rather than cytoplasmic staining of survivin predicted DSS as a single marker with high levels of survivin being associated with better PFS and DSS upon adjuvant chemotherapy ($p = 0.0138$ and $p = 0.001$, respectively). These results were validated by the quantitation of *BIRC5* mRNA by PCR ($p = 0.0004$ and $p = 0.0508$, respectively). Interestingly, nuclear staining of survivin protein was positively associated with *BIRC5* mRNA, while cytoplasmic staining was inversely related, indicating that the translocation of survivin protein into the nucleus occurred at a discrete, higher level of its mRNA. Combining survivin/*BIRC5* levels based on molecular subtype being assessed by *KRT20* expression improved the predictive value, with tumors having low survivin/*BIRC5* and *KRT20* mRNA levels having the best survival (75% vs. 20% vs. 10% 5-year DSS, $p = 0.0005$), and these values were independent of grading, node status, and tumor stage in multivariate analysis ($p = 0.0167$). Macrophage infiltration dominated in basal tumors and was inversely related with the luminal subtype marker gene expression. The presence of macrophages in survivin-positive or *ERBB2*-positive tumors was associated with worse DSS. Conclusions: For muscle-invasive bladder cancer patients, the proliferative activity as determined by the nuclear staining of survivin or RT-qPCR on the basis of molecular subtype characteristics outperforms single marker detections and single technology approaches. Infiltration by macrophages detected by IHC or PCR is associated with worse outcome in defined subsets of tumors. The limitations of this study are the retrospective nature and the limited number of patients. However, the number of molecular markers has been restricted and based on predefined assumptions, which resulted in the dissection of muscle-invasive disease into tumor–biological axes of high prognostic relevance, which warrant further investigation and validation.

Keywords: survivin; BIRC5; macrophage; KRT20; ERBB2; MIBC; prediction; RT-qPCR; adjuvant chemotherapy; survival; bladder cancer

---

1. Introduction

Bladder cancer is the fifth most frequent cancer in Europe. In 2018, its incidence and annual mortality rate were estimated to reach 197,105 and 64,966 cases, respectively [1]. Approximately 30% of these patients suffered from muscle-invasive bladder cancer (MIBC) at the time of initial diagnosis [2]. Radical cystectomy (RC) is the gold standard to treat these patients. Compared to patients with non-muscle-invasive bladder cancer (NMIBC), MIBC patients are subject to a high risk of cancer-related death.

In order to remedy this unsatisfactory situation, serious efforts have recently focused on new therapeutic strategies regarding the application of neoadjuvant and adjuvant chemotherapies [3]. A better risk assessment of patients has been recommended by developing novel predictive/prognostic models [4]. In clinical practice, the therapeutic management of these patients has so far been performed almost exclusively on the basis of clinical data and classical pathological TNM criteria but with few reliable results [4]. It is hoped that the identification of new molecular tissue biomarkers could help to stratify risk groups and determine patients who could have a benefit from adjuvant strategies after surgery [5]. In the last decades, many different markers (nucleic acid or protein based) have been identified to add more information on risk assessment. A subset of different markers was selected and further investigated in this study.

Survivin, also known as baculoviral IAP repeat containing 5 (BIRC5), is a member of the inhibitor of apoptosis family and has an important role in cell cycle regulation [6]. The protein survivin is present in different tumor tissues; it occurs in cytoplasm, but also in nuclei [7,8]. The protein is very rarely present in normal tissue [9]. Survivin acts as an apoptosis suppressor in cytoplasm and nuclei and influences cell division [8]. If the stress signal is high enough, survivin is released into cytoplasm, which leads to the inhibition of different caspases [10]. The relevance of *BIRC5* mRNA expression has been less studied in detail. However, its high prognostic impact for certain bladder cancer stages has been shown in the prospective UROMOL trial, wherein it belongs to a 12 gene signature with an adverse effect on survival for NMIBC [11].

CD68 is the most frequently used pan-macrophage marker. Its function is still unknown, but it has been considered to play a role in the phagocytic activities of tissue macrophages [12]. Common lymphatic endothelial and vascular endothelial receptor-1 (CLEVER-1, also known as stabilin-1 or STAB1) is a multifunctional immunosuppressive scavenger receptor expressed by lymphatic and vascular endothelial cells and tissue macrophages [13]. Its prognostic significance in bladder cancer is not clear, but there is evidence that high CLEVER-1-positive macrophage count associates with chemoresistance [14] in neoadjuvant-treated bladder cancer patients. The monoclonal antibody MAC387 detects an epitope on the calcium-binding protein MRP14/S100A9 present in the cytosol of monocytes and granulocytes [15]. It is the exclusive arachidonic acid-binding protein in human neutrophils and is thereby involved in the calcium-dependent cellular signal of lipid second messengers during inflammatory and metabolic changes of tumor-associated macrophages [16].

The molecular subtyping of bladder cancer has been well accepted after its initial introduction in 2014 [17–19]. Therein, the quantitation of *KRT5* and *KRT20* on mRNA level and/or their recapitulation on protein level by immunohistochemistry (IHC) have been identified as exemplary biomarkers for the molecular subtyping of basal and luminal tumors, respectively. In our previous work, we could show that *KRT20* is strongly associated with adverse outcome for pT1 NMIBC [20].

ERBB2 belongs to the key bladder cancer genes as recently defined in an international consensus paper [21]. Belonging to the EGFR-related receptor tyrosine kinase family, it is a key driver and well-established drug target in breast and gastric cancer. In our previous work, we showed that *ERBB2* mRNA expression is superior to the WHO grading of 1973 when dissecting the remaining risk in pT1 NMIBC exhibiting centrally confirmed grade 3 [22], with high *ERBB2* mRNA levels indicating inferior outcome (90% vs. 50% 5-year PFS, $p < 0.0001$). Higher levels are also associated with worse outcome in MIBC not being treated by adjuvant or neoadjuvant chemotherapy [23], with *ERBB2*-positive tumors above median mRNA expression having worse prognosis (20% vs. 60% 4-year DSS, $p = 0.009$). *ERBB2* mRNA is associated with luminal subtypes of bladder cancer [17–19].

However, the prognostic role of these markers in MIBC patients receiving adjuvant chemotherapy is unknown. The aim of the present study was to evaluate the prognostic role of the above-mentioned fundamental bladder cancer markers in the adjuvant situation and to test their clinical usefulness when assessed by IHC or PCR in context with clinical parameters to provide real-world evidence for the respective tumor biological motifs. The herein presented work served as a pilot study for validation of the above-mentioned biomarker assessment and moreover allowing the formulation of a working hypothesis for subsequent prospective non-interventional validation studies in the future. These studies are currently being planned and ultimately may lead to prospective interventional study designs.

2. Results

2.1. Patient Population

Clinical characteristics are presented in Table 1. The total study cohort consisted of 50 MIBC tumor patients diagnosed from 1996 to 2006 at a single institution. Median age was 65 years, with 76% male patients and 34% female patients; 50% of patients had ECOG status 0, while 34% and 16% were ECOG1 and ECOG2, respectively. Forty-two percent of patients were N0 at initial diagnosis, while 14% were N1 and 44% were N2. Median follow-up was 60.5 months with 54% of patients suffering from disease-specific deaths. Similar clinical characteristics were found in the analysis cohorts as defined in the cohort diagram (Table 1).

Table 1. Clinical characteristics of patients in the total cohort ($n = 50$), and the PCR ($n = 39$) and combined IHC and PCR subcohorts ($n = 28$). IHC: immunohistochemistry.

Cohort	Total Cohort	PCR Cohort	IHC & PCR Cohort
Size (n)	50	39	28
Age (years)			
Average	65	67	68.5
Range	49-80	48–80	48–80
Gender			
Male	38 (76%)	27 (69%)	18 (64%)
Female	12 (24%)	12 (31%)	10 (36%)
ECOG Performance Status			
0	25 (50%)	19 (49%)	11 (39%)
1	17 (34%)	13 (33%)	11 (39%)
2	8 (16%)	7 (18%)	6 (21%)
Lymph Node Metastases before Chemotherapy			
N0	21 (42%)	16 (41%)	10 (36%)
N1	7 (14%)	4 (10%)	2 (7%)
N2	22 (44%)	(19 (49%)	16 (57%)
Clinical outcome after Chemotherapy			
Progression	27 (54%)	21 (54%)	18 (64%)
Overall death	36 (72%)	29 (74%)	23 (82%)
Disease specific death	27 (54%)	21 (54%)	19 (68%)
Overall survival	14 (28%)	10 (26%)	5 (18%)
Response to Chemotherapy			
Complete response	20 (40%)	15 (38%)	8 (29%)
Partial response	3 (6%)	2 (5%)	1 (4%)
No change	25 (50%)	20 (51%)	18 (64%)

2.2. Distribution of Assessed Protein Markers across the Study Cohort

All investigated experimental markers could be determined by IHC or PCR in the same tissue microarray (TMA) samples of urinary bladder cancer transurethral resection of bladder (TURB) biopsies.

2.3. Distribution of Assessed mRNA Markers across the Study Cohort

As depicted in the remark diagram (Figure 1), TURB biopsies from 39 patients could be analyzed, while IHC data were available from 28 TURB biopsies.

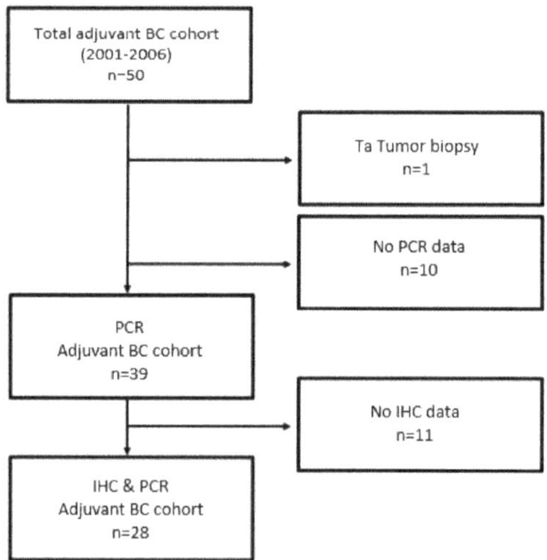

Figure 1. Remark diagram.

Data distribution of immunohistochemical staining of CD68, CLEVER-1, MAC387, and survivin by digital image analysis, visual inspection, or semi-quantitative assessment of cytoplasmic versus nuclear staining indicated a substantial infiltration of macrophages into the TURB biopsies of tumor specimens, while visual inspection reached higher sensitivity than image analysis. The numbers of CD68+ macrophages and CLEVER-1 positive macrophages and vessels were scored from three hotspots (areas with the most macrophages by eye) intratumorally and peritumorally with a 0.0625 mm^2 grid using 40× magnification when scoring macrophages and 20× when scoring lymphatic/blood vessels. The scoring was performed independently by two observers blinded to the clinical information. Cases with an inadequate quality of immunohistochemical staining or tumor morphology were excluded from further statistical analyses. Survivin protein expression could be observed in almost all TURB biopsies with varying extent, while the nuclear staining of survivin could be detected in only 60% of cases (Figure 2a).

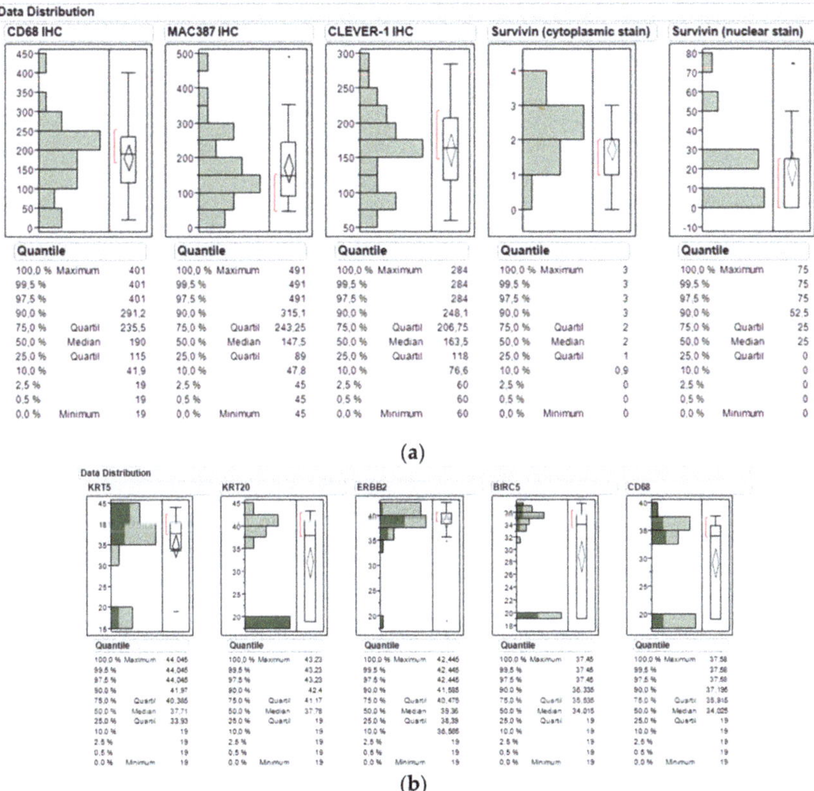

Figure 2. (**a**) Data distribution of immunohistochemical staining of CD68, MAC387, and common lymphatic endothelial and vascular endothelial receptor-1 (CLEVER-1) by visual analysis and survivin by semi-quantitative assessment of cytoplasmic versus nuclear stain; (**b**) Data distribution and box and whisker plot of *KRT5, KRT20, ERBB2, BIRC5,* and *CD68* mRNA levels in the bladder cancer study cohort treated by adjuvant chemotherapy (*n* = 39). Normalized gene expression (40-DCT method) as well as quantile values are depicted in the y-axis. DCT: Delta Cycle Threshold.

RNA expression of the candidate genes *KRT5, KRT20, ERBB2, BIRC5,* and *CD68* could also be detected to a varying extent. While *ERBB2* mRNA levels could be determined in almost all cases (38 of 39 samples), *KRT5* and *KRT20* mRNA were detected in fewer biopsies (31 of 39 and 24 of 39 samples, respectively). Similarly, *BIRC5* and *CD68* were detected in subsets of the TURB tissue dots (24 of 39 samples, each). A comparison of NMIBC and MIBC was possible for only four patients. Marker gene expression was comparable. However, with regard to *KRT20* expression, one MIBC did exhibit a significantly increased expression of the luminal marker *KRT20*.

2.4. Correlation of Protein and mRNA Markers on Basis of Molecular Subtyping and Clinical Variables

A comparison of survivin protein expression in cytoplasm versus nucleus compared to its respective mRNA level revealed that higher mRNA is positively associated to nuclear expression (Spearman rho 0.2949) and negatively associated with cytoplasmic stain (Spearman rho −0.3026), while both associations did not yet reach statistical significance due to small sample size (Figure 3).

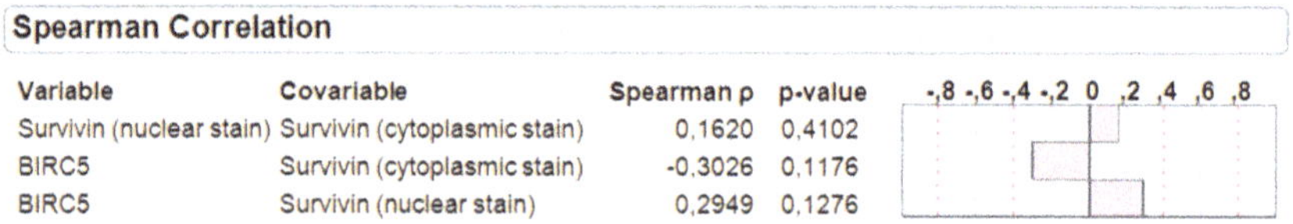

Spearman Correlation

Variable	Covariable	Spearman ρ	p-value	-,8 -,6 -,4 -,2 0 ,2 ,4 ,6 ,8
Survivin (nuclear stain)	Survivin (cytoplasmic stain)	0,1620	0,4102	
BIRC5	Survivin (cytoplasmic stain)	-0,3026	0,1176	
BIRC5	Survivin (nuclear stain)	0,2949	0,1276	

Figure 3. Spearman correlation of IHC staining and semi-quantitative assessment of survivin protein located in cytoplasmic versus nuclear localization with quantitative *BIRC5* (survivin) mRNA levels in the combined PCR and IHC cohort (*n* = 28). Graphical display of Spearman rho values and respective *p*-values are depicted.

As depicted in Figure 4a, Spearman correlation of the intergene RNA expression relations revealed a strong positive association between the two luminal cancer markers *KRT20* and *ERBB2* (Spearman rho 0.6811, *p* < 0.0001) and inverse relation between the luminal *KRT20* and basal *KRT5* marker (Spearman rho −0.3588, *p* = 0.0249) as expected. The negative association between *ERBB2* and *KRT5* was less prominent and not significant (Spearman rho −0.1473, *p* = 0.3709), indicating that several basal-like tumors harbor elevated *ERBB2* expression to some extent. Of note, the proliferation/apoptosis marker *BIRC5* was positively associated with *CD68* mRNA levels (Spearman rho 0.3484, *p* = 0.0156).

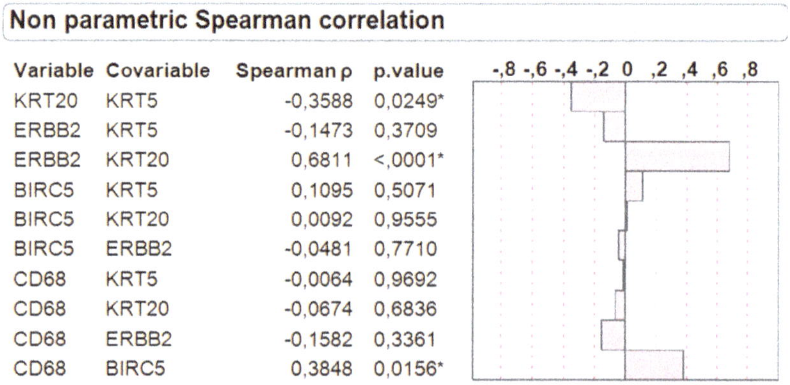

Non parametric Spearman correlation

Variable	Covariable	Spearman ρ	p.value	-,8 -,6 -,4 -,2 0 ,2 ,4 ,6 ,8
KRT20	KRT5	-0,3588	0,0249*	
ERBB2	KRT5	-0,1473	0,3709	
ERBB2	KRT20	0,6811	<,0001*	
BIRC5	KRT5	0,1095	0,5071	
BIRC5	KRT20	0,0092	0,9555	
BIRC5	ERBB2	-0,0481	0,7710	
CD68	KRT5	-0,0064	0,9692	
CD68	KRT20	-0,0674	0,6836	
CD68	ERBB2	-0,1582	0,3361	
CD68	BIRC5	0,3848	0,0156*	

(**a**)

Figure 4. *Cont.*

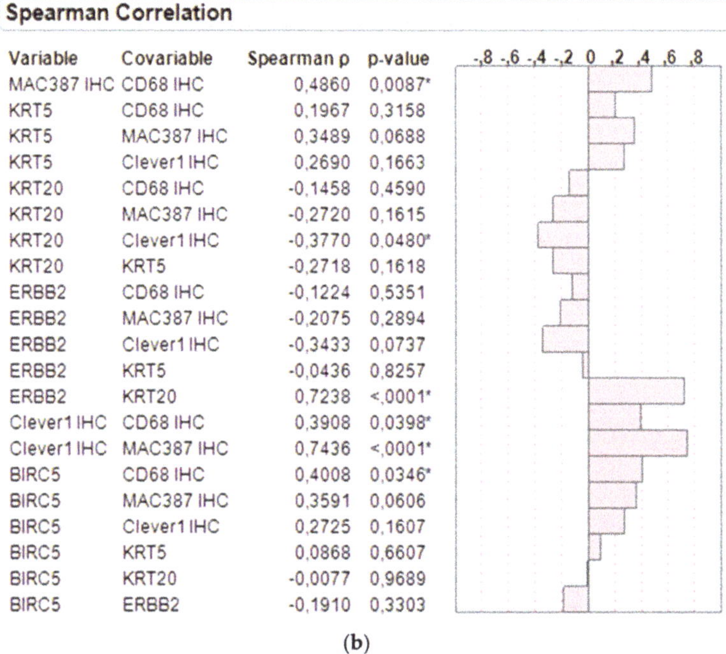

Spearman Correlation

Variable	Covariable	Spearman ρ	p-value
MAC387 IHC	CD68 IHC	0,4860	0,0087*
KRT5	CD68 IHC	0,1967	0,3158
KRT5	MAC387 IHC	0,3489	0,0688
KRT5	Clever1 IHC	0,2690	0,1663
KRT20	CD68 IHC	-0,1458	0,4590
KRT20	MAC387 IHC	-0,2720	0,1615
KRT20	Clever1 IHC	-0,3770	0,0480*
KRT20	KRT5	-0,2718	0,1618
ERBB2	CD68 IHC	-0,1224	0,5351
ERBB2	MAC387 IHC	-0,2075	0,2894
ERBB2	Clever1 IHC	-0,3433	0,0737
ERBB2	KRT5	-0,0436	0,8257
ERBB2	KRT20	0,7238	<,0001*
Clever1 IHC	CD68 IHC	0,3908	0,0398*
Clever1 IHC	MAC387 IHC	0,7436	<,0001*
BIRC5	CD68 IHC	0,4008	0,0346*
BIRC5	MAC387 IHC	0,3591	0,0606
BIRC5	Clever1 IHC	0,2725	0,1607
BIRC5	KRT5	0,0868	0,6607
BIRC5	KRT20	-0,0077	0,9689
BIRC5	ERBB2	-0,1910	0,3303

(**b**)

Figure 4. (**a**) Correlation of normalized *KRT5*, *KRT20*, *ERBB2*, *BIRC5*, and *CD68* mRNA levels in the PCR cohort ($n = 39$) of bladder cancer patients treated with adjuvant chemotherapy. Graphical display of Spearman rho values and respective p-values are depicted. * indicates statistically significant results; (**b**) Correlation of *KRT5*, *KRT20*, *ERBB2*, and *BIRC5* mRNA levels with protein levels of CD68, MAC387, and CLEVER-1 determined by IHC in the combined PCR and IHC cohort ($n = 28$) of bladder cancer patients treated with adjuvant chemotherapy. Graphical display of Spearman rho values and respective p-values are depicted. * indicates statistically significant results.

In line with this, *BIRC5* mRNA was also positively associated with CD68 levels determined by IHC (Spearman rho 0.4008, $p = 0.0346$; Figure 4b). Interestingly, infiltration by macrophages as determined by IHC of CD68 and MAC387 tended to be negatively associated with luminal tumors as determined by *KRT20* (Spearman rho −0.2720 and −0.1458) and positively with basal tumors as determined by *KRT5* (Spearman rho 0.1967 and 0.3489).

Pearson correlation of *KRT5*, *KRT20*, *ERBB2*, *BIRC5*, and *CD68* mRNA levels with clinical variables such as performance status (PS), age, sex, body mass index (BMI), presence of carcinoma in situ (Cis), tumor stage (T-prim), and WHO Grade 1973 (G-prim) levels in the larger PCR cohort (Figure 5a) revealed that luminal tumors determined by *KRT20* mRNA were negatively associated with the presence of Cis and positively associated with higher age and male gender. In contrast, basal tumors determined by *KRT5* were negatively associated with BMI. Interestingly, macrophage infiltration was positively associated with age and Cis, while being negatively associated with grade. *BIRC5* mRNA was comparably associated with Cis. Similar associations were obtained by doing Spearman correlations (Table 2).

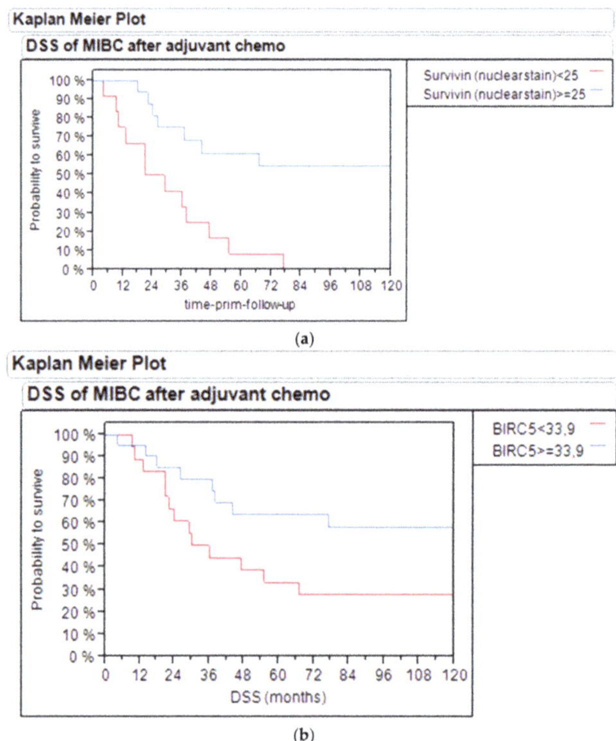

(a)

(b)

Figure 5. (**a**) Disease-specific survival (DSS) of bladder cancer patients treated with adjuvant chemotherapy based on survivin nuclear stain in the PCR and IHC cohort. (**b**) DSS of bladder cancer patients treated with adjuvant chemotherapy based on *BIRC5* mRNA expression in the PCR cohort.

Table 2. Pearson correlation of *KRT5*, *KRT20*, *ERBB2*, *BIRC5*, and *CD68* mRNA levels with performance status (PS), age, sex, body mass index (BMI), presence of carcinoma in situ (Cis), tumor size (T-prim), and WHO Grade 1973 (G-prim) levels in the PCR cohort of bladder cancer patients treated with adjuvant chemotherapy. Blue values indicate positive associations of significance, red values indicate negative associations of significance, and black values indicate insignificant trends.

	KRT5	KRT20	ERBB2	BIRC5	CD68	PS	Age	Sex	BMI	Cis	T-Prim	G-Prim
KRT5	1.0000	−0.1522	−0.0286	0.1052	0.0028	−0.0493	−0.0477	0.1678	−0.2302	−0.0040	−0.1413	0.0691
KRT20	−0.01522	1.0000	0.4266	0.0763	−0.1783	−0.0443	0.2165	0.2627	0.0498	−0.3599	−0.0544	0.1547
ERBB2	−0.0296	0.4266	1.0000	0.1019	0.0507	−0.2721	0.0280	0.3259	−0.0149	−0.0934	−0.1754	−0.0563
BIRC5	0.1052	0.0763	0.1019	1.0000	0.5390	−0.0579	0.2019	0.1273	−0.0553	0.2807	0.1831	0.0858
CD68	0.0028	−0.1783	0.0507	0.5390	1.0000	0.1646	0.3190	−0.0525	−0.1784	0.2361	0.1812	−0.2662
PS	−0.0493	−0.0443	−0.2721	−0.0578	0.1646	1.0000	0.3352	−0.1978	0.0978	−0.1370	0.1196	−0.0217
Age	−0.0477	0.2185	0.0280	0.2019	0.3190	0.3352	1.0000	0.1101	−0.3689	0.1915	−0.1977	−0.0184
Sex	0.1678	0.2827	0.3259	0.1273	−0.0625	−0.1978	0.1101	1.0000	0.0990	−0.0160	−0.1514	−0.0358
BMI	−0.2302	0.0498	−0.0149	−0.0553	−0.1784	0.0978	−0.3689	0.0990	1.0000	−0.2538	0.2724	−0.0904
Cis	−0.0040	−0.3599	−0.0934	0.2007	0.2361	−0.1370	0.1915	−0.0160	−0.2538	1.0000	−0.1852	0.0154
T-prim	−0.1413	−0.0544	−0.1754	0.1831	0.1612	0.1196	−0.1977	−0.1514	0.2724	−0.1852	1.0000	0.2200
G-prim	0.0691	0.1547	−0.0563	0.0858	−0.2662	−0.0217	−0.0184	−0.0356	−0.0904	0.0154	0.2200	1.0000

2.5. Disease-Specific Survival Analysis by Survivin and Macrophage Infiltration in Subtypes

Kaplan–Meier analysis revealed that high levels of survivin protein above the median expression (>25% positive nuclei) in the IHC cohort (n = 28) identified patients with improved disease-specific survival (DSS, 60% vs. 10% 5-year DSS, p = 0.001; Figure 5a) and PFS (60% vs. 10% 5-year PFS, p = 0.0138; Figure S1).

Similarly, in the enlarged PCR cohort (n = 39), high levels of *BIRC5* mRNA (DCT >33.9) identified patients with better outcome (60% vs. 30% 5-year DSS, p = 0.0507; Figure 5b) and progression-free survival (75% vs. 10% 5-year PFS, p = 0.0042; Figure S2).

Combining survivin expression and *KRT20* mRNA for outcome prediction revealed that *KRT20*-positive tumors as well as *BIRC5*-negative tumors had worse outcomes compared to survivin-positive tumors both on the protein level (20% and 10% vs. 75% 5-year DSS, p = 0.0005; Figure 6a) and mRNA level (30% each vs. 75% 5-year DSS, p = 0.0358; Figure 6b). Similarly, the combination of *KRT20* mRNA with *BIRC5* mRNA or survivin protein stain was significant for PFS (p = 0.0181 Figure S3 and p = 0.0209 Figure S4).

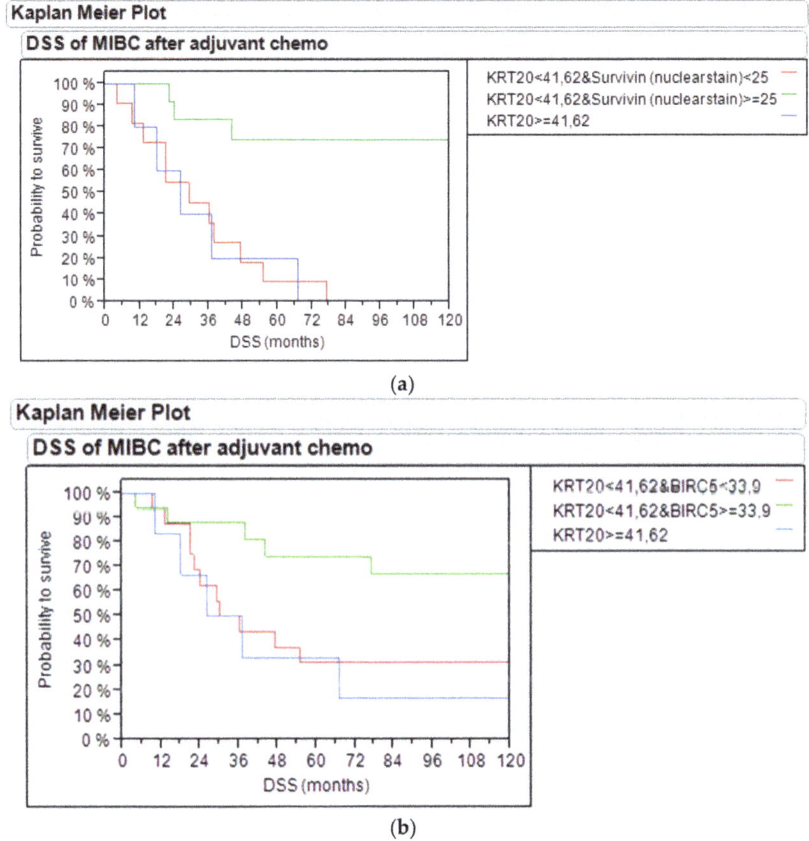

Figure 6. (**a**) DSS of bladder cancer patients treated with adjuvant chemotherapy based on *KRT20* mRNA and survivin nuclear protein stain in the PCR and IHC cohort; (**b**) DSS of bladder cancer patients treated with adjuvant chemotherapy based on *KRT20* and *BIRC5* mRNA expression in the PCR cohort.

Multivariate cox proportional hazard analysis of DSS revealed that the combination of *BIRC5* and *KRT20* mRNA to predict outcome was an independent prognostic factor, when age, sex, BMI, tumor stage, grade, and node status were included in the analysis (p = 0.0167, Table 3).

BMI and node status were also independent prognostic factors in multivariate cox regression. Similarly, multivariate cox proportional hazard analysis revealed that the combination of *BIRC5* and *KRT20* mRNA tended to be an independent prognostic factor for PFS (p = 0.0816; Table 4).

Table 3. Cox regression analysis for DSS by *BIRC5* × *KRT20* mRNA expression and clinicopathological features in the PCR cohort of bladder cancer patients treated with adjuvant chemotherapy. Statistically significant values are highlighted in boldface.

Parameter	Hazard Ratio	95% CI	p-Value
Age	1.07	0.99–1.14	0.0518
Sex	0.89	0.27–2.98	0.8329
BMI	1.16	1.00–1.24	**0.0499**
Node status	1.95	1.15–3.53	**0.0127**
Stage	1.13	0.42–3.16	0.8038
Grade	0.86	0.33–2.29	0.7638
KRT20 × BIRC5 Groups			
KRT20 low & BIRC5 high vs. KRT20 low & BIRC5 low	0.22	0.06–0.75	**0.0144**
KRT20 low & BIRC5 high vs. KRT20 high	0.24	0.06–0.94	**0.0407**
KRT20 low & BIRC5 low vs. KRT20 high	1.09	0.28–4.39	0.8988

Table 4. Cox regression analysis for progression-free survival (PFS) by *BIRC5* × *KRT20* mRNA expression and clinicopathological features in the PCR cohort of bladder cancer patients treated with adjuvant chemotherapy. Statistically significant values are highlighted in boldface.

Parameter	Hazard Ratio	95% CI	p-Value
Age	1.08	0.94–1.25	0.2911
Sex	1.25	0.23–7.45	0.7979
BMI	1.19	0.97–1.47	0.0985
Node status	1.75	0.89–3.87	0.1045
Stage	0.65	0.19–2.11	0.4750
Grade	0.86	0.33–2.29	0.4989
KRT20 × BIRC5 Groups			
KRT20 low & BIRC5 high vs. KRT20 low & BIRC5 low	0.15	0.02–0.79	**0.0252**
KRT20 low & BIRC5 high vs. KRT20 high	0.26	0.02–1.93	0.1908
KRT20 low & BIRC5 low vs. KRT20 high	1.77	0.41–8.92	0.4489

Combining survivin protein with the quantitation of macrophage infiltration based on protein or mRNA level revealed that the presence of macrophages in MIBC treated with adjuvant chemotherapy had an adverse effect on DSS. Tumors with high levels of nuclear survivin protein levels but low *CD68* mRNA levels had the best survival (70% vs. 40% vs. 10% 5-year DSS, p = 0.0083; Figure 7a). Similar results were found for PFS (p = 0.0169, Figure S5).

In line with this, tumors with high levels of nuclear survivin protein levels but low MAC387 protein levels had the best survival (100% vs. 30% vs. 10% 5-year DSS, p = 0.0011; Figure 7b). Similar results were found for PFS (p = 0.0259, Figure S6). Additionally, Figure S7 shows DSS of bladder cancer patients treated with adjuvant chemotherapy based on survivin nuclear protein stain and CLEVER-1 protein in the PCR and IHC cohort. Figure S8 shows PFS of bladder cancer patients treated with adjuvant chemotherapy based on survivin nuclear protein stain and CLEVER-1 protein in the PCR and IHC cohort.

Importantly and in contrast to previous publications, in pT1 NMIBC [22] and MIBC [23] not treated with chemotherapy, the overexpression of *ERBB2* was not related to adverse outcome (data not shown). However, within *ERBB2*-positive tumors (median mRNA expression), the presence of macrophages as determined by RT-qPCR of *CD68* had an adverse effect on the DSS of adjuvant-treated MIBC patients

(70% vs. 20% 5-year DSS, *p* = 0.0280; Figure 8). Similarly, the combination of *ERBB2* and *CD68* tended to predict PFS (*p* = 0.0537, Figure S9).

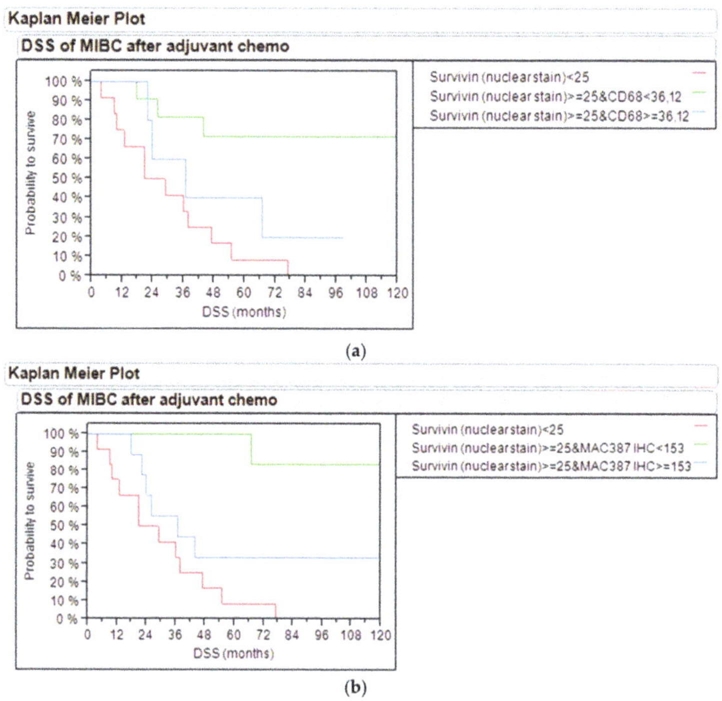

Figure 7. (**a**) DSS of bladder cancer patients treated with adjuvant chemotherapy based on survivin nuclear protein staining and *CD68* mRNA in the PCR and IHC cohort. (**b**) DSS of bladder cancer patients treated with adjuvant chemotherapy based on survivin nuclear protein staining and MAC387 protein in the PCR and IHC cohort.

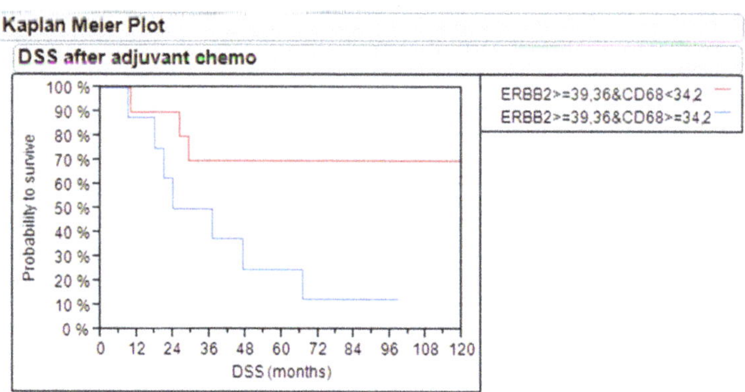

Figure 8. DSS of bladder cancer patients treated with adjuvant chemotherapy based on *ERBB2*-positive tumors in relation to *CD68* mRNA levels in the PCR and IHC cohort.

3. Discussion

High levels of survivin have been associated with poor prognosis in bladder cancer [24]. Survivin has also been described to be a predictor of cisplatin-resistance in gastric cancer, as well as in different cell lines [25,26]. A higher proliferative activity determined by *BIRC5* mRNA expression has been associated with worse outcome in NMIBC [11]. In line with this, a higher WHO 1973 grade was associated with *MKI67* and *ERBB2* mRNA levels [20]. Similarly, *FOXM1* mRNA expression was associated with a higher grade and stage as well as a 6 to 8-fold higher risk of progression in multivariable analysis ($p < 0.03$) of the UROMOL study (n = 488), which could be validated in independent NMIBC cohorts (n = 277) in silico [27]. Further analysis revealed that proliferation as determined by *FOXM1* mRNA expression was predictive for chemotherapy benefit in T1 NMIBC (n = 296) with patients having low *FOXM1* expression having better outcomes, irrespective of instillation therapy, while patients with high *FOXM1* expression benefitted from intravesical chemotherapy with mitomycin C [28]. In addition, meta-analysis revealed survivin protein and RNA to be associated with adverse outcome in NMIBC [29]. However, the predictive or prognostic role of proliferation and particularly of survivin is less clear for MIBC, particularly upon chemotherapeutic intervention targeting proliferative tissues. We showed that a high expression of survivin both on protein and RNA level was associated with good outcome in MIBC patients treated with adjuvant chemotherapy. It has to be noted that the triple chemotherapeutic regimen investigated within this study including taxol in addition to platinum-based chemotherapy is no standard regimen, which has to be taken into account when interpreting the results. However, it is reasonable that highly proliferative tissues do exhibit better response to chemotherapeutic regimen. Moreover, it has to be assumed that adding taxol to the standard chemotherapeutic regimen does not diminish the non-response of tumor tissues with low proliferative activity reflected by low survivin expression. This indicates that survivin might be a good predictive marker for chemotherapy benefit, which should be further investigated in randomized clinical trials. In contrast, low levels of nuclear staining of survivin were associated with the DSS of only 10% of patients after 5 years ($p = 0.001$), which indicates that tumors with low proliferation and apoptotic activity as indicated by survivin expression do require alternative treatment approaches.

In contrast, Als et al. identified survivin as a molecular marker for survival in locally advanced and/or metastatic bladder cancer following cisplatin-based chemotherapy [30]. In their study, multivariate analysis revealed that survivin expression was an independent marker for poor outcome, together with the presence of visceral metastases. In the group of patients without visceral metastases, both markers showed significant discriminating power as supplemental risk factors ($p < 0.0001$). Protein expression assessed by IHC was strongly correlated to response to chemotherapy. Another study on survivin was published by Pollard et al. [31]. This group evaluated an approach that combines genomic, proteomic, and therapeutic outcome datasets to identify novel putative urinary biomarkers of clinical outcome after neoadjuvant application of methotrexate, vinblastine, adriamycin, and cisplatin (MVAC). Using disease-free survival as a marker for clinical outcome, this group evaluated the ability of GGH, emmprin, survivin, and DBI expression in tumor tissue to stratify 27 patients treated with neoadjuvant MVAC. Interestingly, DBI ($p = 0.046$) but not GGH ($p = 0.190$), emmprin ($p = 0.066$), or survivin ($p = 0.393$) successfully stratified patients [31]. Our study revealed an inverse relation of survivin protein in cytoplasmic versus nuclear localization particularly when compared to its mRNA levels. This indicates the need of careful subcellular quantitation and may in part explain conflicting study results with regard to the prognostic and or predictive value of survivin expression, as discussed above.

Importantly, in our study, the proliferative subset of MIBC patients having better survival (i.e., 60% DSS after 5 years) could be further dissected by macrophage infiltration. Tervahartiala et al. [14] found that MAC387+ cells as well as CLEVER-1+ macrophages and vessels are associated with the response after neoadjuvant chemotherapy in bladder cancer patients. High MAC387+ tumor cell density was associated with disease progression after neoadjuvant chemotherapy, whereas the majority of patients with a lower amount of MAC387+ tumor cells exhibited a complete response. Patients with high amounts of CLEVER-1+ macrophages were associated with a poorer response to neoadjuvant chemotherapy, while higher amounts of CLEVER-1+ vessels were associated with a more favorable response [14]. The results of Tervahartiala et al. [14] verified also their previous studies where they could demonstrate that CD68 and MAC387 are associated with poorer survival in bladder cancer patients, whereas CLEVER-1-positive vessels act more as a protective marker [32].

In our study, we could validate that the presence of macrophages as determined by immunohistochemistry of CD68, CLEVER-1, and MAC387 or PCR of *CD68* was associated with worse disease-specific survival, particularly in tumors of high proliferative activity or elevated *ERBB2* mRNA expression.

Macrophages are challenging to investigate by immunohistochemistry due to their nature to cluster. This may lead to variations in results, especially when using TMAs and would require sufficient tissue sampling in routine clinical practice. TMAs are an efficient method in immunohistochemistry, but the results should be interpreted with care when studying clustering particles, e.g., macrophages. RNA quantitation may offer advantages by a more objective and standardized assessment of macrophage infiltration and the opportunity to embed the results in the context of immune infiltrates of diverse sets of T-cells with specified functions such as natural killer cells, helper cells, and regulatory T-cells.

The potential limitations of our study relate to its retrospective design and the impact of factors such as age and comorbidity on the indication of cystectomy and, consequently, on cancer-specific mortality in the elderly patients. The number of patients was limited, but the study included consecutive bladder cancer patients, who received adjuvant chemotherapy after radical cystectomy. Since retrospective designs do not guarantee causality, further prospective studies and the use of an independent series are warranted to prove the prognostic and predictive value of the analyzed marker combinations to robustly stratify the clinical outcome in real-world assessments.

4. Materials and Methods

4.1. Patients

4.1.1. Patient Population

From August 1996 to June 2006, a total of 50 patients diagnosed with bladder cancer were included in the trial. Together, 38 male patients and 12 female patients (average age 65 years, range 49–80 years) were included. Pathohistological T-category and grade for the primary tumors are as follows. The study included for the primary tumors pTaG2 (n = 1), pT1G2 (n = 9), pT1G3 (n = 7), pT2G1 (n = 1), pT2G2 (n = 10), and pT2G3 (n = 22) obtained by transurethral resection under institutional review board-approved protocols. Three patients showed carcinoma in situ (6%). All non-muscle invasive urothelial carcinomas included in the study progressed to muscle-invasive tumors under the follow-up. All patients were treated with radical surgery before chemotherapy. Patient characteristics, including lymph node status before chemotherapy as well as ECOG performance status at the point of starting chemotherapy, are summarized in Table 1. The study population had its origin in one single institution. The analysis of the different markers has been performed at different study sites.

4.1.2. Eligibility

Eligible patients for this trial were required to have either metastatic or locally advanced histologically confirmed transitional cell carcinoma of the urothelial tract. Patients who had received a previous systemic chemotherapy regimen were excluded. Previous radiation therapy was also an exclusion criterion.

Additional eligibility requirements included the following: an ECOG performance status of 0 to 2, a leukocyte count ≥3000/µL, a platelet count ≥100,000/µL, serum bilirubin <1.5 mg/dL, serum creatinine ≤2.5 mg/dL, and age >18 years. Patients with other active malignancies or any other serious or active medical conditions were excluded. Pregnant or lactating females were ineligible. The study protocol was approved by the Research Ethical Board of the Landesärztekammer Brandenburg (AS 25(bB)/2017;

AS 147(bB)/2013) for the German part of the study. For the Finnish part, there was an ethical approval from the Hospital District of Southwestern Finland. All methods in this study were carried out in accordance with relevant guidelines and regulations. The study was conducted in compliance with the current revision of the Declaration of Helsinki, guiding physicians and medical research involving human subjects. All patients were required to provide written informed consent prior to the study enrolment. The study did not affect the patients or their further treatment of follow-up in any way. All the sample collections were done on already existing tissue specimens received during the diagnosis and treatment of these patients.

4.2. Pretreatment Evaluation

Prior to enrollment in this trial, all patients were required to have a complete history, physical examination, complete blood counts, chemistry profile, and urine analysis. In addition, patients underwent computed tomography scans of the chest, abdomen, and pelvis with appropriate tumor measurements.

4.3. Assessment of Treatment Efficacy

All fifty patients received treatment with the following regimen: gemcitabine at a dose of 1000 mg/m^2 as a 30 min intravenous infusion followed by paclitaxel at a dose of 80 mg/m^2 as a 1 h intravenous infusion on days 1 and 8. On day 2, cisplatin at a dose of 50 mg/m^2 was administered as an intravenous infusion and hydration with 2000 mL NaCl 0.9%. The regimen was repeated every 21 days. Patients received standard paclitaxel premedication and antiemetic prophylaxis. Patients were evaluated for response to treatment after the completion of 4 courses (12 weeks). Reevaluation included a repeat of all previously abnormal radiologic studies with a repeat of objective tumor measurement. Patients who achieved an objective response (complete or partial) or stable disease after the completion of four courses of therapy continued treatment with this regimen. Treatment was continued for a total of six courses. None of the patients received neoadjuvant therapy before cystectomy.

Thirty-four patients who completed 6 courses and remained in remission were followed with further treatment of a single dose of gemcitabine at a dose of 1000 mg/m^2 as a 30 min intravenous infusion repeating every 28 days. This following treatment was continued for at least two years.

Two patients received the second-line chemotherapy (methotrexate, epirubicin and cisplatin chemotherapy (MEC)) because of rapid progression after a three-drug regimen with gemcitabine, paclitaxel, and cisplatin or during gemcitabine monotherapy.

4.4. Dose Modifications

All patients received full doses of all 3 agents on day 1 of the first course of treatment. Subsequent doses were based on hematologic and non-hematologic toxicity observed. Dose modifications for myelosuppression were determined by the blood counts measured on the day of scheduled treatment. Nadir blood counts were not used as a basis for dose reduction.

On day 1 of each course, full doses of all drugs were administered if the leukocyte count was ≥3000/µL and the platelet count was >100,000/µL. If the leukocyte count was <3000/µL or the platelet count was <100,000/µL, treatment was delayed for one or two days.

All patients with an ECOG performance status of 2 or with renal insufficiency in the stage of compensated retention received reduced doses of 50% to 70%. In case of good tolerance of the therapy, we applicated higher doses for following cycles.

4.5. Criteria for Follow-Up

The follow-up consisted of clinical examination, ultrasound of abdomen, and computed tomography scans of the chest, abdomen, and pelvis with appropriate tumor measurements every 6 months. Progression was defined as new metastatic disease or local progress during follow-up. Chemotherapy response was defined as absence of recurrence, progression, or death from the disease during follow-up. Responses were defined using the Response Evaluation criteria in Solid Tumors (RECIST). A complete response (CR) required the total disappearance of all clinically and radiographically detected tumors for at least 4 weeks. Patients had partial response (PR) if treatment produced a reduction of at least 30% in the sum of the longest diameter, with no evidence of new disease. No change (NC) was defined as patients who showed no visible reduction or even progress less than 20%. Patients who had the appearance of any new lesions or who had an increase of at least 20% in the size of any existing lesions had progressive disease (PD).

4.6. Clinical Follow-Up and Treatment Efficacy

Among the 50 cases analyzed, 26 progressed (52%), and 34 patients died (68%). Tumor-related death is 27 in total (54%). Twenty-one patients (42%) achieved complete response, three patients achieved partial response (6%), and for twenty-five patients (50%), no change was documented (Table 1).

The median time interval from diagnosis at the point of the first transurethral resection of the primary tumor and the date of death (or last follow-up) of all patients was 36.5 months (range: 8.0–221.0). The median time interval between the point of radical operation of the muscle-invasive tumor and the date of death (or last follow-up) of all patients was 49.0 months (range: 7.0–175.0). The median time interval between the point of chemotherapy and the date of death (or last follow-up) of all patients was 23.0 months (range: 3.0–171.0). The median time between primary resection and muscle-invasive tumor at the point of radical operation of all patients was 8.0 months (range: 6.0–58.0). The median time to progress between radical operation and the progressive disease of all patients was 13 months (range: 6.0–32.0).

4.7. Procedure

For each case, the most representative formalin-fixed, paraffin-embedded tissue block was selected for analysis. Sections (5 µm thickness) were deparaffinized with xylene and rehydrated with a graded alcohol series.

4.8. Immunostaining for CD68, MAC387, and CLEVER-1

The primary antibodies used were mouse monoclonal IgG1 antiCD68 (KP1) (concentration 1:5; ab845, Abcam, U.K.) and mouse monoclonal IgG1 antiMAC387 (concentration 1:500; ab22506, Abcam, U.K.), which detects the myclomonocytic L1 molecule calprotectin. CLEVER-1 (common lymphatic endothelial and vascular endothelial receptor-1, also known as STAB1 and FEEL-1) positive type 2 macrophages and vessels were detected with the rat IgG 2-7 antibody (concentration 1:5) [33,34]. The antibodies 3G6 (mouse IgG1 antibody against chicken T cells) [35] and MEL-14 [rat IgG2a antibody against mouse L-selectin (CD62L)] (Exbio, Czech Republic) were used as negative controls. The primary immunoreaction was performed with using the mouse/rat Vectastain Elite ABC Kit (Vector Laboratories). Sections for CD68 and MAC387 staining were heat pre-treated in citric acid (0.01 M, pH 6.0) in a 97 °C water bath for 20 min. Antigen retrieval for CLEVER-1-stained sections was performed with proteinase K (Dako, Glostrup, Denmark) (10 min at 37 °C), and the slides were washed three times with PBS after the pre-treatment. Endogenous peroxidase was blocked with 0.1% H_2O_2 for 30 min. Non-specific sites were blocked with horse (CD68 and MAC387) or rabbit (CLEVER-1) normal serum at room temperature for 20 min. Sections were incubated with primary antibodies overnight at 4 °C and then treated with biotinylated secondary antibody solution according to the manufacturer's instructions. After washing with PBS, Vectastain Elite ABC Reagent was added (30 min at room temperature), the slides were washed, and immunoreactions were detected using 3,3′-diaminobenzidine as a substrate. Slides were counterstained with hematoxylin, dehydrated, re-fixed in xylene, mounted with distyrene plasticizer xylene (DPX). The whole tumor and surrounding peritumoral area were screened by light microscopy. A detailed description of that scoring process has already been published by Boström et al. [32]. These experiments have been performed at University Hospital Turku (Finland).

4.9. Immunostaining for Survivin

Survivin antibody was provided by the Department of Molecular Medicine at the Institute for Prevention and Occupational Medicine of the German Social Accident Insurance in Bochum, Germany. A detailed description of recombinant survivin and antibody production as well as the analytical specificity of the survivin antibody can be found at Gleichenhagen et al. [36]. We used this method for survivin in a regular immunohistochemistry procedure. In this study, we are one of the first centers who evaluated this survivin antibody by immunohistochemistry. Reproducibility of the new survivin antibody as a component of an ELISA was investigated and published by Gleichenhagen et al. [36]. The experiments for immunostaining for survivin have been performed and evaluated at University Hospital Charité Berlin (Germany). Examples of immunohistochemical stainings are visible in Figures S10–S13.

4.10. Isolation of Tumor RNA

For RNA extraction from FFPE tissue, tissue dots (1.5 mm diameter, 5 µm cuts) from tissue microarray material were picked by stamp technology and further processed according to a commercially available bead-based extraction method (XTRACT kit; STRATIFYER Molecular Pathology GmbH, Cologne, Germany). RNA was eluted with 100 µL elution buffer, and then, RNA eluates were stored at −80 °C until use.

4.11. Gene Expression by RT-qPCR

The mRNA expression levels of *KRT5, KRT20, ERBB2, BIRC5* and *CD68* as well as one reference gene (REF), namely *CALM2*, were determined by RT-qPCR, which involves the reverse transcription of RNA and subsequent amplification of cDNA executed successively as a 1-step reaction using inventoried validated TaqMan Gene Expression Assays (MP002, MP015, MP452, MP089, MP120 and MP501, STRATIFYER Molecular Pathology GmbH, Köln, Germany). The robustness and usefulness of *CALM2* as a housekeeping gene for diverse candidate genes as well as comparability to diverse IHC assessments such as CK20/KRT20, MKI67/Ki67, and PDL1, when used as a single reference gene, have been demonstrated in several of our own publications [20,37,38] and resulted in the introduction of *CALM2* as a housekeeping gene in CE-certified IVD products such as Endopredict [39] and MammaTyper [40]. Each patient sample or control was analyzed with each assay mix in triplicate. The experiments were run on a Siemens Versant (Siemens, Germany) according to the following protocol: 5 min at 50 °C, 20 Sec at 95 °C, followed by 40 cycles of 15 Sec at 95 °C and 60 Sec at 60 °C. Forty amplification cycles were applied, and the cycle quantification threshold (Cq) values of three markers and one reference gene for each sample (S) were estimated as the median of the triplicate measurements. The final values were generated using ΔCT from the total number of cycles (40-DCT) to ensure that the normalized gene expression obtained by the test was proportional to the corresponding mRNA expression levels. This part of the work has been measured and analyzed at STRATIFYER Molecular Pathology, Cologne (Germany). Examples of immunostaining for survivin, CD68, CLEVER-1, and MAC387 are shown in Figures S11–S13.

4.12. Statistical Analysis

The Kaplan–Meier method, log-rank testing, and Cox proportional hazards regression models were used to analyze the associations between IHC and outcome. Partitioning tests were used to identify appropriate cut-off values for dichotomization of the continuous variables for Kaplan–Meier analysis. In the Cox proportional hazards regression models, the markers were evaluated as continuous variables. Outcome measures included DSS and OS. The survival time was calculated from the date of surgery to the date of the last follow-up or death. Any death due to bladder cancer (BC) or with metastatic BC was defined as cancer-specific mortality. All statistical tests were two-sided, and p-values <0.05 were considered statistically significant. All tests and calculations were performed using the software R, version 3.1.2 (R Development Core Team 2014) or JMP 9.0.0 (SAS Institute Inc, 100 SAS Campus Drive Cary, NC 27513-2414, USA).

5. Conclusions

Markers that are validated to predict poor prognosis in NMIBC and MIBC not being treated with chemotherapy, such as survivin and potentially *ERBB2*, exhibit inverse outcome relation upon adjuvant chemotherapeutic treatment, indicating their potential as being predictive for chemotherapy benefit. In addition, macrophage infiltration seems to have a key role in high-risk tumors that could be attributed to its potential of modulating the activity of infiltrating T-cells particularly under circumstances of the chemotherapeutic destruction of tumor cells and subsequent antigen presentation. The findings of the study are limited by the small size of the stud group and its retrospective character, but based on its results, we could demonstrate that further prospective studies with a higher number of patients might be worth pursuing. The combination of immunohistochemical and robust molecular methods being applicable in clinical routine situation harbors the promise of predicting the outcome of patients and serving as valuable pathological tools to better select patients for specific therapeutic interventions.

Supplementary Materials: Supplementary Materials can be found at http://www.mdpi.com/1422-0067/21/19/7420/s1. Figure S1: PFS of bladder cancer patients treated with adjuvant chemotherapy based on survivin nuclear stain in the PCR and IHC cohort. Figure S2: PFS of bladder cancer patients treated with adjuvant chemotherapy based on *BIRC5* mRNA expression in the PCR cohort. Figure S3: PFS of bladder cancer patients treated with adjuvant chemotherapy based on *KRT20* mRNA and survivin nuclear protein stain in the PCR and IHC cohort. Figure S4: PFS of bladder cancer patients treated with adjuvant chemotherapy based on *KRT20* and *BIRC5* mRNA expression in the PCR cohort. Figure S5: PFS of bladder cancer patients treated with adjuvant chemotherapy based on survivin nuclear protein stain and *CD68* mRNA in the PCR and IHC cohort. Figure S6: PFS of bladder cancer patients treated with adjuvant chemotherapy based on survivin nuclear protein stain and MAC387 protein in the PCR and IHC cohort. Figure S7: DSS of bladder cancer patients treated with adjuvant chemotherapy based on survivin nuclear protein stain and CLEVER-1 protein in the PCR and IHC cohort. Figure S8: PFS of bladder cancer patients treated with adjuvant chemotherapy based on survivin nuclear protein stain and CLEVER-1 protein in the PCR and IHC cohort. Figure S9: PFS of bladder cancer patients treated with adjuvant chemotherapy based on ERBB2 positive tumors in relation to *CD68* mRNA levels in the PCR and IHC cohort. Figure S10: Immunohistochemical staining of survivin. Figure S11: immunohistochemical staining of CD68. Figure S12: Immunohistochemical staining of CLEVER-1. Figure S13: immunohistochemical staining of MAC387.

Author Contributions: T.H.E. designed and performed study and cooperation, data collection, and drafted the manuscript. A.K., E.K., F.F., T.S., A.R., and K.J. performed and supervised experiments for survivin. P.B., M.T., and P.T. performed and supervised experiments for CLEVER-1, CD68 and MAC387. J.G., G.J. and T.B. performed survivin experiments. S.K. and J.R. helped collect the samples and supervised clinical data collection. R.M.W. defined candidate genes, performed and supervised experiments for nucleic acid extraction from tissue microarray dots and subsequent RT-qPCR of *KRT5*, *KRT20*, *ERBB2*, *CD68*, *BIRC5*. All authors have read and agreed to the published version of the manuscript.

Funding: This research received no external funding.

Conflicts of Interest: R.M.W. is employee of STRATIFYER Molecular Pathology GmbH. All authors declare no conflict of interest.

Abbreviations

BC	bladder cancer
BIRC5	baculoviral IAP repeat containing 5 (BIRC5)
BMI	body mass index
BRCA1	breast cancer 1
Cis	carcinoma in situ
CLEVER-1	common lymphatic endothelial and vascular endothelial receptor-1
CR	complete response
DCT	Delta Cycle Threshold (gene expression based on difference of thereshold passing of individual genes when using qPCR)
DPX	distyrene plasticizer xylene
DSS	disease-specific survival
GC	gemcitabine and cisplatin chemotherapy
IHC	immunohistochemistry
N	lymph node status
MEC	methotrexate, epirubicin and cisplatin chemotherapy
MIBC	muscle-invasive bladder cancer
M	metastases status
MVAC	methotrexate, vinblastine, adriamycin and cisplatin chemotherapy
MVEC	methotrexate, vinblastine, epirubicin and cisplatin chemotherapy
NC	no change
NGS	next generation sequencing
NMIBC	non-muscle invasive bladder cancer
OS	overall survival
PCG	paclitaxel, cisplatin and gemcitabine chemotherapy
PCR	polymerase chain reaction
PD	progressive disease
PFS	progression-free survival
PR	partial response
RC	radical cystectomy
RECIST	Response Evaluation criteria in Solid Tumors
TMA	tissue microarray
TURB	transurethral resection of bladder

References

1. Ferlay, J.; Colombet, M.; Soerjomataram, I.; Mathers, C.; Parkin, D.M.; Piñeros, M.; Znaor, A.; Bray, F. Estimating the global cancer incidence and mortality in 2018: GLOBOCAN sources and methods. *Int. J. Cancer* **2018**, *144*, 1941–1953. [CrossRef]
2. Witjes, J.A.; Compérat, E.; Cowan, N.C.; De Santis, M.; Gakis, G.; Lebret, T.; Ribal, M.J.; Van Der Heijden, A.G.; Sherif, A. EAU Guidelines on Muscle-invasive and Metastatic Bladder Cancer: Summary of the 2013 Guidelines. *Eur. Urol.* **2014**, *65*, 778–792. [CrossRef]
3. Alfred Witjes, J.; Lebret, T.; Comperat, E.M.; De Santis, M.; Gakis, G.; Lebret, T.; Ribal, M.J.; Van der Heiden, M.J.; Sherif, A. Updated 2016 EAU Guidelines on Muscle-invasive and Metastatic Bladder Cancer. *Eur. Urol.* **2017**, *71*, 462–475. [CrossRef]
4. Kluth, L.A.; Black, P.C.; Bochner, B.H.; Catto, J.; Lerner, S.P.; Stenzl, A.; Sylvester, R.; Vickers, A.J.; Xylinas, E.; Shariat, S.F. Prognostic and Prediction Tools in Bladder Cancer: A Comprehensive Review of the Literature. *Eur. Urol.* **2015**, *68*, 238–253. [CrossRef] [PubMed]
5. Hoffmann, A.-C.; Wild, P.; Leicht, C.; Bertz, S.; Danenberg, K.D.; Danenberg, P.V.; Stöhr, R.; Stöckle, M.; Lehmann, J.; Schuler, M.; et al. MDR1 and ERCC1 Expression Predict Outcome of Patients with Locally Advanced Bladder Cancer Receiving Adjuvant Chemotherapy. *Neoplasia* **2010**, *12*, 628–636. [CrossRef] [PubMed]
6. Garg, H.; Suri, P.; Gupta, J.C.; Talwar, G.; Dubey, S. Survivin: A unique target for tumor therapy. *Cancer Cell Int.* **2016**, *16*, 49. [CrossRef] [PubMed]

7. Engels, K.; Knauer, S.; Metzler, D.; Simf, C.; Struschka, O.; Bier, C.; Mann, W.; Kovács, A.; Stauber, R.; Knauer, S.; et al. Dynamic intracellular survivin in oral squamous cell carcinoma: Underlying molecular mechanism and potential as an early prognostic marker. *J. Pathol.* **2007**, *211*, 532–540. [CrossRef] [PubMed]

8. Li, F.; Yang, J.; Ramnath, N.; Javle, M.M.; Tan, N. Nuclear or cytoplasmic expression of survivin: What is the significance? *Int. J. Cancer* **2005**, *114*, 509–512. [CrossRef]

9. Uren, A.G.; Wong, L.; Pakusch, M.; Fowler, K.J.; Burrows, F.J.; Vaux, D.L.; Choo, K. Survivin and the inner centromere protein INCENP show similar cell-cycle localization and gene knockout phenotype. *Curr. Boil.* **2000**, *10*, 1319–1328. [CrossRef]

10. Dohi, T.; Beltrami, E.; Wall, N.R.; Plescia, J.; Altieri, D.C. Mitochondrial survivin inhibits apoptosis and promotes tumorigenesis. *J. Clin. Investig.* **2004**, *114*, 1117–1127. [CrossRef]

11. Dyrskjøt, L.; Reinert, T.; Algaba, F.; Christensen, E.; Nieboer, D.; Hermann, G.G.; Mogensen, K.; Beukers, W.; Marquez, M.; Segersten, U.; et al. Prognostic Impact of a 12-gene Progression Score in Non-muscle-invasive Bladder Cancer: A Prospective Multicentre Validation Study. *Eur. Urol.* **2017**, *72*, 461–469. [CrossRef] [PubMed]

12. Holness, C.L.; Simmons, D.L. Molecular cloning of CD68, a human macrophage marker related to lysosomal glycoproteins. *Blood* **1993**, *81*, 1607–1613. [CrossRef] [PubMed]

13. Kzhyshkowska, J.; Gratchev, A.; Goerdt, S. Stabilin-1, a homeostatic scavenger receptor with multiple functions. *J. Cell Mol. Med.* **2006**, *10*, 635–649. [CrossRef] [PubMed]

14. Tervahartiala, M.; Taimen, P.; Mirtti, T.; Koskinen, I.; Ecke, T.; Jalkanen, S.; Boström, P.J. Immunological tumor status may predict response to neoadjuvant chemotherapy and outcome after radical cystectomy in bladder cancer. *Sci. Rep.* **2017**, *7*, 12682. [CrossRef]

15. Goebeler, M.; Roth, J.; Teigelkamp, S.; Sorg, C. The monoclonal antibody MAC387 detects an epitope on the calcium-binding protein MRP14. *J. Leukoc. Boil.* **1994**, *55*, 259–261. [CrossRef]

16. Netea-Maier, R.T.; Smit, J.; Netea, M.G. Metabolic changes in tumor cells and tumor-associated macrophages: A mutual relationship. *Cancer Lett.* **2018**, *413*, 102–109. [CrossRef]

17. The Cancer Genome Atlas Research Network; Cancer Genome Atlas Research Network Comprehensive molecular characterization of urothelial bladder carcinoma. *Nature* **2014**, *507*, 315–322. [CrossRef]

18. Choi, W.; Porten, S.; Kim, S.; Willis, D.; Plimack, E.R.; Hoffman-Censits, J.; Roth, B.; Cheng, T.; Tran, M.; Lee, I.-L.; et al. Identification of distinct basal and luminal subtypes of muscle-invasive bladder cancer with different sensitivities to frontline chemotherapy. *Cancer Cell* **2014**, *25*, 152–165. [CrossRef]

19. Damrauer, J.S.; Hoadley, K.A.; Chism, D.D.; Fan, C.; Tignanelli, C.; Wobker, S.E.; Yeh, J.J.; Milowsky, M.I.; Iyer, G.; Parker, J.S.; et al. Intrinsic subtypes of high-grade bladder cancer reflect the hallmarks of breast cancer biology. *Proc. Natl. Acad. Sci. USA* **2014**, *111*, 3110–3115. [CrossRef]

20. Breyer, J.; Wirtz, R.M.; Otto, W.; Erben, P.; Kriegmair, M.C.; Stoehr, R.; Eckstein, M.; Eidt, S.; Denzinger, S. In stage pT1 non-muscle-invasive bladder cancer (NMIBC), high KRT20 and low KRT5 mRNA expression identify the luminal subtype and predict recurrence and survival. *Virchows Arch.* **2017**, *470*, 267–274. [CrossRef]

21. Kamoun, A.; De Reyniès, A.; Allory, Y.; Sjödahl, G.; Robertson, A.G.; Seiler, R.; Hoadley, K.A.; Groeneveld, C.S.; Al-Ahmadie, H.; Choi, W.; et al. A Consensus Molecular Classification of Muscle-invasive Bladder Cancer. *Eur. Urol.* **2020**, *77*, 420–433. [CrossRef] [PubMed]

22. Breyer, J.; Wirtz, R.M.; Otto, W.; Laible, M.; Schlombs, K.; Erben, P.; Kriegmair, M.C.; Stoehr, R.; Eidt, S.; Denzinger, S.; et al. Predictive value of molecular subtyping in NMIBC by RT-qPCR of ERBB2, ESR1, PGR and MKI67 from formalin fixed TUR biopsies. *Oncotarget* **2017**, *8*, 67684–67695. [CrossRef] [PubMed]

23. Kriegmair, M.; Wirtz, R.; Worst, T.; Breyer, J.; Ritter, M.; Keck, B.; Boehmer, C.; Otto, W.; Eckstein, M.; Weis, C.; et al. Prognostic Value of Molecular Breast Cancer Subtypes based on Her2, ESR1, PGR and Ki67 mRNA-Expression in Muscle Invasive Bladder Cancer. *Transl. Oncol.* **2018**, *11*, 467–476. [CrossRef] [PubMed]

24. Akhtar, M.; Gallagher, L.; Rohan, S. Survivin: Role in Diagnosis, Prognosis, and Treatment of Bladder Cancer. *Adv. Anat. Pathol.* **2006**, *13*, 122–126. [CrossRef] [PubMed]

25. Tran, J.; Master, Z.; Yu, J.L.; Rak, J.; Dumont, D.J.; Kerbel, R.S. A role for survivin in chemoresistance of endothelial cells mediated by VEGF. *Proc. Natl. Acad. Sci. USA* **2002**, *99*, 4349–4354. [CrossRef]

26. Nakamura, M.; Tsuji, N.; Asanuma, K.; Kobayashi, D.; Yagihashi, A.; Hirata, K.; Torigoe, T.; Sato, N.; Watanabe, N. Survivin as a predictor of cis-diamminedichloroplatinum sensitivity in gastric cancer patients. *Cancer Sci.* **2004**, *95*, 44–51. [CrossRef]

27. Rinaldetti, S.; Wirtz, R.; Worst, T.S.; Hartmann, A.; Breyer, J.; Dyrskjøt, L.; Erben, P. FOXM1 predicts disease progression in non-muscle invasive bladder cancer. *J. Cancer Res. Clin. Oncol.* **2018**, *144*, 1701–1709. [CrossRef]

28. Breyer, J.; Wirtz, R.M.; Erben, P.; Rinaldetti, S.; Worst, T.S.; Stoehr, R.; Eckstein, M.; Sikic, D.; Denzinger, S.; Burger, M.; et al. FOXM1 overexpression is associated with adverse outcome and predicts response to intravesical instillation therapy in stage pT1 non-muscle-invasive bladder cancer. *BJU Int.* **2018**, *123*, 187–196. [CrossRef]

29. Jeon, C.; Kim, M.; Kwak, C.; Kim, H.H.; Ku, J.H. Prognostic Role of Survivin in Bladder Cancer: A Systematic Review and Meta-Analysis. *PLoS ONE* **2013**, *8*, e76719. [CrossRef]

30. Als, A.B.; Von Der Maase, H.; Koed, K.; Mansilla, F.; Toldbod, H.E.; Jensen, J.L.; Jensen, K.M.; Dyrskjøt, L.; Ulhøi, B.P.; Sengeløv, L.; et al. Emmprin and Survivin Predict Response and Survival following Cisplatin-Containing Chemotherapy in Patients with Advanced Bladder Cancer. *Clin. Cancer Res.* **2007**, *13*, 4407–4414. [CrossRef]

31. Pollard, C.; Nitz, M.; Baras, A..; Williams, P.; Moskaluk, C.; Theodorescu, D. Genoproteomic mining of urothelial cancer suggests {gamma}-glutamyl hydrolase and diazepam-binding inhibitor as putative urinary markers of outcome after chemotherapy. *Am. J. Pathol.* **2009**, *175*, 1824–1830. [CrossRef] [PubMed]

32. Boström, M.M.; Irjala, H.; Mirtti, T.; Taimen, P.; Kauko, T.; Ålgars, A.; Jalkanen, S.; Boström, P.J. Tumor-Associated Macrophages Provide Significant Prognostic Information in Urothelial Bladder Cancer. *PLoS ONE* **2015**, *10*, e0133552. [CrossRef] [PubMed]

33. Palani, S.; Maksimow, M.; Miiluniemi, M.; Auvinen, K.; Jalkanen, S.; Salmi, M. Stabilin-1/CLEVER-1, a type 2 macrophage marker, is an adhesion and scavenging molecule on human placental macrophages. *Eur. J. Immunol.* **2011**, *41*, 2052–2063. [CrossRef] [PubMed]

34. Irjala, H.; Elima, K.; Johansson, E.-L.; Merinen, M.; Kontula, K.; Alanen, K.; Grénman, R.; Salmi, M.; Jalkanen, S. The same endothelial receptor controls lymphocyte traffic both in vascular and lymphatic vessels. *Eur. J. Immunol.* **2003**, *33*, 815–824. [CrossRef]

35. Salmi, M.; Jalkanen, S. A 90-kilodalton endothelial cell molecule mediating lymphocyte binding in humans. *Science* **1992**, *257*, 1407–1409. [CrossRef]

36. Gleichenhagen, J.; Arndt, C.; Casjens, S.; Meinig, C.; Gerullis, H.; Raiko, I.; Bruning, T.; Ecke, T.; Johnen, G. Evaluation of a New Survivin ELISA and UBC((R)) Rapid for the Detection of Bladder Cancer in Urine. *Int. J. Mol. Sci.* **2018**, *19*, 226. [CrossRef]

37. Eckstein, M.; Wirtz, R.M.; Pfannstil, C.; Wach, S.; Stoehr, R.; Breyer, J.; Erlmeier, F.; Gunes, C.; Nitschke, K.; Weichert, W.; et al. A multicenter round robin test of PD-L1 expression assessment in urothelial bladder cancer by immunohistochemistry and RT-qPCR with emphasis on prognosis prediction after radical cystectomy. *Oncotarget* **2018**, *9*, 15001–15014. [CrossRef]

38. Eckstein, M.; Strissel, P.; Strick, R.; Weyerer, V.; Wirtz, R.; Pfannstiel, C.; Wullweber, A.; Lange, F.; Erben, P.; Stoehr, R.; et al. Cytotoxic T-cell-related gene expression signature predicts improved survival in muscle-invasive urothelial bladder cancer patients after radical cystectomy and adjuvant chemotherapy. *J. Immunother. Cancer* **2020**, *8*, e000162. [CrossRef]

39. Filipits, M.; Dafni, U.; Gnant, M.; Polydoropoulou, V.; Hills, M.; Kiermaier, A.; De Azambuja, E.; Larsimont, D.P.; Rojo, F.; Viale, G.; et al. Association of p27 and Cyclin D1 Expression and Benefit from Adjuvant Trastuzumab Treatment in HER2-Positive Early Breast Cancer: A TransHERA Study. *Clin. Cancer Res.* **2018**, *24*, 3079–3086. [CrossRef]

40. Sinn, H.-P.; Schneeweiss, A.; Keller, M.; Schlombs, K.; Laible, M.; Seitz, J.; Lakis, S.; Veltrup, E.; Altevogt, P.; Eidt, S.; et al. Comparison of immunohistochemistry with PCR for assessment of ER, PR, and Ki-67 and prediction of pathological complete response in breast cancer. *BMC Cancer* **2017**, *17*, 124. [CrossRef]

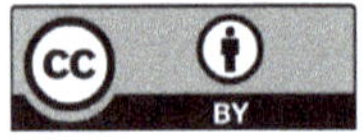

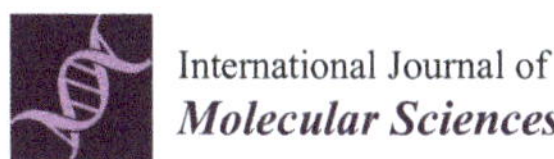

International Journal of
Molecular Sciences

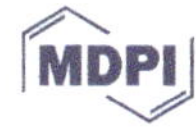

Article

Histone Demethylase KDM7A Regulates Androgen Receptor Activity, and Its Chemical Inhibitor TC-E 5002 Overcomes Cisplatin-Resistance in Bladder Cancer Cells

Kyoung-Hwa Lee [1,†], Byung-Chan Kim [1,†], Seung-Hwan Jeong [2], Chang Wook Jeong [1], Ja Hyeon Ku [1], Hyeon Hoe Kim [1] and Cheol Kwak [1,3,*]

[1]   Department of Urology, Seoul National University Hospital, Seoul 03080, Korea;
      lee12042@snu.ac.kr (K.-H.L.); dalkyal12@gmail.com (B.-C.K.); drboss@gmail.com (C.W.J.);
      randyku@hanmail.net (J.H.K.); hhkim@snu.ac.kr (H.H.K.)
[2]   Graduate School of Medical Science and Engineering, Korea Advanced Institute of Science and
      Technology (KAIST), Daejeon 34052, Korea; 11shjeong@gmail.com
[3]   Department of Urology, Seoul National University College of Medicine, Seoul 03080, Korea
*   Correspondence: mdrafael@snu.ac.kr; Tel.: +822-2072-0817
†   These authors contributed equally to this work.

Received: 21 July 2020; Accepted: 4 August 2020; Published: 6 August 2020

Abstract: Histone demethylase KDM7A regulates many biological processes, including differentiation, development, and the growth of several cancer cells. Here, we have focused on the role of KDM7A in bladder cancer cells, especially under drug-resistant conditions. When the *KDM7A* gene was knocked down, bladder cancer cell lines showed impaired cell growth, increased cell death, and reduced rates of cell migration. Biochemical studies revealed that KDM7A knockdown in the bladder cancer cells repressed the activity of androgen receptor (AR) through epigenetic regulation. When we developed a cisplatin-resistant bladder cancer cell line, we found that AR expression was highly elevated. Upon treatment with TC-E 5002, a chemical inhibitor of KDM7A, the cisplatin-resistant bladder cancer cells, showed decreased cell proliferation. In the mouse xenograft model, KDM7A knockdown or treatment with its inhibitor reduced the growth of the bladder tumor. We also observed the upregulation of KDM7A expression in patients with bladder cancer. The findings suggest that histone demethylase KDM7A mediates the growth of bladder cancer. Moreover, our findings highlight the therapeutic potential of the KMD7A inhibitor, TC-E 5002, in patients with cisplatin-resistant bladder cancer.

Keywords: bladder cancer; KDM7A; histone demethylase; TC-E 5002; androgen receptor; drug resistance

---

1. Introduction

Bladder cancer (BCa) is one of the most common cancers in men, resulting in a reported 8470 new cases and over 17,670 deaths in the United States in 2019 [1]. BCa has a high prevalence of recurrence and metastatic spread, and the 5-year survival rate has remained relatively low, despite the advances in various surgical and chemotherapeutic treatment options [2]. The incidence of BCa is three times higher in men than women, and is the 4th and 11th most common cancer in men and women, respectively [3]. The variation in prevalence depending on gender has prompted a number of studies into the role of sex hormone receptors in BCa. Notably, emerging evidence has supported a role for the androgen receptor (AR) in BCa [4]. AR is a well-known transcription factor that responds to male sex hormones, and controls prostate cancer development and metastasis [5,6]. Recently, many studies have highlighted its role in other cancer types, including colon [7], breast [8], stomach [9], and bladder cancer [10–13]. A reduced incidence of N-butyl-N-(4-hydroxybutyl)-nitrosamine (BBN)-induced BCa has been reported in both full-body [14] as well as urothelial-specific [15] AR knock-out mice models. Recent preclinical studies have suggested that the androgen-mediated AR signaling promotes bladder cancer progression, and blocking this signaling with enzalutamide can strongly impair bladder cancer cell growth [16–18]. Another recent study has shed light on the role of the AR in cisplatin-resistant bladder cancer [19]. It is also reported that the anti-androgenic drug hydroxyflutamide increased cisplatin sensitivity in cisplatin-resistant bladder cancer cell line T24.

Since AR is a transcription factor, controlling its transcriptional activity can be a major target for anti-cancer drug development. Among the mechanisms known to regulate transcriptional activity, epigenetic regulation, including DNA methylation and histone modification, plays a key role in cancer development [20,21]. Specifically, histone methylation on lysine residues of histone H3 or H4 are known to modify transcriptional activity, depending on the residues modified. Methylation on lysine 4 (H3K4) or 36 (H3K36) is usually associated with transcriptional activation, while H3K9 and H3K27 methylation are frequently linked with gene silencing, and are hallmarks of chromatin condensation [22,23]. Each methylase and demethylase has specific target promoters; therefore, inhibitors can be used for targeting the regulation of a specific gene. Since the epigenetic modifications play important roles in cancer formation, malignancy, and metastasis, targeting the epigenetic enzymes would be a promising approach in cancer therapy. Indeed, epigenetic processes which control AR activity have been reported to play a role in prostate cancer development [24,25]. For the regulation of histone methylation on its target promoters, AR is known to interact with several enzymes, including LSD1, KDM4B, KDM5B, EZH2, SMYD3, PRMT5, and KDM7A [26–32].

Among the histone modifying enzymes, the enzyme KDM7A belongs to a family of plant homeodomain finger proteins, that contain a plant homeodomain (PHD) and a JmjC domain. The methyl groups of the lysine at positions 9 and 27 in histone 3 can be removed by the JmjC domain-containing family of proteins [33]. Since the methylation of H3K9 and H3K27 represent the repression of gene expression, their demethylation activates target gene transcription. Previous studies have shown that KDM7A regulates bone development, adipogenesis, inflammation, as well as the development of various types of cancers [34–36]. A recently published paper from our research group described the H3K27 demethylase activity of KDM7A on the response elements of AR target genes in prostate cancer [32]. The study presents a detailed account of the physical interaction of KDM7A with AR, using the immune-precipitation method. Furthermore, we found that KDM7A directly binds to the androgen response element (ARE) sequences of AR target genes, including KLK3, KLK2, and TMPRSS2. An increase in the histone H3K27 di-methylation of those ARE sequences and a decrease in the AR activity was also observed in KDM7A knockdown prostate cells. The existence of a KDM7A chemical inhibitor further highlighted the value of this data, owing to its clinical application as an anti-cancer drug.

In the present study, we have further investigated the role of KDM7A in the epigenetic regulation of AR in BCa, with a focus on the regulation of AR activity in the cisplatin-resistant bladder cancer cells.

2. Results

2.1. KDM7A Regulates AR Transcription Activity in Bladder Cancer Cells

In order to investigate the possible role of KDM7A demethylase in the functioning of AR in bladder cancer cells, we first compared the AR expression levels in various bladder cancer cell lines, including 253J, RT4, T24, and J82. As expected, the levels of AR mRNA and protein in bladder cancer cells were quite low compared to that in LNCaP prostate cancer cells (Supplemental Figure S1A,B). Nonetheless, we were able to detect AR mRNA and protein in the bladder cancer cells that we tested, with the levels found to be comparable among them. Since a previous study has reported the development of cisplatin-resistant T24 cells [19], we selected this cell line for our experiments. We also included another bladder cancer cell line, J82, in order to demonstrate data reproducibility. To analyze the function of KDM7A histone demethylase in bladder cancer cells, we produced KDM7A knock-down bladder cell lines (T24 and J82), using a lenti-viral shRNA expression system. After antibiotics selection, efficient knock-down of the gene expression was confirmed by Western blotting and reverse transcriptase quantitative PCR (RT-qPCR) (Figure 1A). Since KDM7A is known to regulate AR activity in prostate cancer cells [32], we speculated that it may control AR activity as an epigenetic regulator in bladder cancer cells. Our studies showed that the levels of both AR mRNA and protein were regulated by KDM7A, before and after dihydrotestosterone (DHT) induction (Figure 1B, Supplemental Figure S2), even though we had expected changes only in the protein activity. A possible explanation could be the autoregulatory effect of AR on its own promoter [37]. In order to measure AR activity in KDM7A knock-down cells, the expression of previously reported downstream target genes of AR was screened using RT-qPCR [38–43]. The relative mRNA levels of these genes, compared with those of LNCaP, are listed in Supplemental Figure S1C. The PCR signals of six genes (*KLK3, TMPRSS2, KLK4, IGF1R, VEGF,* and *MYC*) were successfully amplified in bladder cancer cell lines. The mRNA levels of these AR target genes were elevated after DHT treatment, and this induction was reduced in KDM7A knock-down stable cells (Figure 1C).

2.2. KDM7A Regulates AR Transcription Activity via Epigenetic Regulation of AR Target Gene Promoters

Next, we analyzed the histone methylation status in KDM7A knock-down cells. The cell extracts from each of the cell lines were analyzed with specific antibodies for diverse histone methylation sites (Figure 2A). Among the sites tested, only H3K27 di-methylated lysine was elevated in KDM7A knock-down cells. The AR activity can be measured as the extent of binding of AR onto target promoters. We, therefore, analyzed the binding efficiency of AR to its target promoters, using the chromatin immunoprecipitation (ChIP) experiment. The T24 bladder cancer cells expressing control or KDM7A shRNA were treated with DHT, sonicated, and the chromatin was precipitated with AR antibody. The promoter binding by AR on the indicated genes was detected with IP PCR. The precise location of the PCR primers for each of the gene promoters is described in Supplemental Figure S3. Induction with DHT was shown to increase the binding of AR to these promoters, while this induction was abolished in the KDM7A knock-down cells (Figure 2B). We next attempted to investigate methylation statuses on AR responsive promoters in the KDM7A knock-down cells. Based on the changes in methylation (Figure 2A), we used H3K27 di-methyl-specific histone antibodies for immunoprecipitations, and H3K27 methylation was found to be increased in KDM7A knock-down bladder cells, before and after DHT induction (Figure 2C). Our data confirmed the molecular function of KDM7A on AR transcription factor activity in bladder cancer cells.

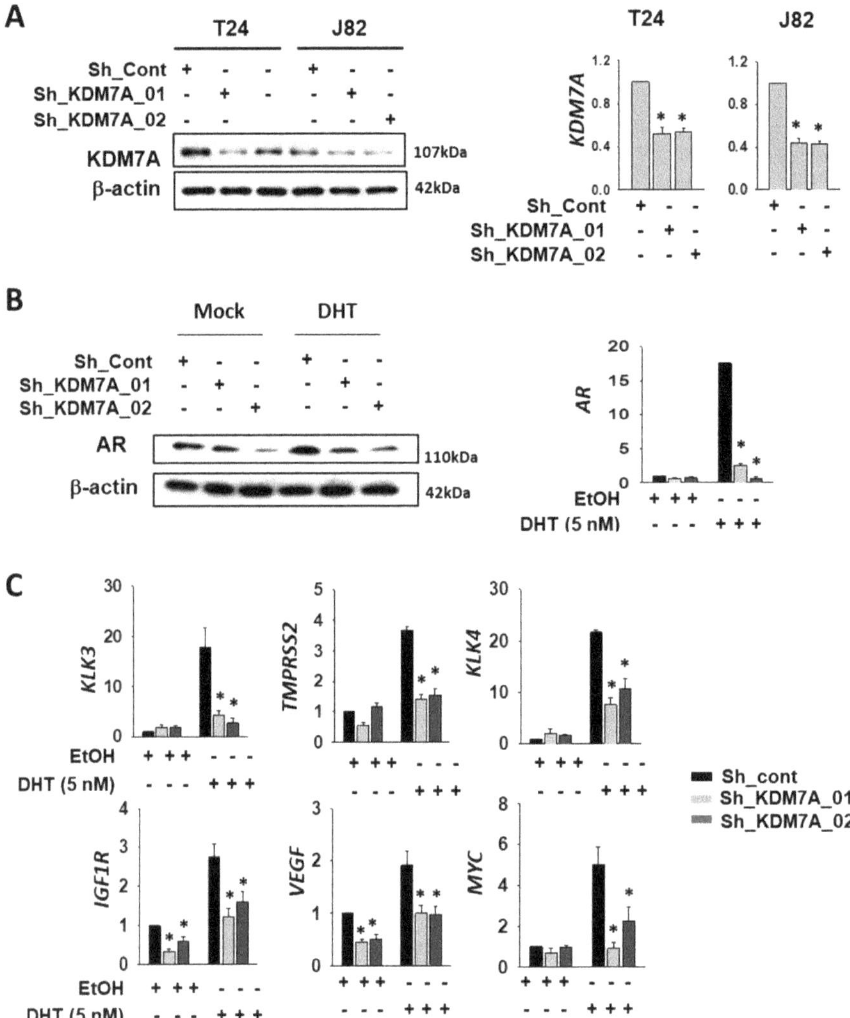

Figure 1. Histone demethylase KDM7A is required for AR activity in bladder cancer cells. (**A**) The efficiency of KDM7A knock-down was measured by comparing protein levels of KDM7A in the indicated cell lines, expressing control or two different shRNAs. Whole-cell lysates were analyzed with the indicated antibodies (left). The mRNA levels of KDM7A were measured by RT-qPCR method in the KDM7A knock-down cell lines (right graphs). Bars represent the means ± SD of three independent experiments, and * denotes $p < 0.05$ (student *t*-test) versus the control shRNA (sh-cont) group. (**B**) The AR protein levels in KDM7A knock-down T24 cells treated with dihydrotestosterone (DHT) were analyzed with indicated antibodies (left). The mRNA levels of AR in T24 cells after DHT induction were measured by RT-qPCR (right graph). Bars represent the means ± SD of three independent experiments, and * denotes $p < 0.05$ (student *t*-test) versus the control shRNA (sh-cont) group. (**C**) The mRNA levels of AR downstream genes were measured by RT-qPCR method in KDM7A knock-down T24 cell lines. Bars represent mean ± SD of three independent experiments. * $p < 0.05$ (Student's *t*-test), versus the control shRNA (sh-cont) group.

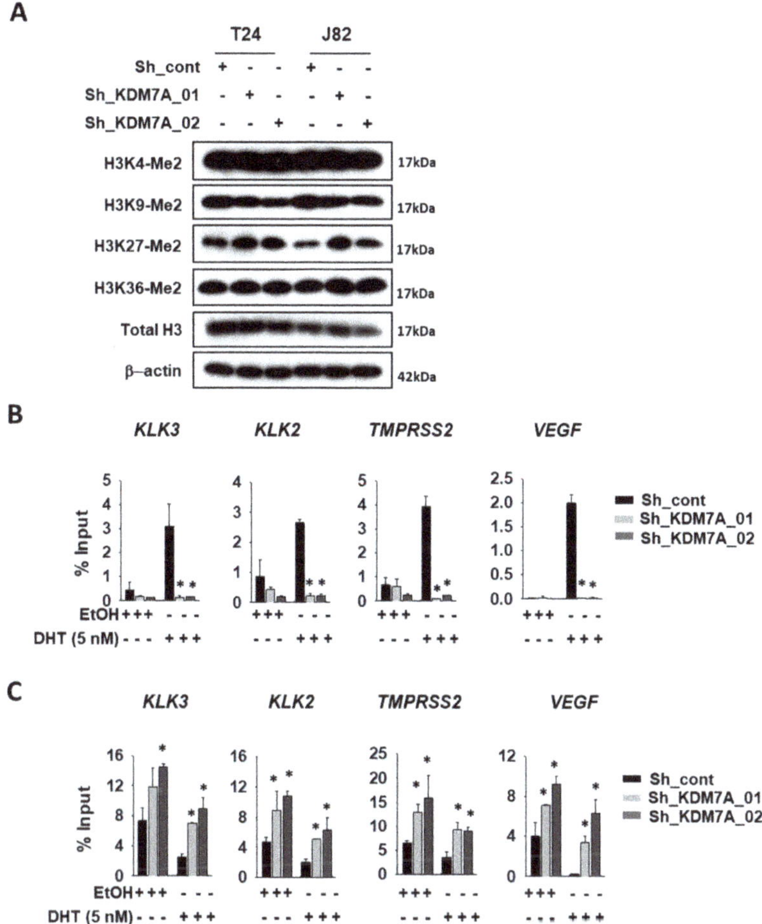

Figure 2. KDM7A directly binds on androgen receptor (AR) downstream gene promoters, and regulates H3K27 methylation. (**A**) Histone methylation status in KDM7A knock-down cells was analyzed with the indicated antibodies. T24 cells expressing control or KMD7A shRNA were treated with 5 nM DHT for 1 day, and the sonicated chromatins were immune-precipitated with anti-AR (**B**) or anti-H3K27 di-methyl (**C**) antibody. Immunoprecipitated DNAs were subjected to qPCR with the indicated gene promoter sequence primers. Bars represent means ± SD of three independent experiments. * $p < 0.05$ (Student's *t*-test), versus the control shRNA (sh-cont) group.

2.3. KDM7A is Required for Bladder Cancer Cell Growth and Apoptosis Inhibition

Since AR is known to be essential for cell growth in many cancers, we treated AR siRNA or enzalutamide, to confirm the growth inhibition effect on bladder cancer cell growth (Supplemental Figure S4). Next, we measured cell proliferation in both control and KDM7A knock-down cells. Although the morphology of KDM7A knock-down cells was not different from control cells (Supplemental Figure S5), the rate of cell proliferation in KDM7A knock-down bladder cancer cells was reduced compared to that of control shRNA-expressing cells (Figure 3A). When we seeded the same number of cells in cell culture dishes, knock-down cells showed a reduction in colony numbers and size compared to control cells (Figure 3B). We next observed the expression levels of cell cycle proteins in KDM7A knock-down cells (Figure 3C). Previous studies have reported that AR regulates cell cycle by controlling cyclin D1 [44], and cyclin B1 is a direct target of AR [45]. We observed a decrease in the cyclin B1 protein levels in KDM7A knock-down bladder cancer cells, which is consistent with the cell proliferation rate difference data in Figure 3A,B. It was observed that the decrease in cyclin D1 is not as obvious as that in cyclin B1 in our experimental conditions. Since AR is known to inhibit apoptosis induced by cytotoxic stimuli [46], we measured the levels of apoptotic proteins in KDM7A knock-down cells treated with the anti-cancer drug cisplatin (Figure 3D). We observed an increase in the PARP and caspase 3 cleavage products compared to control shRNA-expressing cells. These results strongly suggest that KDM7A regulates the rate of cell proliferation and drug-induced apoptosis in bladder cancer cells.

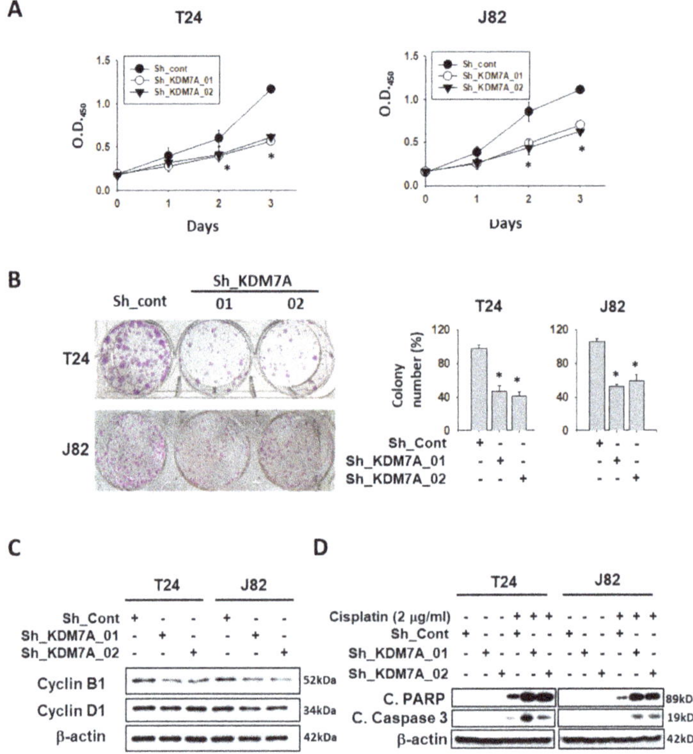

Figure 3. Histone demethylase KDM7A is required for the cell proliferation and apoptosis inhibition in bladder cancer cell lines. (**A**) The time dependent viability changes of control shRNA and KDM7A shRNA expressing bladder cancer cell lines were measured using EZ-Cytox solution. Bars represent means ± SD of three independent experiments. * $p < 0.05$ (Student's *t*-test) versus the control shRNA (sh-cont) group. (**B**) Crystal violet staining for colonies from the same number of indicated shRNA-expressing stable cells. The average number of colonies is shown in the right panel. Bars represent means ± SD of three independent experiments. * $p < 0.05$ (Student's *t*-test) versus the sh-cont group. (**C**) The levels of cell cycle-related proteins were measured from the whole cell extracts of control and KDM7A knock-down cells. (**D**) The apoptotic proteins were detected in the cisplatin-treated KDM7A knock-down bladder cells. Whole-cell lysates were analyzed with the indicated antibodies.

2.4. KDM7A Facilitates Migration and Invasion of Bladder Cancer Cells

One of the major functions of AR in cancer progression is to facilitate cell migration and metastasis. It was observed that AR inhibition by enzalutamide affected the migration of bladder cancer cells

(Supplemental Figure S6). To verify the effect of KDM7A in bladder cancer cell migration and metastasis, we measured migration and invasion in KDM7A knock-down T24 and J82 bladder cancer cells. One day after scratch, KDM7A knock-down cells showed decreased mobility when compared to control cells (Figure 4A). We demarcated the wound margin with a yellow line for better visualization, and added the original pictures and quantification of remaining scratched areas after the indicated times in Supplemental Figure S7. The cell invasion assay using Matrigel Transwell showed the decreased invasion of KDM7A knock-down cells compared to control cells (Figure 4B). To elucidate the molecular mechanism of this decrease in cell migration, we measured the expression of several epithelial-mesenchymal transition (EMT) markers in KDM7A knock-down cells. Although a decrease in the protein levels of N-cadherin and vimentin, the epithelial markers, was observed only in J82 cells (Figure 4C, Supplemental Figure S8), the mRNA expression levels of them were reduced in both T24 and J82 cells (Figure 4D). The protein and mRNA levels of mesenchymal marker E-cadherin were elevated in KDM7A knock-down cells in both T24 and J82 cells (Figure 4C,D, Supplemental Figure S8). The findings suggest that KDM7A is required for cell migration and EMT transition in bladder cancer cells.

2.5. Enzalutamide and a KDM7A Inhibitor Decrease the Proliferation of Cisplatin-resistant Bladder Cancer Cells

The effect of AR induction on the cisplatin resistance process of bladder cancer has been previously reported [19]. Therefore, we wanted to explore the possibility of AR regulation as a target for overcoming the drug resistance of bladder cancer. Initially, we established a cisplatin-resistant T24 (CR-T24) bladder cancer cell line. After 2 months of exposure to increasing concentrations of cisplatin, we obtained T24 cells that survived in 2 μM cisplatin (Figure 5A). To compare the AR protein levels between original and CR-T24 cells, we compared their nuclear extracts, since the active form of AR protein occurs only in the nuclear fraction. We used the Lamin B1 antibody as the loading control of the nuclear extract, and for establishing the purity of the fraction, while GAPDH acted as the loading control of the cytosolic fraction. In addition to an increase in the total AR protein level, our study found that the level of active AR protein was higher in the nuclear fraction of CR-T24 when compared to the parental cells (Figure 5B). The protein level of KDM7A in CR-T24 cells decreased in the cytosolic fraction, but remained the same in nuclear fraction. The AR protein level in CR-T24 cells was found to be elevated before and after DHT treatment (Figure 5C), as reported previously [19]. The mRNA levels of several AR target genes also showed an increase, when compared to the parental T24 cells before and after DHT treatment (Figure 5D), suggesting that the elevated AR has functional activity. After confirming an increase in AR activity in CR-T24 cells, we utilized the KDM7A inhibitor TC-E 5002, in conjunction with AR antagonist enzalutamide, to evaluate the role of KDM7A on bladder cancer growth and drug resistance in terms of the AR pathway. Cell viability was tested in parental and CR-T24 cells in the presence of enzalutamide and/or TC-E 5002 (Figure 5E). In order to obtain a clearer picture of the changes in cell viability, we used a non-toxic dose and time of enzalutamide or TC-E 5002 when treated to parental T24 cells. CR-T24 cells were found to be more sensitive to a single treatment with enzalutamide or TC-E 5002 than parental cells. Moreover, when CR-T24 cells were treated with both enzalutamide and TC-E 5002, fewer cells survived compared to the single drug treatments. The anti-cancer effect of this co-treatment was significantly greater in CR-T24 compared to the parental T24 cells. Finally, we investigated the involvement of cellular signaling pathways involved in the anti-cancer effect of AR and/or KDM7A inhibitors on CR-T24 cells. Of the several pathways tested, Akt signaling pathway molecules were significantly decreased upon treatment with AR and/or KDM7A inhibitor. In our experiments, the total and phosphorylated protein levels of Akt and mTOR in T24 cells were decreased after enzalutamide and/or TC-E 5002 treatment. The changes were more significant in CR-T24 compared to the parental cells, and the effect was synergistically increased in co-treatment (Figure 5F; Supplemental Figure S9A). Upon cisplatin treatment, we observed the synergistic effect of two drugs on apoptosis signaling induction in the parental T24 cells, although the resistant cells did not show the apoptosis induction (Supplemental Figure S9B). For studying the changes in cell migration ability in CR-T24 cells, we performed a wound healing assay using both the cell lines treated with AR and/or KDM7A inhibitors (Supplemental Figure S10). The findings showed a decrease in the migration of cells upon treatment with AR and/or KDM7A inhibitors, in both original as well as CR-T24 cells.

2.6. KDM7A Knock-Down Attenuated Tumor Growth in Orthotopic Bladder Cancer Xenograft Model

To investigate the role of KDM7A in bladder tumor growth in vivo, we stably incorporated a luciferase-expressing vector into KDM7A shRNA-expressing bladder cancer cell lines and control cell line. After their inoculation into the bladders of NOD scid gamma (NSG) immune-deficient mice, the growth of the cancer cells was monitored using luciferase signal. The growth of bladder tumors was consistently higher in control cells compared to KMD7A knock-down cells (Figure 6A, Supplemental Figure S11). On the day of sacrifice, the tumors were extracted and the luminescence in control tumors was seen to be significantly higher than in KDM7A knock-down tumors (Figure 6B). Immunostaining of proliferation marker Ki-67 was used to evaluate the aggressiveness of the tumor (Figure 6C). The control tumor was positive for Ki-67, while the KDM7A knock-down tumor was found to be negative. The expression of vascular endothelial growth factor (VEGF) was detected in control tumor, but not in KDM7A knock-down tumors. These results implied that the growth and migration capability of bladder tumor is highly affected by the expression of KDM7A in vivo.

2.7. TC-E 5002 Treatment of Xenografted Bladder Tumors Reduced the Tumor Size

In the prostate study, we found that the KDM7A inhibitor TC-E 5002 effectively reduced tumor cell growth and migration in vitro [32]. In order to assess the in vivo effect of TC-E 5002 on bladder cancer development, we subcutaneously injected the T24 cells in the flanks of the NSG mice. After the tumor volume had reached 200 mm^3, the mice were divided into 2 groups and injected with the vehicle or TC-E 5002 intraperitoneally daily for 8 days. After day 8, we observed a difference in the tumor sizes between the two groups (Figure 7A). The tumors excised from mice treated with TC-E 5002 weighed lesser than those excised from control mice (Figure 7B). Suppression of the AR activity by TC-E 5002 treatment was evident from the protein and mRNA expression levels of AR-dependent genes in the individual tumors (Figure 7 C,D). In tumors treated with TC-E 5002, the expression of the cell-cycle marker Ki-67 and VEGF protein were decreased, while the expression of the apoptotic DNA-fragmentation marker TUNEL was increased (Figure 7E). Our data exemplified the potential applications of TC-E 5002 in bladder cancer treatment in vivo.

2.8. KDM7A Protein and mRNA Level Were Elevated in Bladder Cancer Patients

In order to analyze KDM7A expression in bladder cancer patients, we performed immunohistochemistry (IHC) of KDM7A using tissue microarray. The results showed a higher level of KMD7A in tumor tissues compared to normal bladder tissue (Figure 8A). In the next step, patient tissue samples were collected, and the KDM7A protein and mRNA levels were analyzed. The protein (Figure 8B, Table 1) and mRNA (Figure 8C, Table 1) levels were significantly higher in tumor samples compared to normal bladder tissue from the same patients. Upon quantification of the signal from Western blot for KDM7A and its comparison with the tumor stages, the results were not statistically significant, which might be due to the small sample size (Supplemental Figure S12). Next, we evaluated the correlation between mRNA expression level of KDM7A and clinical outcome using a Kaplan–Meier plotter in public database (www.kmplot.com). We examined the prognostic value of KDM7A expression at each tumor stage, and in both men and women, in the bladder cancer database using KDM7A as the 'key gene' for data mining. High *KDM7A* mRNA expression was associated with significantly worse overall survival (OS) in men with stage 2 bladder cancer (Figure 8D). However, we were not able to identify a correlation in other stages of male cancer patients (Supplemental Figures S13 and S14), or in any stages of female patients.

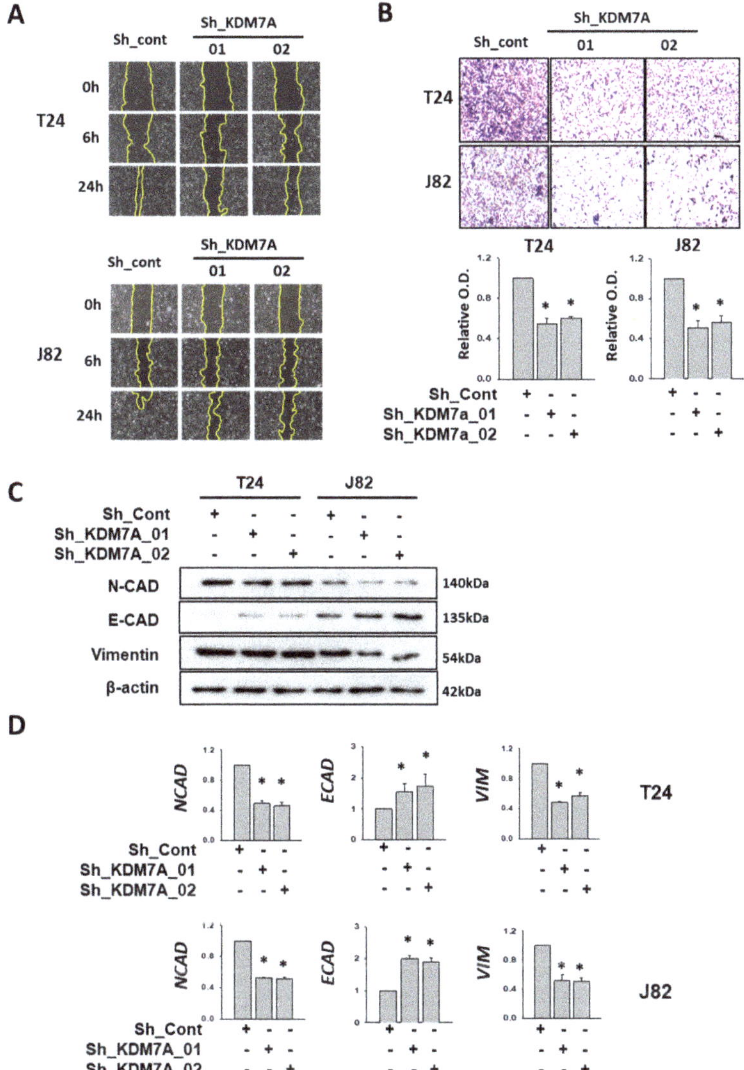

Figure 4. KDM7A knock-down reduced cell mobility and EMT-related gene expressions in bladder cancer cells. (**A**) Scratch-wounding cell migration assay of the control and KDM7A shRNA-expressing cells was performed for the indicated time. The wound margin is marked with a yellow line. (**B**) The Transwell assay of the same number of control and KDM7A shRNA-expressing cells. At 48 h after plating, cells that had migrated to the underside of the filters were fixed and stained with crystal violet. Photographs were taken and the relative cell migration was determined by measuring OD_{495} after extraction. Bars represent means ± SD of three independent experiments. * $p < 0.05$ (Student's *t*-test) versus the control shRNA (sh-cont) group. (**C**) The protein levels of indicated EMT markers were measured from the whole cell extracts of control or KDM7A knock-down cells. (**D**) The mRNA levels of the indicated EMT marker genes were measured from cell lines with control or KDM7A shRNA expression. Bars represent means ± SD of three independent experiments * $p < 0.05$ (Student's *t*-test) versus the sh-cont group.

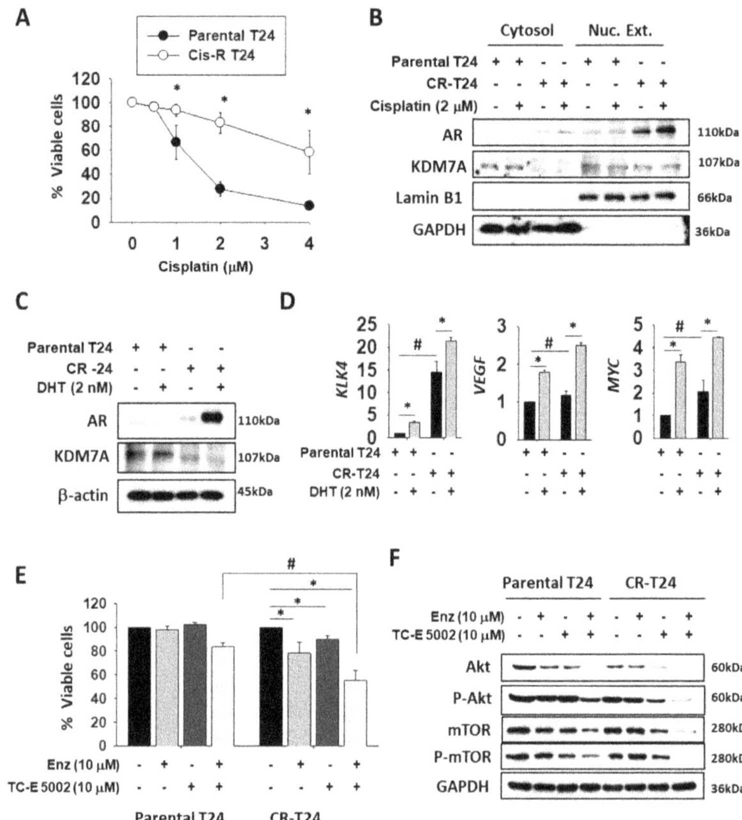

Figure 5. Nuclear localization and activity of AR were elevated in cisplatin-resistant T24 (CR-T24) cells, and treatment with enzalutamide and KDM7A inhibitor reduced the growth of CR-T24 bladder cancer cells. (**A**) Viability of parental and CR-T24 cells after treatment with the indicated concentrations of cisplatin for 3 days. Bars represent means ± SD of three independent experiments. * $p < 0.05$ (Student's *t*-test) versus parental cells. (**B**) Western blots of the indicated proteins from parental and CR-T24 cells. The cytosolic and nuclear fractions from each cell line were extracted and blotted with the indicated antibodies. Lamin B1 immunostaining served as the nuclear protein loading control and GAPDH immunostaining as cytoplasmic control. (**C**) Western blots of AR and KDM7A proteins from parental and CR-24 cells, before and after 5α-dihydrotestosterone (DHT) treatment. (**D**) mRNA levels of the indicated genes were measured from parental and CR-T24 cells. Bars represent means ± SD of three independent experiments. * $p < 0.05$ (Student's *t*-test), versus the mock-treated group. # $p < 0.05$ (Student's t-test) versus parental T24 cells. (**E**) Cell viability changes after 3 days of treatment with the indicated drugs on parental or CR-T24 cells. Bars represent means ± SD of three independent experiments. * $p < 0.05$ (Student's *t*-test) versus the mock-treated group. # $p < 0.05$ (Student's *t*-test) versus parental T24 cells. (**F**) Levels of the indicated proteins were measured from whole cell extracts of parental and CR-T24 cells, treated with either enzalutamide and/or TC-E 5002 for 2 days.

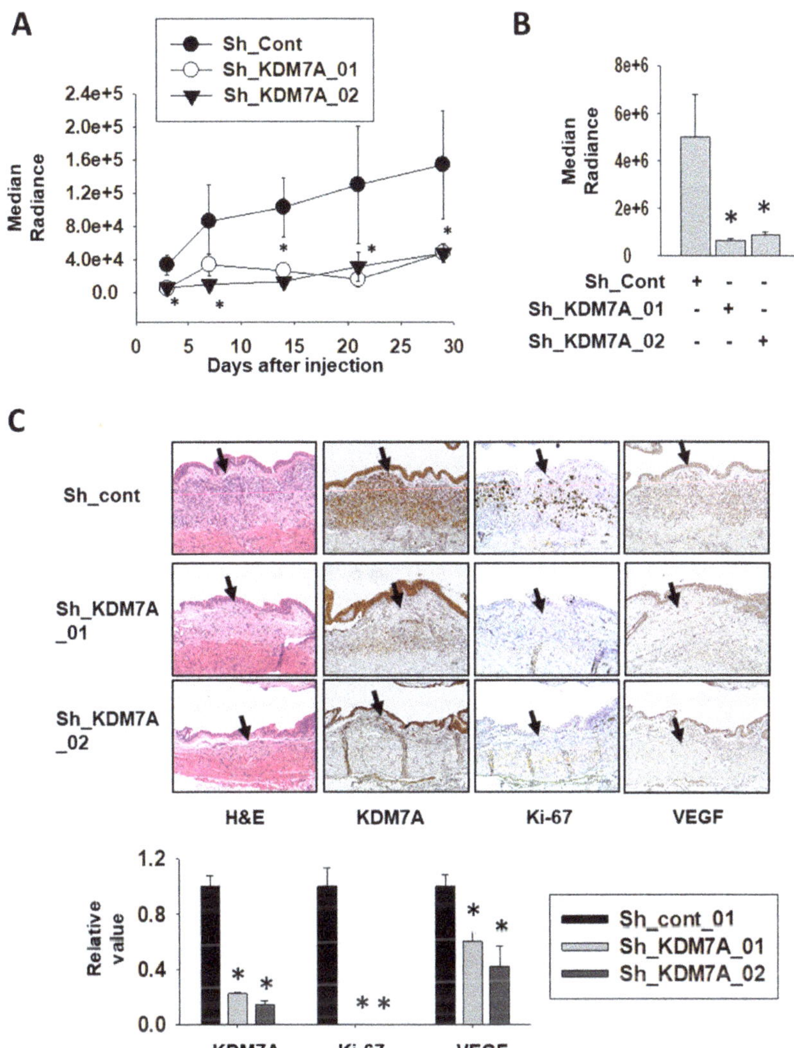

Figure 6. Attenuation of KDM7A expression reduces bladder tumor growth in orthotopic xenograft model. (**A**) Bioluminescent flux plot quantifying tumors in response to control or KDM7A shRNA-expressing T24 cells xenografted into mouse bladder. Error bars represent means ± SEM of each group ($n = 5$). * $p < 0.05$ (Student's t-test) versus the control shRNA (sh-cont) group. (**B**) Bioluminescent flux plot from the extracted bladder from each group. Error bars represent means ± SEM of each group ($n = 5$). * $p < 0.05$ (Student's t-test) versus the sh-cont group. (**C**) Representative hematoxylin-eosin staining and immunohistochemistry images of the orthotopically implanted bladder tumors. Arrow indicates tumor area of the mouse bladder. Positive signal was calculated from at least 3 independent areas, and relative values were plotted. Error bars represent means ± SEM of each group ($n = 5$). * $p < 0.05$ (Student's t-test) versus the sh-cont group.

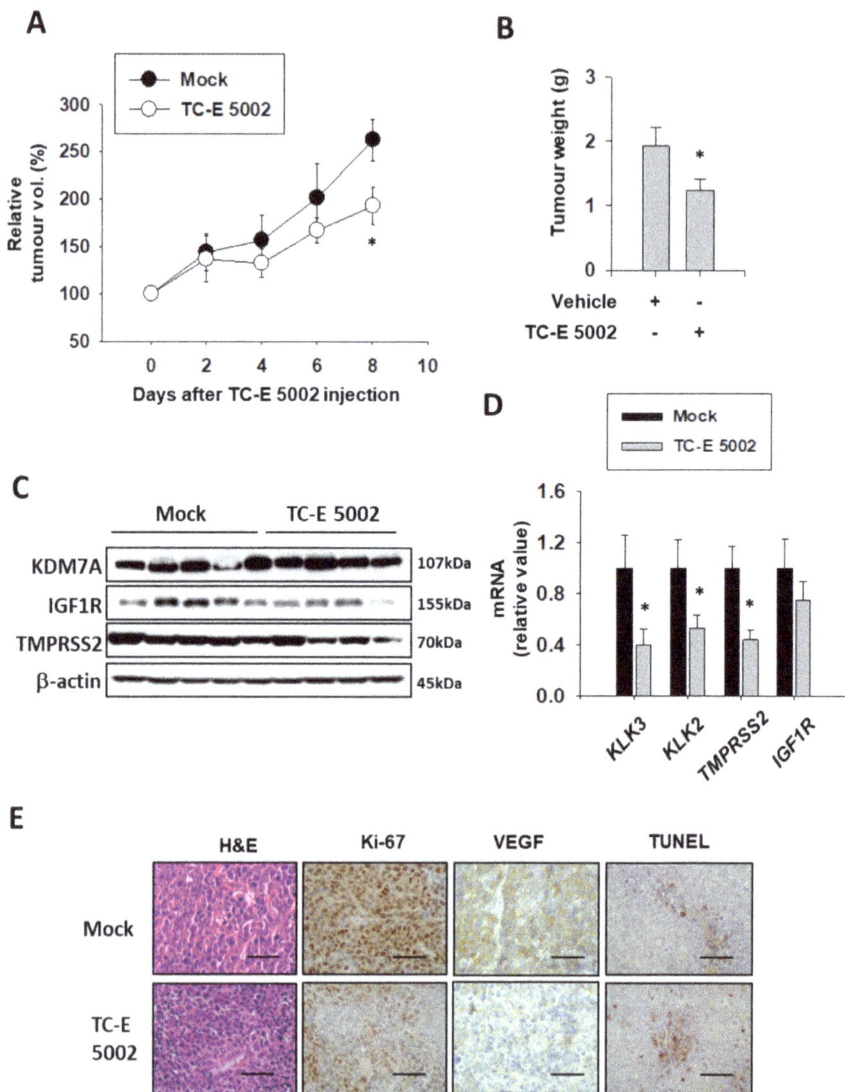

Figure 7. Effect of TC-E 5002 treatment on bladder tumor growth in the xenograft model in NSG mice. (**A**) Relative tumor volume in animals treated with vehicle or TC-E 5002 (10 mg/kg per day). Intraperitoneal drug treatment was started when the average tumor volume reached 200 mm^3 and continued every day for 8 days. Error bars represent means ± SEM for each group ($n = 5$). * $p < 0.05$ (Student's *t*-test) versus the vehicle-treated group. (**B**) Weight of tumors excised from animals treated with the vehicle or TC-E 5002. Error bars represent means ± SEM for each group ($n = 5$). * $p < 0.05$ (Student's *t*-test) versus the vehicle-treated group. (**C**) Total protein was extracted from each xenografted tumor, and Western blotting was performed using the indicated antibodies. (**D**) Total RNA was extracted from each xenografted tumor, and the indicated mRNA levels were measured. Bars represent means ± SEM for each group ($n = 5$). * $p < 0.05$ (Student's *t*-test) versus the vehicle-treated group. (**E**) Representative hematoxylin-eosin staining and immunohistochemistry images of the excised tumors. Scale bar is 20 μm.

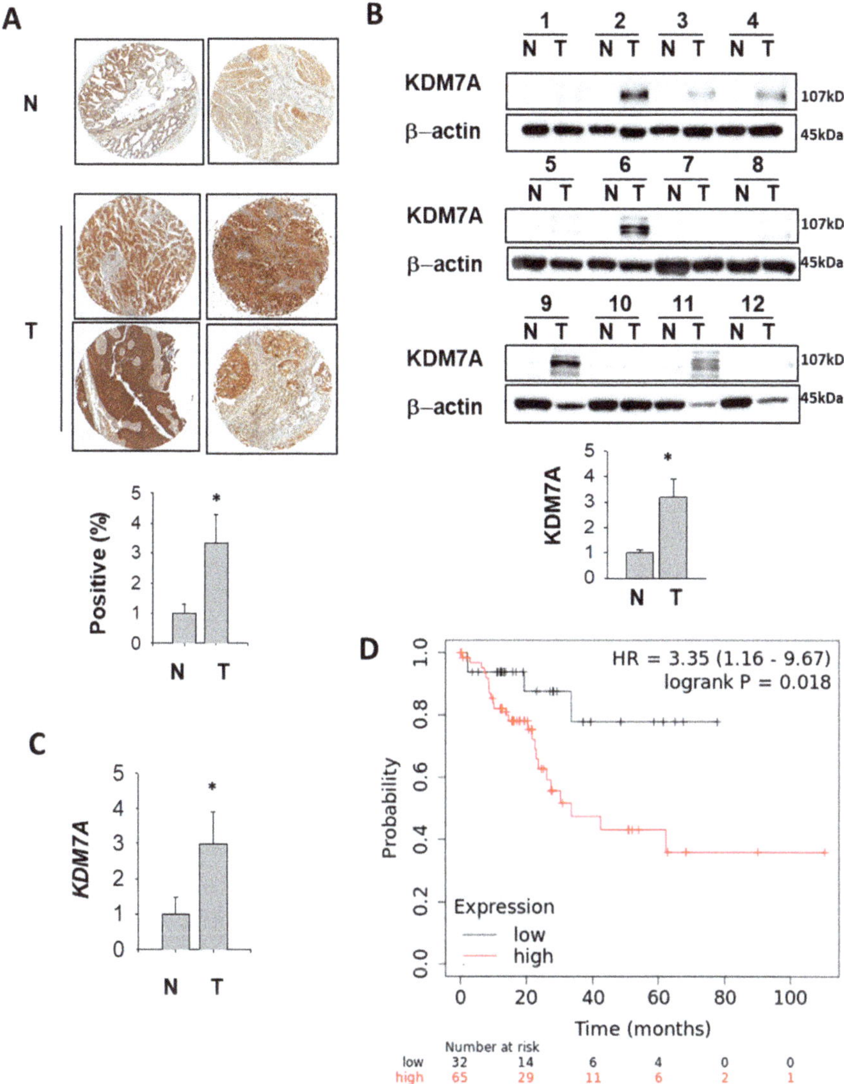

Figure 8. KDM7A is up-regulated in bladder cancer patients (**A**) Representative images of KDM7A expression in bladder tumor and normal tissue arrays (upper figures). N, normal bladder tissue; T, bladder tumor tissue. The expression level of KDM7A from 25 different bladder tumors and 6 normal tissues were calculated and plotted (below graph). * $p < 0.05$ (Student's *t*-test) between two groups. (**B**) Bladder tumor (T) and adjacent normal (N) tissues were subjected to Western blotting using the KDM7A and beta actin antibodies. Protein bands were analyzed densitometrically and protein levels normalized to beta actin levels were plotted in the lower graph. * $p < 0.05$ (Student's *t*-test) between two groups. (**C**) Comparison of KDM7A mRNA expression levels between normal and tumor bladder tissues. * $p < 0.05$ (Student's t-test) between two groups. (**D**) A survival curve was plotted for male bladder cancer patients with cancer stage 2 ($n = 97$). Data were analyzed using the Kaplan–Meier Plotter (www.kmplot.com). Patients with expression above the median are indicated in red line, and patients with expressions below the median in black line. HR means hazard ratio.

Table 1. Demographics of patients used for tissue extract.

No.	Age	Sex	T Stage
1	66	M	T2bN0(0/21) LVI necrosis
2	73	F	T2aN0(0/16)
3	58	M	TaN0(0/25) CIS
4	56	F	T1N0(0/37)
5	84	M	T4aN0(0/1) LVI, Perineural invasion
6	67	M	TaN0(0/26)
7	64	M	T3aN2(2/7) LVI, Perineural invasion
8	75	M	T3bN1(1/17), Perineural invasion
9	72	M	T2aN0(0/14)
10	70	M	T3aN0(0/15) Lymphatic invasion
11	61	M	T4aN2(3/17), LVI Perineural invasion, necrosis
12	63	M	T3aN0(0/13)

3. Discussion

Although the epigenetic regulation of AR has been extensively studied in prostate cancer, a growing body of evidence has suggested a role for AR in other cancers, including colon, breast, and bladder cancer. Because anti-cancer drugs targeting AR have been well-characterized in prostate cancer, existing drugs can be explored as potential treatment options for other AR-positive cancers as well. In this paper, we focused on the AR function in bladder cancer, because of its high malignant character, which is known to be related to AR malfunction.

KDM7A histone demethylase is known to act on H3K27 residues, which function as repressive marks of transcription. Consequently, lowering KDM7A activity results in H3K27 methylation on chromatin and reduced gene transcription. We had previously showed that AR binding to KLK3, KLK2, and TMPRSS2 gene promoters was decreased in KDM7A knock-down prostate cells, and the expression levels of these genes were also reduced. More importantly, the effect of the KDM7A inhibitor TC-E 5002 on prostate cancer cell proliferation was analyzed, and we observed that prostate cancer cell growth was reduced on treatment with TC-E 5002 treatment. In the present study, we found that the bladder cancer cells expressing KDM7A shRNA also showed decreased cell proliferation. As expected, the AR expression in bladder cancer cells was lower than that of prostate cells (Supplemental Figure S1). Therefore, the effect of KDM7A knockdown was not as dramatic as in prostate cells. However, the reduction of bladder cancer cell growth, migration and metastatic abilities was found to be statistically significant. On the other hand, when we used TC-E 5002, a chemical inhibitor of KDM7A, we detected a relatively small effect on T24 bladder cancer cell growth (Figure 5E) compared to the inhibition effect of KDM7A knock-down (Figure 3A). This could be because the selected TC-E 5002 treatment time and concentration were not high enough to kill the original T24 cells, since we wanted to see the effect of TC-E 5002 and/or enzalutamide on CR-T24 cells. When we continued TC-E 5002 treatment for longer durations and using higher doses, more cell death was achieved. Since many in vitro studies have shown the anti-cancer effect of enzalutamide in bladder cancer, including drug-resistant conditions [16–19], co-treatment of TC-E 5002 together with enzalutamide was performed to study the effect on cisplatin-resistant bladder cancer cells. As we can see in the right part of graph in Figure 5E, CR-T24 cells, which had elevated AR expression, died more efficiently upon TC-E 5002 treatment. In addition to cisplatin-resistant T24 [19], gemcitabine-resistant T24 has also been reported to show increased AR expression [17]. Therefore, it would be interesting to investigate whether treatment of gemcitabine-resistant cells with TC-E 5002 has the same effect. In particular, the effect of co-treatment with enzalutamide and TC-E 5002 on CR-T24 bladder cancer cell line could be useful for understanding the value of this treatment in drug-resistant bladder cancer. In addition to testing TC-E 5002 in vitro in cell culture, our in vivo data using the xenograft bladder tumors illustrated the future possibility of applying the drug clinically.

Although we focused only on demonstrating the role of KDM7A in regulating AR activity, we cannot rule out the possibility that KDM7A acts on other factors, regulating the cell cycle, or that our results are owing to the non-specific knockdown effect of KDM7A. This is because the AR expression level of the cell lines that we used was notably lower than that of prostate cancer, and the repressive effect on neoplasia was relatively strong. Factors other than AR may include KLF4 and c-MYC, which were found to be involved in breast cancer stem cell maintenance [34]. The use of only two bladder cell lines with undifferentiated character may also limit the universality of our data. Therefore, it would be interesting to study the function of KDM7A in other differentiated cancer cells.

Our finding that the protein and mRNA levels of KDM7A are increased in bladder cancer tissues (Figure 8) may point to elevated AR activity in the cancer. Based on our results, it is possible that KDM7A controls AR activity as an epigenetic co-activator during cancer progression. Most importantly, the KDM7A protein level increased in tumor tissues compared to matching normal tissues (Figure 8B). However, the correlation of KDM7A expression level with each cancer stage was not statistically significant, perhaps due to the small number of cases for each stage (Supplemental Figure S12). Nonetheless, the fact that we identified a correlation between high KDM7A mRNA levels and cancer-dependent deaths only in men (Figure 8D), but not in women, may explain the AR dependency of this effect. Interestingly, this correlation was lost in men with higher grades of cancer (grade 3 and 4; Supplement Supplement Figures S13 and S14), which may be due to the AR loss-of-function during the progression of bladder cancer. Given that this phenomenon is widely reported in prostate cancer, a similar mechanism may exist in bladder cancer. For the early stage male bladder cancer patients, it would be interesting to explore whether an AR antagonist can be used as an anti-cancer drug upon screening KMD7A expression levels. In addition, the regulation of other transcription factors besides AR, which are under the control of KDM7A, should be considered.

An increasing number of histone-modifying enzymes have been shown to be important for bladder cancer development. Among them, the knock-down of LSD1 was found to effectively repress bladder cancer growth, and this effect was confirmed to be associated with AR activity regulation [47]. Additionally, it has been shown that the up-regulation of histone methyl transferase SMYD3 promotes bladder cancer progression. It is worth noting that, although the authors demonstrated that SMYD3 physically interacted with the BCLAF1 promoter [48], it is possible that SMYD3 may regulate bladder cancer growth *via* AR, because of its previously reported interaction with the receptor [30]. Our data point to the possibility that KDM7A may regulate AR in bladder cancer together with the above-mentioned co-regulators. Investigating potential interactions of the above mentioned co-factors with KDM7A on the AR-regulated gene promoters would lead to a better understanding of the mechanism.

The anti-cancer effect of many histone methylase or demethylase inhibitors have been reported in bladder cancer, and many of them are presently being developed for cancer treatment [49]. Based on our data, we suggest that KDM7A inhibitor TC-E 5002 could be added to this list. Although further in-depth research is needed to validate the results of our study, our findings suggest that KDM7A could be a new target for treating bladder cancer and overcoming drug resistance, in conjunction with an AR inhibitor.

4. Materials and Methods

4.1. Materials

RPMI-1640, DMEM, trypsin, anti-biotics, Trizol and Lipofectamine 2000 were purchased from Invitrogen (Carlsbad, CA, USA). Fetal bovine serum and culture media were obtained from HyClone Laboratories Inc. (South Logan, UT, USA). The detailed information of all primary antibodies is listed in Supplemental Table S1.

4.2. Cell Lines, Plasmids, Virus Production and Infection

The T24, J82, and 293T cell lines were purchased from the American Type Culture Collection (Rockville, MD). T24 and J82 cells were cultured in RPMI-1640, and 293T cells for lentiviral package were cultured in DMEM medium at 37 °C in 5% CO_2, which was supplemented with 10% fetal bovine serum. For gene silencing, the control or KDM7A shRNA expressing lenti-virus packaging and stable cell line establishment were performed as described [32]. The oligo sequence used for KDM7A shRNA 01 cloning is 5′-CCGGTGGATTTGATGTCCCTATTATCTCGAGATAATAGGGACATCAAATCCAT TTTT-3′, and for shRNA 02 sequence is 5′-CCGGTTAGACCTGGACACCTTATTACTCGAGTAATAA GGTGTCCAGGTCTAATTTTT-3′. The oligo sequence for control shRNA cloning is 5′-CCGGCGTGA TCTTCACCGACAAGATCTCGAGATCTTGTCGGTGAAGATCACGTTTTT-3′. FUGW-luc vector (from the Molecular Imaging and Neurovascular Research Laboratory, Dongguk University Ilsan Hospital, Goyang, Korea) expressing cells were produced as described below. FUGW-luc vector was cut with XhoI enzyme and transfected into the T24 cell line, expressing either control vector or KMD7A shRNA vector. The cells with FUGW-luc incorporation were sorted with GFP channel using BD FACSAria II (BD Biosciences, Franklin Lakes, NJ, USA).

4.3. Colony Formation Assay and Cell Viability Assay

For the colony formation assay, 1000 cells were plated in 6-well plates. The cells were cultured for 14 days and stained with 0.1% crystal violet. The cell colonies were photographed, and the number of colonies comprising more than 50 individual cells was counted using SZX7 stereo microscope (Olympus, Tokyo, Japan). For the cell viability assay, cells (2000 to 3000 cells/well) were dispensed in 100 µL culture medium in a 96-well plate, and incubated for the indicated time. EZ-Cytox cell viability kit (Daeil-Lab, Seoul, Korea) solution (10 µL) was mixed with the culture medium in each well of the plate. Samples were incubated for 1 h at 37 °C, and the absorbance of each sample at 450 nm was measured using a microplate reader (PerkinElmer, Waltham, MA, USA).

4.4. RNA Isolation and the Real-Time Quantitative Polymerase Chain Reaction (RT-qPCR)

The total cellular RNA was extracted using the Trizol reagent (Ambion, Austin, TX, USA), according to the manufacturer's instructions. For the induction of AR activity, 5 nM 5α-dihydrotestosterone (DHT) was added after one day of serum deprivation. For each reverse-transcription reaction, 1 µg of total RNA was used for cDNA synthesis, using the MultiScribe Reverse Transcription Kit from Life Technologies (Carlsbad, CA, USA). RT-qPCR was performed using the EvaGreen qPCR Master Mix Kit from Applied Biological Materials Inc. (Richmond, BC, Canada) and a StepOne™ Real-Time PCR System (Applied Biosystems, Foster City, CA, USA). The quantity of 18S ribosomal RNA was measured as an internal control. The sequences of the primers used for RT-qPCR are listed in Supplemental Table S2.

4.5. Wound Healing and Cell Invasion Assays

The wound healing assay was performed on 100% confluent cells, plated into 6-well culture plates. Straight scratches were made by using a pipette tip. The cells were washed twice to remove debris, followed by the addition of fresh medium. The cells were incubated in a 5% CO_2 environment at 37 °C, and observed using a SZX7 stereo microscope at the indicated time. The scratched areas were measured using ImageJ program (ver. 1.43u; www.rsb.info.nih.gov/ij). For the invasion assay, cells (5×10^4/well) were plated in the upper chambers of Transwells without serum, using Matrigel-coated polycarbonate membranes (Corning, Big Flats, NY, USA). The basal medium containing 10% fetal bovine serum was added into the lower chambers, as a chemoattractant for cell migration. After 48-h, non-migrated cells were removed from the upper chambers, while cells that migrated through chambers were fixed using 10% ethanol (Sigma-Aldrich). After cells were stained with the 0.01% crystal violet solution (Sigma-Aldrich), migrated cells were randomly counted in five different microscopic fields at 20× magnification.

4.6. Human Ethics Approval and Collection of Human Tissues

The frozen tissues from bladder cancer patients were collected from Seoul Nation University Hospital Tissue Bank, with the approval of Institutional Review Board No. H-1004-037-315 (Date of approval: 06/11/2010). The demographic data of each patient are shown in Table 1. Tumor tissues and matching normal tissues from the same patient were identified from the pathology results. For Western blotting, 50–200 mg of tissues was ground in liquid nitrogen and lysed with RIPA buffer.

4.7. Animal Studies and In Vivo Bioluminescent Imaging

All animal experiments were performed in accordance with the Seoul National University Hospital institutional guidelines, under IACUC protocol No.16-0167-C2A0 (Date of approval: 07/20/2018). NOD scid gamma (NSG) mice were bred and maintained under specific pathogen-free (SPF) conditions. For generating orthotopic tumors, 1×10^5 T24 human bladder cells expressing the indicated shRNA and Luciferase expression vector were injected into the bladder of six-week-old male NSG mice ($n = 5$ for each group). For injection, the cells were suspended with 100 µL of 50 % Matrigel (BD Biosciences) in complete media. The mice from each group were injected intraperitoneally with 150 mg/kg D-luciferin (Promega, Madison, WI, USA), 15 min before acquiring the image. After anesthetizing the mice using 1–3% isoflurane, the photons emitted from the tumor were detected with Xenogen IVIS imaging system 200 (Alameda, CA, USA) as described. The image acquisition period was 1 s. Living Image (Version 2.20, Xenogen) was used to quantify signals emitted from the regions of interest. The mice were sacrificed after 30 days of tumor implantation, and bladder tumor was fixed in 4% paraformaldehyde at 4 °C and embedded in paraffin. The specimens were subjected to IHC with the indicated antibodies. For subcutaneous xenografting, six-week-old male NSG mice were injected, in their lower flanks, with 1×10^7 T24 cells in 100 µL of 50% (*v/v*) Matrigel ($n = 5$ for each group). When the average tumor volume reached 200 mm^3, mice were randomly assigned into two groups and injected intraperitoneally everyday with vehicle (0.05 mL; 90% corn-oil and 10% DMSO (*v/v*)) or 10 mg/kg TC-E 5002 in the same vehicle, respectively. The tumors were measured every other day, and at the end of 8 days of treatment, the mice were sacrificed, and the tumors were excised, weighed, and either frozen or fixed in formalin for further analyses.

4.8. Western Blotting

The cells (5×10^6) and ground tissue (50–200 mg) were lysed in 1ml RIPA buffer (150 mM NaCl, 50 mM Tris-HCl [pH 7.2], 0.5% NP-40, 1% Triton X-100, and 1% sodium deoxycholate), containing a protease/phosphatase inhibitor cocktail (Sigma-Aldrich, St. Louis, MO, USA). For the induction of AR activity, 5 nM 5α-dihydrotestosterone (DHT) was added after one day of serum deprivation. The cell lysates were separated on sodium dodecyl sulfate-polyacrylamide gels and transferred to an Immobilon-P membrane (Millipore, Darmstadt, Germany). The membranes were blocked with 5% skim milk in 0.1% Tween-20 for 1 h, followed by overnight incubation at 4 °C with the indicated primary antibodies. The membranes were incubated with a horseradish peroxidase-conjugated secondary antibody (1:5000) for 1 h and developed using the ECL-Plus Kit (Thermo Scientific, Rockford, IL, USA).

4.9. Immunohistochemical Staining and Analysis

Bladder cancer tissue microarrays purchased from SuperBioChips Laboratories (Seoul, Korea) were stained with an anti-KDM7A antibody. The slides were incubated with an anti-Rabbit IgG secondary antibody and hematoxylin and eosin (nuclear staining dye). The expression level of KDM7A from 25 different bladder tumors and 6 normal tissues was calculated and plotted. The expression of KDM7A positive cells was evaluated using the Cytoplasmic V2.0 algorithm in Aperio ImageScope software (Leica, Nussloch, Germany), and logistic regression analysis was used to compare the expression patterns between groups. Mouse tumor tissues were fixed in paraffin after formaldehyde fixation. Mouse tissue slides were deparaffinized and stained with indicated antibodies, and the slides were photographed under a Leica microscope (Wetzlar, Germany). Positive signals were counted from at least 3 different fields of the same area, and relative values were calculated.

4.10. The Kaplan–Meier Plotter

The prognostic significance of the mRNA expression of KDM7A was evaluated using the Kaplan–Meier plotter (www.kmplot.com), an online database comprising gene expression data and clinical data. In order to assess the prognostic value of the KDM7A gene, the patient samples were divided into two cohorts according to the median expression level of the gene (high vs. low expression). We analyzed overall survival (OS) of bladder cancer patients by the Kaplan–Meier survival plot. KDM7A gene was uploaded into the database to obtain the Kaplan–Meier survival plot, in which the number-at-risk was shown below the main plot. Log rank p-value and hazard ratio (HR) with 95% confidence intervals were calculated and displayed on the webpage. We exported the plot data as a PowerPoint file.

4.11. Statistical Analyses

All data were analyzed using Microsoft Excel 2010 software, unless otherwise stated. Continuous variables were analyzed using Student's *t*-test if the data were normally distributed. All statistical tests were two-sided. Differences were considered significant in cases where *p* values were <0.05.

Supplementary Materials: Supplementary materials can be found at http://www.mdpi.com/1422-0067/21/16/5658/s1. Figure S1. AR expression in bladder cell lines. Figure S2. AR expression levels in KDM7A knockdown J82 cells. Figure S3. The primer positions for ChIP-qPCR in the indicated gene promoters are illustrated. Figure S4. AR inhibition reduced cell viability of bladder cancer cells. Figure S5. T24 and J82 bladder cancer cells expressing KDM7A shRNAs or treated with TC-E 5002 photographed under phase contrast microscope. Figure S6. Enzalutamide treatment reduced cell mobility in bladder cancer cells. Figure S7. KDM7A knock-down reduced cell mobility in bladder cancer cells. Figure S8. Protein bands from Figure 4C were analyzed densitometrically and protein levels were normalized to beta-actin levels. Figure S9. The enzalutamide and TC-E 5002 treatment reduces cell growth and increased apoptosis in cisplatin resistant T24 cells. Figure S10. Enzalutamide and TC-E 5002 treatment reduced cell mobility in bladder cancer cells. Figure S11. IVIS images demonstrating tumor formation on the day of sacrifice. Figure S12. KDM7A protein expression in human bladder tumor tissues and normal tissues from the same patient. Figure S13. Survival curve was plotted for male bladder cancer patients with cancer stage 3. Figure S14. A survival curve was plotted for male bladder cancer patients with cancer stage 4. Table S1. The company and catalog numbers of antibodies. Table S2. Oligonucleotide sequences for RT-PCR and ChIP-PCR.

Author Contributions: Conceptualization, K.-H.L. and C.K.; Data curation, K.-H.L. and B.-C.K.; Funding acquisition, K.-H.L. and C.K.; Writing—original draft, K.-H.L.; Writing—review and editing, S.-H.J., C.W.J., J.H.K., H.H.K. and C.K. All authors have read and agreed to the published version of the manuscript.

Funding: This work was supported by a Basic Science Research Program through the National Research Foundation of Korea (NRF), funded by the Ministry of Education (NRF-2018R1A2B6001317), and by (NRF-2018R1D1A1B07041191).

Conflicts of Interest: The authors declare no conflict of interest.

Abbreviations

AR	androgen receptor
BCa	bladder cancer
CBP	CREB-binding protein
ChIP	chromatin immunoprecipitation
DHT	dihydrotestosterone
ECAD	E-cadherin
EMT	epithelial-mesenchymal transition
EZH2	enhancer of zeste homolog 2

HAT	histone acetyltransferase
IGF1R	insulin-like growth factor 1 receptor
KDM	lysine demethylase
KLK	kallikrein related peptidase
LSD1	lysine-specific histone demethylase 1
NCAD	N-cadherin
PCAF	P300/CBP-associated factor
PSA	prostate specific antigen
PHD	plant homeodomain
SET	su(var)3-9, enhancer-of-zeste and trithorax
SRC	steroid receptor coactivator proteins
VEGF	vascular endothelial growth factor

References

1. Siegel, R.L.; Miller, K.D.; Jemal, A. Cancer statistics, 2019. *CA Cancer J. Clin.* **2019**, *69*, 7–34. [CrossRef] [PubMed]
2. Sievert, K.D.; Amend, B.; Nagele, U.; Schilling, D.; Bedke, J.; Horstmann, M.; Hennenlotter, J.; Kruck, S.; Stenzl, A. Economic aspects of bladder cancer: What are the benefits and costs? *World J. Urol.* **2009**, *27*, 295–300. [CrossRef] [PubMed]
3. Dobruch, J.; Daneshmand, S.; Fisch, M.; Lotan, Y.; Noon, A.P.; Resnick, M.J.; Shariat, S.F.; Zlotta, A.R.; Boorjian, S.A. Gender and Bladder Cancer: A Collaborative Review of Etiology, Biology, and Outcomes. *Eur. Urol.* **2016**, *69*, 300–310. [CrossRef] [PubMed]
4. Chen, J.; Cui, Y.; Li, P.; Liu, L.; Li, C.; Zu, X. Expression and clinical significance of androgen receptor in bladder cancer: A meta-analysis. *Mol. Clin. Oncol.* **2017**, *7*, 919–927. [CrossRef]
5. Claps, M.; Petrelli, F.; Caffo, O.; Amoroso, V.; Roca, E.; Mosca, A.; Maines, F.; Barni, S.; Berruti, A. Testosterone Levels and Prostate Cancer Prognosis: Systematic Review and Meta-analysis. *Clin. Genitourin. Cancer* **2018**, *16*, 165–175. [CrossRef]
6. Sumanasuriya, S.; De Bono, J. Treatment of Advanced Prostate Cancer-A Review of Current Therapies and Future Promise. *Cold Spring Harb. Perspect. Med.* **2018**, *8*, a030635. [CrossRef]
7. Roshan, M.H.; Tambo, A.; Pace, N.P. The role of testosterone in colorectal carcinoma: Pathomechanisms and open questions. *EPMA J.* **2016**, *7*, 22. [CrossRef]
8. Ricciardelli, C.; Bianco-Miotto, T.; Jindal, S.; Butler, L.M. The Magnitude of Androgen Receptor Positivity in Breast Cancer is Critical for Reliable Prediction of Disease Outcome. *Clin. Cancer Res.* **2018**, *24*, 2328–2341 [CrossRef]
9. Zhang, B.G.; Du, T.; Zang, M.D.; Chang, Q.; Fan, Z.Y.; Li, J.F.; Yu, B.Q.; Su, L.P.; Li, C.; Yan, C.; et al. Androgen receptor promotes gastric cancer cell migration and invasion via AKT-phosphorylation dependent upregulation of matrix metalloproteinase 9. *Oncotarget* **2014**, *5*, 10584–10595. [CrossRef]
10. Li, Y.; Izumi, K.; Miyamoto, H. The role of the androgen receptor in the development and progression of bladder cancer. *Jpn. J. Clin. Oncol.* **2012**, *42*, 569–577. [CrossRef]
11. Zhuang, Y.H.; Blauer, M.; Tammela, T.; Tuohimaa, P. Immunodetection of androgen receptor in human urinary bladder cancer. *Histopathology* **1997**, *30*, 556–562. [CrossRef] [PubMed]
12. Boorjian, S.; Ugras, S.; Mongan, N.P.; Gudas, L.J.; You, X.; Tickoo, S.K.; Scherr, D.S. Androgen receptor expression is inversely correlated with pathologic tumor stage in bladder cancer. *Urology* **2004**, *64*, 383–388. [CrossRef] [PubMed]
13. Boorjian, S.A.; Heemers, H.V.; Frank, I.; Farmer, S.A.; Schmidt, L.J.; Sebo, T.J.; Tindall, D.J. Expression and significance of androgen receptor coactivators in urothelial carcinoma of the bladder. *Endocr.-Relat. Cancer* **2009**, *16*, 123–137. [CrossRef] [PubMed]
14. Miyamoto, H.; Yang, Z.; Chen, Y.-T.; Ishiguro, H.; Uemura, H.; Kubota, Y.; Nagashima, Y.; Chang, Y.-J.; Hu, Y.-C.; Tsai, M.-Y.; et al. Promotion of Bladder Cancer Development and Progression by Androgen Receptor Signals. *JNCI J. Natl. Cancer Inst.* **2007**, *99*, 558–568. [CrossRef] [PubMed]
15. Hsu, J.-W.; Hsu, I.; Xu, D.; Miyamoto, H.; Liang, L.; Wu, X.-R.; Shyr, C.-R.; Chang, C. Decreased Tumorigenesis and Mortality from Bladder Cancer in Mice Lacking Urothelial Androgen Receptor. *Am. J. Pathol.* **2013**, *182*, 1811–1820. [CrossRef]

16. Kawahara, T.; Ide, H.; Kashiwagi, E.; El-Shishtawy, K.A.; Li, Y.; Reis, L.O.; Zheng, Y.; Miyamoto, H. Enzalutamide inhibits androgen receptor-positive bladder cancer cell growth. *Urol. Oncol.* **2016**, *34*, e15–e23. [CrossRef]

17. Kameyama, K.; Horie, K.; Mizutani, K.; Kato, T.; Fujita, Y.; Kawakami, K.; Kojima, T.; Miyazaki, T.; Deguchi, T.; Ito, M. Enzalutamide inhibits proliferation of gemcitabine-resistant bladder cancer cells with increased androgen receptor expression. *Int. J. Oncol.* **2017**, *50*, 75–84. [CrossRef]

18. Kawahara, T.; Inoue, S.; Kashiwagi, E.; Chen, J.; Ide, H.; Mizushima, T.; Li, Y.; Zheng, Y.; Miyamoto, H. Enzalutamide as an androgen receptor inhibitor prevents urothelial tumorigenesis. *Am. J. Cancer Res.* **2017**, *7*, 2041–2050. [CrossRef]

19. Kashiwagi, E.; Ide, H.; Inoue, S.; Kawahara, T.; Zheng, Y.; Reis, L.O.; Baras, A.S.; Miyamoto, H. Androgen receptor activity modulates responses to cisplatin treatment in bladder cancer. *Oncotarget* **2016**, *7*, 49169–49179. [CrossRef]

20. Baylin, S.B. DNA methylation and gene silencing in cancer. *Nat. Clin. Pract. Oncol.* **2005**, *2*, S4–S11. [CrossRef]

21. Dompe, C.; Janowicz, K.; Hutchings, G.; Moncrieff, L.; Jankowski, M.; Nawrocki, M.J.; Józkowiak, M.; Mozdziak, P.; Petitte, J.; Shibli, J.A.; et al. Epigenetic Research in Stem Cell Bioengineering-Anti-Cancer Therapy, Regenerative and Reconstructive Medicine in Human Clinical Trials. *Cancers* **2020**, *12*, 1016. [CrossRef] [PubMed]

22. Black, J.C.; Van Rechem, C.; Whetstine, J.R. Histone lysine methylation dynamics: Establishment, regulation, and biological impact. *Mol. Cell* **2012**, *48*, 491–507. [CrossRef] [PubMed]

23. Greer, E.L.; Shi, Y. Histone methylation: A dynamic mark in health, disease and inheritance. *Nat. Rev. Genet.* **2012**, *13*, 343–357. [CrossRef] [PubMed]

24. Kooistra, S.M.; Helin, K. Molecular mechanisms and potential functions of histone demethylases. *Nat. Rev. Mol. Cell Biol.* **2012**, *13*, 297–311. [CrossRef]

25. Baumgart, S.J.; Haendler, B. Exploiting Epigenetic Alterations in Prostate Cancer. *Int. J. Mol. Sci.* **2017**, *18*, 1017. [CrossRef]

26. Kahl, P.; Gullotti, L.; Heukamp, L.C.; Wolf, S.; Friedrichs, N.; Vorreuther, R.; Solleder, G.; Bastian, P.J.; Ellinger, J.; Metzger, E.; et al. Androgen receptor coactivators lysine-specific histone demethylase 1 and four and a half LIM domain protein 2 predict risk of prostate cancer recurrence. *Cancer Res.* **2006**, *66*, 11341–11347. [CrossRef]

27. Coffey, K.; Rogerson, L.; Ryan-Munden, C.; Alkharaif, D.; Stockley, J.; Heer, R.; Sahadevan, K.; O'Neill, D.; Jones, D.; Darby, S.; et al. The lysine demethylase, KDM4B, is a key molecule in androgen receptor signalling and turnover. *Nucleic Acids Res.* **2013**, *41*, 4433–4446. [CrossRef]

28. Han, M.; Xu, W.; Cheng, P.; Jin, H.; Wang, X. Histone demethylase lysine demethylase 5B in development and cancer. *Oncotarget* **2017**, *8*, 8980–8991. [CrossRef]

29. Deb, G.; Thakur, V.S.; Gupta, S. Multifaceted role of EZH2 in breast and prostate tumorigenesis. *Epigenetics* **2013**, *8*, 464–476. [CrossRef]

30. Liu, C.; Wang, C.; Wang, K.; Liu, L.; Shen, Q.; Yan, K.; Sun, X.; Chen, J.; Liu, J.; Ren, H.; et al. SMYD3 as an oncogenic driver in prostate cancer by stimulation of androgen receptor transcription. *J. Natl. Cancer Inst.* **2013**, *105*, 1719–1728. [CrossRef]

31. Mounir, Z.; Korn, J.M.; Westerling, T.; Lin, F.; Kirby, C.A.; Schirle, M.; McAllister, G.; Hoffman, G.; Ramadan, N.; Hartung, A.; et al. ERG signaling in prostate cancer is driven through PRMT5-dependent methylation of the Androgen Receptor. *Elife* **2016**, *5*, e13964. [CrossRef] [PubMed]

32. Lee, K.H.; Hong, S.; Kang, M.; Jeong, C.W.; Ku, J.H.; Kim, H.H.; Kwak, C. Histone demethylase KDM7A controls androgen receptor activity and tumor growth in prostate cancer. *Int. J. Cancer* **2018**, *143*, 2849–2861. [CrossRef] [PubMed]

33. Tsukada, Y.; Fang, J.; Erdjument-Bromage, H.; Warren, M.E.; Borchers, C.H.; Tempst, P.; Zhang, Y. Histone demethylation by a family of JmjC domain-containing proteins. *Nature* **2006**, *439*, 811–816. [CrossRef] [PubMed]

34. Meng, Z.; Liu, Y.; Wang, J.; Fan, H.; Fang, H.; Li, S.; Yuan, L.; Liu, C.; Peng, Y.; Zhao, W.; et al. Histone demethylase KDM7A is required for stem cell maintenance and apoptosis inhibition in breast cancer. *J. Cell. Physiol.* **2020**, *235*, 932–943. [CrossRef] [PubMed]

35. Yang, X.; Wang, G.; Wang, Y.; Zhou, J.; Yuan, H.; Li, X.; Liu, Y.; Wang, B. Histone demethylase KDM7A reciprocally regulates adipogenic and osteogenic differentiation via regulation of C/EBPalpha and canonical Wnt signalling. *J. Cell. Mol. Med.* **2019**, *23*, 2149–2162. [CrossRef]

36. Higashijima, Y.; Matsui, Y.; Shimamura, T.; Nakaki, R.; Nagai, N.; Tsutsumi, S.; Abe, Y.; Link, V.M.; Osaka, M.; Yoshida, M.; et al. Coordinated demethylation of H3K9 and H3K27 is required for rapid inflammatory responses of endothelial cells. *EMBO J.* **2020**, *39*, e103949. [CrossRef] [PubMed]

37. Grad, J.M.; Le Dai, J.; Wu, S.; Burnstein, K.L. Multiple Androgen Response Elements and a Myc Consensus Site in the Androgen Receptor (AR) Coding Region Are Involved in Androgen-Mediated Up-Regulation of AR Messenger RNA. *Mol. Endocrinol.* **1999**, *13*, 1896–1911. [CrossRef]

38. Blackburn, J.; Vecchiarelli, S.; Heyer, E.E.; Patrick, S.M.; Lyons, R.J.; Jaratlerdsiri, W.; van Zyl, S.; Bornman, M.S.R.; Mercer, T.R.; Hayes, V.M. TMPRSS2-ERG fusions linked to prostate cancer racial health disparities: A focus on Africa. *Prostate* **2019**, *79*, 1191–1196. [CrossRef]

39. Kim, J.; Coetzee, G.A. Prostate specific antigen gene regulation by androgen receptor. *J. Cell. Biochem.* **2004**, *93*, 233–241. [CrossRef]

40. Lai, J.; Myers, S.A.; Lawrence, M.G.; Odorico, D.M.; Clements, J.A. Direct Progesterone Receptor and Indirect Androgen Receptor Interactions with the Kallikrein-Related Peptidase 4 Gene Promoter in Breast and Prostate Cancer. *Mol. Cancer Res.* **2009**, *7*, 129. [CrossRef]

41. Schayek, H.; Seti, H.; Greenberg, N.M.; Sun, S.; Werner, H.; Plymate, S.R. Differential regulation of insulin-like growth factor-I receptor gene expression by wild type and mutant androgen receptor in prostate cancer cells. *Mol. Cell. Endocrinol.* **2010**, *323*, 239–245. [CrossRef] [PubMed]

42. Eisermann, K.; Broderick, C.J.; Bazarov, A.; Moazam, M.M.; Fraizer, G.C. Androgen up-regulates vascular endothelial growth factor expression in prostate cancer cells via an Sp1 binding site. *Mol. Cancer* **2013**, *12*, 7. [CrossRef] [PubMed]

43. Gao, L.; Schwartzman, J.; Gibbs, A.; Lisac, R.; Kleinschmidt, R.; Wilmot, B.; Bottomly, D.; Coleman, I.; Nelson, P.; McWeeney, S.; et al. Androgen receptor promotes ligand-independent prostate cancer progression through c-Myc upregulation. *PLoS ONE* **2013**, *8*, e63563. [CrossRef]

44. Xu, Y.; Chen, S.Y.; Ross, K.N.; Balk, S.P. Androgens induce prostate cancer cell proliferation through mammalian target of rapamycin activation and post-transcriptional increases in cyclin D proteins. *Cancer Res.* **2006**, *66*, 7783–7792. [CrossRef]

45. Li, Y.; Zhang, D.Y.; Ren, Q.; Ye, F.; Zhao, X.; Daniels, G.; Wu, X.; Dynlacht, B.; Lee, P. Regulation of a novel androgen receptor target gene, the cyclin B1 gene, through androgen-dependent E2F family member switching. *Mol. Cell. Biol.* **2012**, *32*, 2454–2466. [CrossRef] [PubMed]

46. Frezza, M.; Yang, H.; Dou, Q.P. Modulation of the tumor cell death pathway by androgen receptor in response to cytotoxic stimuli. *J. Cell. Physiol.* **2011**, *226*, 2731–2739. [CrossRef]

47. Kauffman, E.C.; Robinson, B.D.; Downes, M.J.; Powell, L.G.; Lee, M.M.; Scherr, D.S.; Gudas, L.J.; Mongan, N.P. Role of androgen receptor and associated lysine-demethylase coregulators, LSD1 and JMJD2A, in localized and advanced human bladder cancer. *Mol. Carcinog.* **2011**, *50*, 931–944. [CrossRef]

48. Shen, B.; Tan, M.; Mu, X.; Qin, Y.; Zhang, F.; Liu, Y.; Fan, Y. Upregulated SMYD3 promotes bladder cancer progression by targeting BCLAF1 and activating autophagy. *Tumour Biol. J. Int. Soc. Oncodev. Biol. Med.* **2016**, *37*, 7371–7381. [CrossRef]

49. Song, Y.; Wu, F.; Wu, J. Targeting histone methylation for cancer therapy: Enzymes, inhibitors, biological activity and perspectives. *J. Hematol. Oncol.* **2016**, *9*, 49. [CrossRef]

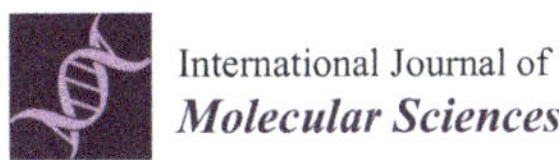

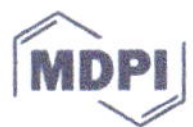

International Journal of
Molecular Sciences

Article

Urinary MicroRNAs as Potential Markers for Non-Invasive Diagnosis of Bladder Cancer

Kati Erdmann [1,2,†], Karsten Salomo [1,†], Anna Klimova [2,3], Ulrike Heberling [1], Andrea Lohse-Fischer [1], Romy Fuehrer [1], Christian Thomas [1], Ingo Roeder [2,3], Michael Froehner [1], Manfred P. Wirth [1] and Susanne Fuessel [1,*]

[1] Department of Urology, Technische Universität Dresden, 01307 Dresden, Germany; kati.erdmann@uniklinikum-dresden.de (K.E.); karsten.salomo@googlemail.com (K.S.); ulrike.heberling@uniklinikum-dresden.de (U.H.); andrea.lohse-fischer@uniklinikum-dresden.de (A.L.-F.); romy.fuehrer@uniklinikum-dresden.de (R.F.); christian.thomas@uniklinikum-dresden.de (C.T.); michael.froehner@ediacon.de (M.F.); manfred.wirth@uniklinikum-dresden.de (M.P.W.)
[2] National Center for Tumor Diseases (NCT), 01307 Dresden, Germany; anna.klimova@nct-dresden.de (A.K.); ingo.roeder@tu-dresden.de (I.R.)
[3] Institute for Medical Informatics and Biometrics, Technische Universität Dresden, 01307 Dresden, Germany
* Correspondence: susanne.fuessel@uniklinikum-dresden.de; Tel.: +49-351-45814544
† These authors contributed equally to this work.

Received: 5 May 2020; Accepted: 26 May 2020; Published: 27 May 2020

Abstract: Currently, voided urine cytology (VUC) serves as the gold standard for the detection of bladder cancer (BCa) in urine. Despite its high specificity, VUC has shortcomings in terms of sensitivity. Therefore, alternative biomarkers are being searched, which might overcome these disadvantages as a useful adjunct to VUC. The aim of this study was to evaluate the diagnostic potential of the urinary levels of selected microRNAs (miRs), which might represent such alternative biomarkers due to their BCa-specific expression. Expression levels of nine BCa-associated microRNAs (miR-21, -96, -125b, -126, -145, -183, -205, -210, -221) were assessed by quantitative PCR in urine sediments from 104 patients with primary BCa and 46 control subjects. Receiver operating characteristic (ROC) curve analyses revealed a diagnostic potential for miR-96, -125b, -126, -145, -183, and -221 with area under the curve (AUC) values between 0.605 and 0.772. The combination of the four best candidates resulted in sensitivity, specificity, positive and negative predictive values (NPV), and accuracy of 73.1%, 95.7%, 97.4%, 61.1%, and 80.0%, respectively. Combined with VUC, sensitivity and NPV could be increased by nearly 8%, each surpassing the performance of VUC alone. The present findings suggested a diagnostic potential of miR-125b, -145, -183, and -221 in combination with VUC for non-invasive detection of BCa in urine.

Keywords: miRNA; quantitative PCR; tumor marker; urothelial carcinoma; voided urine cytology

1. Introduction

Bladder cancer (BCa) was the 10th most common malignancy worldwide with 550,000 new cases and an estimated 200,000 deaths in 2018 [1,2]. The highest BCa incidence rates in the world were reported for Southern and Western Europe and North America. In men, who are four times more frequently affected than women, BCa ranks sixth of all newly diagnosed cancers and is the ninth most deadly cancer worldwide [2]. Initial BCa diagnostic steps include voided urine cytology (VUC), as the current standard for non-invasive BCa detection, and cystoscopy, an invasive procedure. Tissue specimens obtained during transurethral resection of the bladder (TUR-B) undergo histopathological examination for assessment of the putative tumor grade and stage [3]. The same approach is used for regular follow-up after treatment to detect BCa recurrence and progression. Among other factors, these life-long, frequent, and cost-intensive surveillance procedures make BCa one of the most expensive tumor entities [4,5].

VUC is an observer-dependent method and characterized by a high specificity of 78–100%. While it displays a moderate sensitivity of 34–84% for high-grade tumors, its sensitivity for low-grade tumors is very low at 12–26% [6]. Even though several alternative biomarker-based tests for non-invasive BCa detection in urine exist, none of them is recommended for routine use in clinical practice due to their inadequate performance [3,7]. The sensitivity of most alternative BCa tests is higher compared to VUC, but their specificity is not able to reach that of VUC so far [8,9]. Therefore, the search for cost-efficient, highly specific, and sensitive biomarkers for non-invasive BCa diagnosis, screening, and follow-up, which eventually allow reducing the number of invasive, inconvenient, and expensive cystoscopies, is ongoing.

Numerous studies have been aimed at the identification of mRNA expression signatures in tumor tissues and tumor-derived urine specimens that reflect the presence and aggressiveness of BCa and additionally characterize the most powerful predictive biomarker combinations [10–12]. In recent years, microRNAs (miRNAs or miRs) emerged as potential diagnostic and prognostic biomarkers due to their tissue- and tumor-specific expression. miRNAs are small, endogenous, non-coding RNAs that function as post-transcriptional regulators of specific target genes via mRNA degradation or inhibition of the translation [13,14]. As regulators of many cellular processes such as differentiation, proliferation, apoptosis or cell cycle control, miRNAs also play an important role in different deregulated, pathological pathways such as tumor onset and progression, making them promising candidates as tumor markers [13–15].

BCa-associated miRNA signatures were investigated by microarray, next-generation sequencing (NGS), and quantitative PCR (qPCR) analyses in malignant and non-malignant bladder tissue specimens, as well as in urine samples from BCa patients and control subjects. Several promising miRNA candidates showing a differential expression and/or an association with BCa aggressiveness emerged from these studies [16–20]. Additionally, the proven involvement of many of these miRNAs in tumor-related pathways deems them worthy of evaluation as potential biomarkers for diagnosis of BCa [21]. On the basis of a literature search comprising single reports, systematic reviews, and meta-analyses, nine miRNAs fulfilling the abovementioned criteria were selected for an independent validation study as putative biomarkers for non-invasive BCa detection in urine specimens: miR-21, -96, -125b, -126, -145, -183, -205, -210, and -221 [22–32] (for details, see also Supplementary Table S1). Using urine sediments from BCa patients and control subjects, the expression levels of these miRNAs determined by qPCR were assessed individually and in combination with regard to their diagnostic potential. In order to determine a potential diagnostic improvement, their diagnostic performance was also evaluated as an adjunct to VUC.

2. Results

2.1. Characteristics of BCa Patients and Control Subjects

A total of 104 patients with histologically-proven BCa at TUR-B were included in the present study (Table 1). This cohort consisted of 83 male and 21 female patients with a median age of 70 years (range 50 to 85 years). The relative distribution of pTa, pT1, pTis, and ≥pT2 tumors was 48.1%, 21.2%, 14.4%, and 16.3%. Since all of the 15 pTis tumors occurred concomitantly with other tumors, the most severe tumor stage was coded. In doing so, patients with non-muscle-invasive BCa (NMIBC; pTa and pT1) and concomitant pTis were allocated to the pTis group (10 of the 15 pTis cases; 9.6% of all BCa). The remaining five patients with muscle-invasive BCa (MIBC) and concomitant pTis were allocated to the group ≥pT2, resulting in a total of 22 patients with MIBC with or without concomitant pTis (21.1% of all BCa). Multifocal tumors occurred in 32 patients (30.8%).

Table 1. Demographic, clinical, and histopathological characteristics of the BCa patients (n = 104). The table shows the absolute and relative distribution of gender, age, and clinicopathological parameters.

Parameter	Category	Number (n)	Percentage (%)
gender	male	83	79.8
	female	21	20.2
age [1] (years)	≤70.0	54	51.9
	>70.0	50	48.1
tumor stage	pTa	50	48.1
	pT1	22	21.2
	pTis	15	14.4
	pTis only	*0*	*0.0*
	pTis + pTa	*3*	*2.9*
	pTis + pT1	*7*	*6.7*
	pTis + ≥ pT2a	*5*	*4.8*
	≥ pT2a	17	16.3
tumor grade (WHO 1973)	G1	14	13.5
	G2	52	50.0
	G3	38	36.5
tumor grade (WHO 2004)	low-grade	17	16.3
	high-grade	87	83.7
multifocality	unifocal	72	69.2
	multifocal	32	30.8
voided urine cytology	positive	80	76.9
	negative	24	23.1

[1] Age was dichotomized at the median (70.0 years).

Using the WHO grading system from 1973, 13.5% G1, 50.0% G2, and 36.5% G3 BCa were reported. According to the WHO grading system from 2004, 83.7% of the BCa patients displayed high-grade tumors, whereas only 16.3% had low-grade tumors.

Moreover, the control group consisted of eight subjects, who underwent a TUR-B without histopathological evidence of BCa and 38 patients with urolithiasis (Table 2).

Table 2. Demographic, clinical, and histopathological characteristics of the control subjects. The control group was comprised of 46 subjects in total, whereupon eight patients were histopathologically negative for BCa at TUR-B and 38 patients had urolithiasis. The table shows the absolute and relative distribution of gender, age and clinicopathological parameters.

Parameter	Category	Number (n)	Percentage (%)
gender	male	30	65.2
	female	16	34.8
age [1] (years)	<64.5	23	50.0
	≥64.5	23	50.0
diagnosis	BCa-negative TUR-B	8	17.4
	urolithiasis	38	82.6
voided urine cytology	positive	0	0.0
	negative	46	100.0

[1] Age was dichotomized at the median (64.5 years).

2.2. Correlations between the Analyzed miRNAs

Relative expression levels of the selected miRNAs (determined by qPCR and normalized to the geometric mean of the reference RNAs RNU44 and RNU48) were analyzed in detail in BCa-derived and control urine sediments. Some of the analyzed miRNAs showed significant correlations with each other as assessed by the pairwise calculation of Spearman's rank correlation coefficients. Most prominent significant positive correlations ($p < 0.01$) were observed between the miRNAs miR-21, -125b, -205, -210, and -221 with correlation coefficients between 0.566 (miR-210 vs. miR-221) and 0.825 (miR-125b vs. miR-221). Significant positive correlations ($p < 0.01$) were also seen between miR-96 and miR-183 ($r_s = 0.557$), miR-96 and miR-126 ($r_s = 0.311$), and miR-126 and miR-183 ($r_s = 0.483$). Finally, miR-145 correlated negatively ($p < 0.01$) with miR-205 ($r_s = -0.433$) and miR-210 ($r_s = -0.483$).

2.3. Associations of Urinary miRNA Transcript Levels and Histopathological Features

The expression levels of miR-125b ($r_s = -0.434$, $p < 0.01$) and miR-205 ($r_s = -0.206$, $p < 0.05$) in the tumor-derived urine samples decreased with increasing tumor stage, whereas those of miR-96 and miR-183 showed a weak positive correlation with tumor stage ($r_s = 0.238$ and 0.246, $p < 0.05$). A weak, but significant negative correlation ($p < 0.01$) with tumor grade according to the WHO classification from 1973 was detected for miR-125b, miR-205, and miR-210 (r_s between -0.309 and -0.334), whereas miR-145 displayed a weak, but significant positive correlation with tumor grade ($r_s = 0.266$, $p < 0.01$). A similar trend of dependence on tumor grade assessed according to the WHO classification from 2004 could only be observed for miR-125b and -210. The inverse relationships between the miR-125b expression levels in urine and tumor stage, as well as with tumor grade are exemplarily shown in Figure 1. Significant differences in relative miR-125b levels were found between the controls and all tumor stages, as well as between pTa tumors and higher tumor stages. Moreover, relative miR-125b levels differed significantly between the controls and G2/G3 or high-grade BCa, as well as between G1 and G2/G3 or low-grade and high-grade tumors (Figure 1). None of the miRNAs displayed substantial alterations between urine samples from patients with unifocal and multifocal BCa.

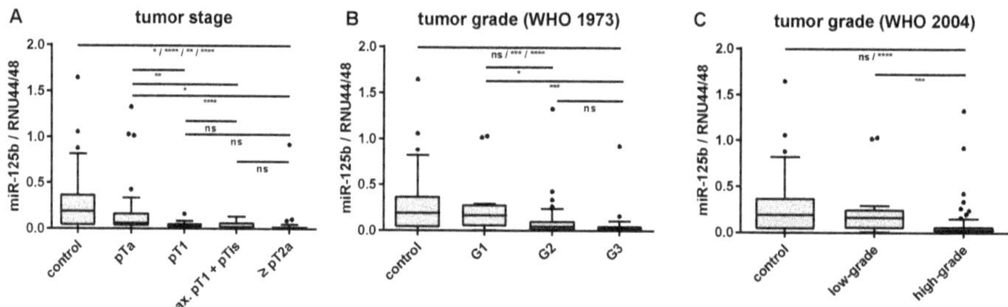

Figure 1. Dependence of the relative miR-125b expression levels (normalized to the geometric mean of the reference RNAs RNU44 and RNU48) in urine sediments on histopathological factors. The relationships between urinary miR-125b expression levels and tumor stage (**A**), as well as tumor grade according to the WHO classifications from 1973 (**B**) and from 2004 (**C**) are shown. Differences were tested by the Mann–Whitney U test. ns, not significant; * $p < 0.05$; ** $p < 0.01$; *** $p < 0.001$; **** $p < 0.0001$.

2.4. Evaluation of the Single miRNAs as Potential Markers for BCa Detection

Next, the relative miRNA expression levels were compared between the urine samples from the eight control patients without histopathological evidence of BCa at TUR-B and from the 38 controls patients with urolithiasis. None of the nine analyzed miRNAs showed significant differences in relative expression levels between both control subgroups (Mann–Whitney U test: $p > 0.05$). Therefore, data from both subgroups were combined, constituting the final control group of 46 subjects.

In comparison to these controls, statistically significant different relative miRNA expression levels were observed in urine sediments from BCa patients for miR-96, -125b, -126, -145, -183, and -221. After Bonferroni's correction for multiple comparisons (Table 3 and Figure 2), the significance was retained for these miRNAs except for miR-96 ($p = 0.05$). While the miRNAs miR-96, -126, and -183 displayed higher relative expression levels in the BCa-derived urine sediments, the miRNAs miR-125b, -145, and -221 were downregulated in these specimens compared to the control group (Table 3). Receiver operating characteristic (ROC) curve analyses also revealed a diagnostic potential for these six miRNAs with area under the curve (AUC) values ranging from 0.605 ($p = 0.369$) for miR-96 to 0.772 ($p < 0.001$) for miR-221 (Table 3 and Figure 3). The remaining three miRNAs miR-21, -205, and -210 did not show significant differences between tumor and control subjects (Table 3).

Table 3. Comparison of the relative miRNA expression levels in urine sediments from the BCa and control groups (Mann–Whitney U test) and assessment of the diagnostic power by ROC curve analyses. All *p*-values were adjusted by Bonferroni's correction for multiple comparisons.

miRNA	Regulation in BCa	Mann–Whitney U Test (*p*-Value)	ROC Curve Analysis AUC	*p*-Value
miR-21	not different	=1.000	0.581	=1.000
miR-96	up	=0.050	0.605	=0.369
miR-125b	down	<0.001	0.714	<0.001
miR-126	up	<0.01	0.667	<0.01
miR-145	down	<0.01	0.687	<0.01
miR-183	up	<0.001	0.720	<0.001
miR-205	not different	=1.000	0.537	=1.000
miR-210	not different	=1.000	0.526	=1.000
miR-221	down	<0.0001	0.772	<0.0001

95% CI, 95% confidence interval; AUC, area under the curve; ROC, receiver operating characteristic.

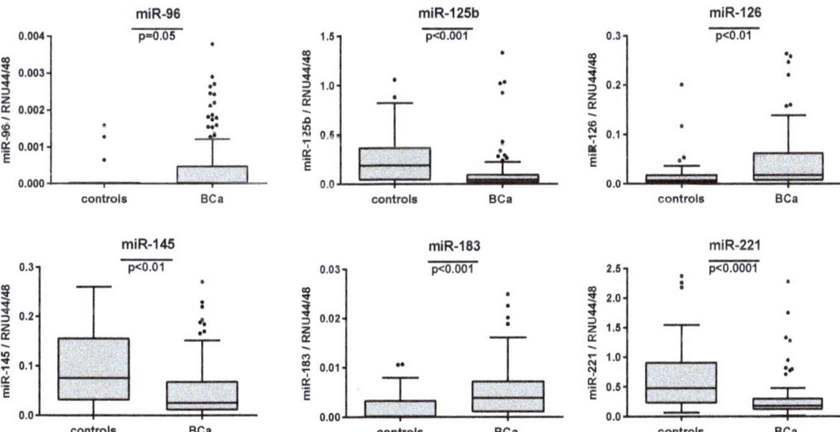

Figure 2. The distribution of the relative expression levels of the significantly altered miRNAs in urine sediments from controls and BCa patients is presented by box plots. Differences in the relative expression levels of the miRNAs (normalized to the geometric mean of the reference RNAs RNU44 and RNU48) were assessed using the Mann–Whitney U test followed by Bonferroni's correction for multiple comparisons.

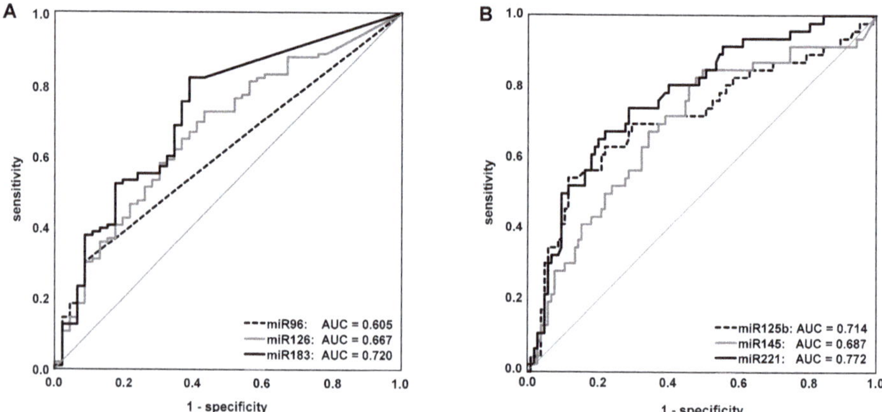

Figure 3. The diagnostic value assessed by ROC curve analysis of the six most promising miRNAs, which were significantly up- (**A**) or down-regulated (**B**) in urine sediments from BCa patients in comparison with controls. AUC, area under the curve; ROC, receiver operating characteristic.

2.5. Comparison of Diagnostic Performance of miRNA Transcript Levels and Voided Urine Cytology

To assess the diagnostic power of the single miRNAs, VUC, and combinations thereof, different statistical approaches were applied. The first approach was based on the simple classification of the measured relative miRNA expression levels and of the results of VUC assessment into positive ("1") and negative ("0") indicators of tumor detection. The diagnostic parameters calculated on this basis were assessed with regard to the best performing single BCa marker. The nine analyzed miRNAs displayed only moderate diagnostic value with accuracy rates between 48.7% for miR-96 and 78.0% for miR-125b (Table 4). None of these single miRNAs could surpass the performance of VUC, which displayed a relatively high sensitivity of 76.9% at a specificity of 100% and an accuracy of 84.0% (Table 4) in our cohort.

Table 4. Diagnostic performance of the miRNAs and VUC as single markers.

Parameter	miR-21	-96	-125b	-126	-145	-183	-205	-210	-221	VUC
SNS	0.865	0.298	0.885	0.885	0.500	0.817	0.779	0.663	0.779	0.769
SPC	0.304	0.913	0.543	0.217	0.848	0.609	0.435	0.500	0.674	1.000
PPV	0.738	0.886	0.814	0.719	0.881	0.825	0.757	0.750	0.844	1.000
NPV	0.500	0.365	0.676	0.455	0.429	0.596	0.465	0.397	0.574	0.657
pLR	1.244	3.428	1.938	1.130	3.286	2.089	1.378	1.327	2.388	n.d.
nLR	0.442	0.769	0.212	0.531	0.590	0.300	0.509	0.673	0.328	0.231
ACC	0.693	0.487	0.780	0.680	0.607	0.753	0.673	0.613	0.747	0.840

ACC, accuracy; n.d., not determinable (division by zero); nLR, negative likelihood ratio; NPV, negative predictive value; pLR, positive likelihood ratio; PPV, positive predictive value; SNS, sensitivity; SPC, specificity.

In the next step, the tumor detection values ("1" or "0") for the six miRNAs with substantially different relative expression levels between urine samples from BCa patients and controls were totaled and evaluated with regard to the best separation of these sums. In doing so, the detection of at least four of these six miRNAs as an indicator of the tumor yielded a sensitivity of 73.1%, a specificity of 93.5%, and an accuracy of 79.3% (Table 5). The combination of only the four miRNAs with the highest AUC values in ROC curve analyses (miR-125b, -145, -183, and -221) and the use of at least three positive miRNAs as a BCa indicator resulted in a slightly better diagnostic performance compared to the combination of six miRNAs and to all single miRNAs (Tables 4 and 5).

Table 5. Diagnostic performance of combinations of selected miRNAs with each other and with VUC.

Parameter	6 miRs 96/125b/126/145/183/221 0-3/4-6 pos. Markers	4 miRs 125b/145/183/221 0-2/3-4 pos. Markers	6 miRs + VUC 96/125b/126/145/183/221 0-3/4-7 pos. Markers	4 miRs + VUC 125b/145/183/221 0-2/3-5 pos. Markers
SNS	0.731	0.731	0.808	0.846
SPC	0.935	0.957	0.935	0.957
PPV	0.962	0.974	0.966	0.978
NPV	0.606	0.611	0.683	0.733
pLR	11.205	16.808	12.385	19.462
nLR	0.288	0.281	0.206	0.161
ACC	0.793	0.800	0.847	0.880

ACC, accuracy; nLR, negative likelihood ratio; NPV, negative predictive value; pos., positive; pLR, positive likelihood ratio; PPV, positive predictive value; SNS, sensitivity; SPC, specificity.

The inclusion of VUC in both miRNA combinations led to a further increase of the diagnostic power and revealed the combination of the four miRNAs with VUC as the best approach with a sensitivity of 84.6%, a specificity of 95.7%, and an accuracy of 88.0% (Table 5). This combination was able to outperform VUC as a single marker with a 4% increase in accuracy, but at the expense of specificity in the same magnitude. However, it also resulted in a gain of nearly 8% each in sensitivity and NPV.

In the second statistical approach, the diagnostic power was analyzed using penalized linear regression applied to standardized miRNA values. This regression analysis (Figure 4) indicated that miR-210, -125b, and -221 had the strongest diagnostic power, while the influence of miR-145 and -205 was much weaker and the one of miR-21, -126, and -183 the weakest. In 10,000 simulations, each performed for a sample set of 20 patients from the original dataset, the penalized regression model correctly classified the tumor status in about 75% of the cases.

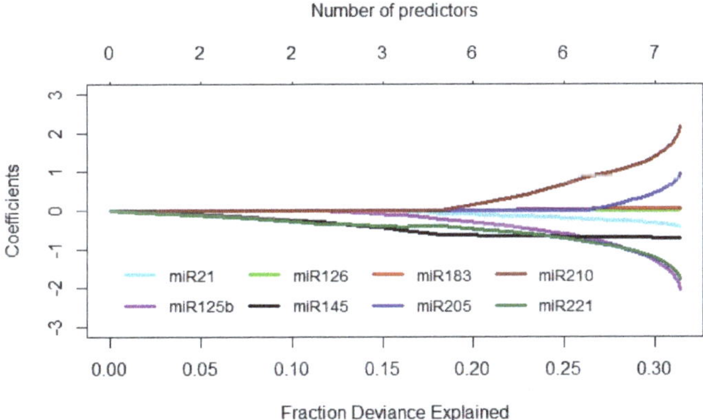

Figure 4. Diagnostic value of the miRNAs assessed by penalized linear regression. The deviance profile plot corresponding to standardized miRNAs as predictor variables in the *glmnet* model is shown. The slope of each path changes each time as another miRNA enters the model. The miRNAs, which explain a larger fraction of deviance, play a more important role in the prediction of the tumor status.

The order of importance of the miRNAs (miR-125b, -221, -145, -183, -205, -126, -210, -21) obtained using the random forest method as the third statistical approach was in concordance with the results of penalized linear regression. The percentage of cases correctly classified with this approach was 82.6%. The classification error in the random forest analysis was 20% (based on 100 simulations). Because of too many observed zero values for miR-96 in the control group, this variable was excluded from the analyses with *glmnet* and *randomForest*. In the overview of all statistical evaluation methods used herein, the miRNAs miR-125b, -145, -183, and -221 appeared to serve as well-suited biomarkers for the non-invasive detection of BCa in urine sediments independent of the chosen approach.

3. Discussion

The early and reliable detection of BCa is one of the biggest challenges to identify and treat patients at risk and to commence treatment in a timely manner. Many efforts have been made in recent years to implement new diagnostic approaches in clinical routine for the non-invasive detection of BCa using urine [6,8,9] and to replace VUC as the current gold standard. Nevertheless, none of these new biomarkers is thus far recommended for routine use in the early detection or follow-up of BCa or for replacement or reduction of the invasive procedure of cystoscopy [3]. According to current guidelines, such urinary molecular marker tests should provide a very high NPV to predict the absence of tumor reliably and eventually to avoid unnecessary cystoscopies [3]. Moreover, they should amend and strengthen the diagnostic performance of VUC and additionally overcome its main drawback: the low sensitivity, particularly for low-grade BCa [6].

For this purpose, this study focused on the diagnostic capability of miRNAs which are well known to be dysregulated in cellular pathways associated with the onset and progression of tumors including BCa [16,18,20]. Based on an extensive literature search, a number of promising miRNA candidates was selected, which were reported to be differentially expressed in bladder tissues and/or urine specimens from BCa patients and control subjects [22–32]. The diagnostic performance of the altered expression of these miRNAs in urine sediments was evaluated, revealing a certain potential of the miRNAs miR-96, -125b, -126, -145, -183, and -221 as single markers or in combination. The best diagnostic power was finally achieved by the use of four of these miRNAs in combination with VUC by simple classification of the urine samples as positive or negative for the single markers and subsequent allocation according to the total number of altered single markers (0-2 vs. 3-5 positive markers) regardless of which markers were changed. This approach resulted in a sensitivity of 84.6%, an NPV of 73.3%, and an accuracy of 88.0%, all surpassing the corresponding parameters of VUC alone (76.9%/65.7%/84.0%). In the marker combination, this was accompanied by losses of 4% in specificity and 2% in PPV compared to VUC alone where both accounted for 100%. Nevertheless, these losses appeared less severe in the face of the gain of nearly 8% each in sensitivity and NPV.

Thus, the combination of the four miRNAs miR-125b, -145, -183, and -221 with VUC seemed to have a promising potential for reliable diagnosis of BCa in urine samples prior to TUR-B. Accordingly, the diagnostic value of a reduced miR-125b expression in urine to prior tumor resection previously reported by Snowdon et al. [33], Mengual et al. [29], Zhang et al. [32], and Pospisilova et al. [34] could be confirmed in this study. This miRNA displayed a steady decrease with increasing tumor stage and grade, as also observed by Zhang et al. [32], indicating a certain prognostic power. Accordingly, Mengual et al. [29] described a prognostic panel comprising miR-125b and -92a for the identification of high-grade BCa, which was, however, not assessed in our patient cohort.

Another miRNA frequently described to be downregulated in cancer and particularly in BCa is miR-145 [27,28,35,36], which was also one of the best single miRNA markers in this study. Its diagnostic power (AUC = 0.687) herein was comparable to that (AUC = 0.729) determined by Yun et al. [36]. In contrast, Mearini et al. did not observe significant differences in urinary miR-145 levels between urine sediments from BCa patients and control subjects [37].

The miRNAs miR-96 and miR-183 are encoded by the miR-183/96/182 cluster on chromosome 7 and regulated in a concerted manner in different pathologies including BCa and other cancers [27,38–40]. Therefore, their expression behavior appears to be very similar as also reflected by their correlation observed in our measurements. Both miRNAs displayed a substantial elevation in BCa-derived urine samples compared to controls with miR-183 showing the second-best diagnostic potential of all miRNAs investigated herein (AUC = 0.720). Yamada et al. analyzed urinary levels of miR-96 and miR-183 in patients with urothelial carcinoma and revealed a high diagnostic value for both miRNAs reflected by AUC values of 0.831 and 0.817, respectively [41]. Moreover, they observed a positive dependence of miR-96/-183 levels on tumor stage and grade, whereas we could only identify a weak, but significant positive correlation with tumor stage. Considerable diagnostic power with regard to the non-invasive diagnosis of BCa by determination of urinary miR-96 levels was also described in several other studies [42–44]. This miRNA showed a differential expression only with a statistical trend ($p = 0.05$) in our study, but had to be excluded from some statistical approaches due to its low expression levels. miR-183, which was better performing in our cohort than miR-96, also emerged as a possible marker for high-grade NMIBC in the report from Pardini et al., who identified promising diagnostic miRNAs by NGS in cell-free urine supernatants from BCa patients and control subjects [45]. In summary, from these data, miR-96 and/or miR-183 seemed to provide substantial information when analyzing urine specimens for BCa diagnosis.

The diagnostic usability of elevated levels of miR-126 as a urinary marker has been reported by several studies so far [33,44,46]. In 2010, Hanke et al. reported an AUC value of 0.768 for the separation of BCa patients vs. healthy donors and of 0.747 vs. healthy donors and infections for miR-126 detection in urine [46]. Interestingly, miR-126 and -183 showed a significant, but less strong positive correlation with each other than miR-96 and -183, but they were both useful as BCa markers in contrast to miR-96.

Remarkably, miR-221 (our best performing BCa marker (AUC = 0.772)) was not found to be a promising candidate in previous studies despite its reported differential expression in BCa tissues [44,47]. In contrast, the remaining candidates (miR-21, -205, and -210), which did not show differential urinary expression levels in this study, were described as promising urinary BCa markers in selected reports [43,45,48–50]. For example, Michaildi et al. obtained a diagnostic AUC value of 0.845 when comparing miR-205 levels in cell-free urine supernatants from 177 normal donors and 32 BCa patients [50]. This miRNA also seemed promising with regard to the distinction of different BCa subsets as reported by Pardini et al. [45]. In contrast, it did not allow discrimination between patients with and without BCa, neither in the urine sediment, nor in the cell-free urine supernatant, in the study performed by Wang et al. [51]. Kim et al., who selected eight miRNAs (including miR-96, -125b, -145, and -205, like in our study) for urine analyses, observed among others increased levels of miR-205, as well as decreased levels of miR-125b and -145 in BCa-derived urine samples compared to negative controls [52]. We observed strong positive correlations between the miRNAs miR-21, -125b, -205, -210, and -221, but only miR-125b and -221 proved to be useful BCa markers in our study, for which we have no conclusive explanation. At the functional level, all of the five mentioned miRNAs were reported to regulate genes involved in cell cycle control, p53, and growth factor receptor signaling, which would fit with the observed correlations [53,54].

To explain the discrepancies observed between different studies, a variety of reasons can be given. On the one hand, there is a large diversity in the type of urinary components explored for miRNA analysis ranging from whole urine over urine sediment as used herein to cell-free urine supernatant or exosomes (Suppl. Table S1). It was assumed that exfoliated tumor cells were the main constituents of cellular urine sediments from BCa patients, and miRNA levels measured therein directly reflected those of the tumor. Both increased and decreased expression of such miRNAs would indicate the presence of BCa against the background of miRNA patterns in non-malignant cells, which are also part of the urine sediment. On the other hand, the kind of miRNA determination varied from NGS- and microarray-based profiling to different kinds of qPCR with and without miRNA-specific probes and the possible inclusion of a preamplification step. Moreover, the number of included patients and controls, the kind of controls (healthy donors or patients with benign urological diseases, infection, or hematuria), and tumor subtypes (e.g., urothelial carcinoma of the bladder or the upper urinary tract, bilharziasis-associated BCa) profoundly influenced the results obtained.

As revealed in this and many other studies, marker combinations seem to be superior to the analysis of single markers. The diagnostic gain, particularly in comparison to VUC alone, was clearly shown herein by the combination of VUC with the best four miRNAs as discussed above. In analogy, Yamada et al. and Eissa et al. reached an increase in diagnostic power by the combined analysis of

VUC and miR-96 due to a considerable number of non-overlapping cancer patients who were positive only for one of these markers. This was particularly reflected by an increase in sensitivity, NPV, and overall accuracy [41,42]. The same was true for the combination of VUC and more miRNAs, as shown by Eissa et al. for miR-10b/-29c/-210 [47], as well as in our study for miR-125b/-145/-183/-221.

However, it remains to be verified whether the achieved improvement of the diagnostic performance of VUC by combination with miRNA levels in urine sediment would really be sufficient to reduce cystoscopies for the first diagnosis or for surveillance after therapy. Alternatively, other BCa-specific biomarkers could potentially fulfill these requirements. Meanwhile, several promising tests became commercially available that detect altered biomarkers in exfoliated tumor cells such as *Xpert Bladder Cancer Monitor*, *Bladder EpiCheck test*, or *AssureMDx test* (reviewed in [55]). The *Xpert test*, which is based on differential mRNA patterns in BCa cells, delivered a sensitivity of 74% and a specificity of 80% for surveillance of NMIBC patients [56]. This was comparable to the results of the *EpiCheck test*, which reflects altered DNA methylation in BCa cells, with a sensitivity of 68% and a specificity of 88% for the detection of recurrent NMIBC [57]. Similar results were reported by Trenti et al., who directly compared the two tests with VUC in the follow-up of NMIBC patients [58]. The *AssureMDx test* (a combined DNA methylation and mutation urine assay) was reported to serve as a useful diagnostic tool to select patients with hematuria for cystoscopy with a sensitivity of 93% and a specificity of 86%, indicating the highest diagnostic potential among the new commercially available biomarker tests [59,60]. Thus, these tests seemed to provide a similar diagnostic power as our test, but only a head-to-head comparison in defined patient cohorts would deliver conclusive results with regard to first BCa diagnosis or surveillance.

Another factor that decisively determines the significance and predictive power of calculated marker combinations is the kind of statistical analysis methods. First, we compared the simple classification of urine samples as positive or negative for the single markers and subsequent allocation according to the total number of altered single markers regardless of which markers were changed with a penalized linear regression. Interestingly, penalized regression indicated the strongest diagnostic power for miR-210, -125b, and -221, although miR-210 was not identified as a suitable marker by ROC analyses. Nevertheless, the diagnostic accuracy of 79.3% and 80.0% for the combination of six or four miRNAs, respectively, accomplished by the first calculation method was higher than that of 75% yielded by penalized linear regression. The random forest method revealed a comparable accuracy of 82.6% using the same miRNAs as our first classification method. Additional principle component analyses could not further increase the diagnostic performance of different miRNA combinations in our study, but should be kept in mind as a further alternative approach, as well as the decision-tree analyses reported by Snowdon et al. and Pospisilova et al. [33,34].

Finally, the general approach for the selection of miRNAs as potential diagnostic BCa markers seems worthy of discussion, as well. The most comprehensive, but also the most cost- and labor-intensive approach is whole transcriptome profiling by NGS, microarray, or PCR array analyses followed by validation of the best candidates by independent methods such as qPCR in independent cohorts [29,32,34,44,45,48,49]. Several other authors made the choice in the same way as in the present study on the basis of publicly accessible datasets and literature reports on differential miRNA expression in malignant and non-malignant bladder tissues and/or in urine samples from BCa patients and suitable controls [33,36,51]. This approach primarily serves the independent validation of candidates that have already been investigated and shown to be promising, supporting the identification of the best markers. On the basis of our results and the presented literature review (Suppl. Table S1), the miRNAs miR-125b and -183 could represent such promising BCa-associated markers in urine. However, further miRNA candidates with a reported considerable diagnostic potential comprised of miR-99a [32,34,52], miR-146a [61], miR-155 [62], or members of the miR-200 family [30,36,51,52] should be further evaluated in comparative analyses.

Our study was associated with several limitations including the relatively low number of control subjects, since such patients are much less common in our department than BCa patients. However, the implementation of patients with benign urological diseases as done herein seemed to be more suitable than the comparison to healthy controls without any symptoms and with fewer exfoliated cells in urine sediment. Furthermore, the BCa patient cohort analyzed in the present study was comprised of a high percentage of cases with high-grade tumors, which is typical for specialized urological clinics and not comparable to those of private urological practices.

Considering this drawback, we avoided extensive calculations of possible associations with tumor grade. However, studies including more low-grade BCa would be required to assess the usefulness of this approach to identify these patients reliably. The clear advantages of our study were the direct comparison to VUC as the current gold standard for non-invasive BCa detection in urine and the combination of miRNA markers with VUC, which resulted in a superior diagnostic power. Nevertheless, this has to be confirmed in future studies on more BCa patients at different stages and suitable controls.

4. Materials and Methods

4.1. Study Population, Data, and Sample Collection

The present study was approved by the institutional review board of the Medical Faculty at the Technische Universität Dresden. Written informed consent was obtained from every participant. Patients with suspicion of having BCa and control subjects were prospectively recruited between May 2014 and September 2016. The inclusion criteria for the cases were comprised of new-onset BCa diagnosed at TUR-B and an age between 40 and 85 years. Patients diagnosed with papilloma or papillary urothelial neoplasm of low malignant potential (PUNLMP) were not eligible. In total, one-hundred four patients undergoing TUR-B with histologically-proven BCa were included (Table 1).

Eight patients suspected to have BCa, but histopathologically diagnosed as tumor-free, were allocated to the control group. Additionally, thirty-eight patients with urolithiasis were included as controls, finally resulting in a total control group size of 46 subjects (Table 2).

The histopathological examination of the resected bladder specimens, which served as the reference standard for BCa diagnosis, was performed using the UICC TNM classification from 2011 [63]. The tumors were accordingly classified as non-muscle-invasive BCa (NMIBC), comprised of the tumor stages pTa, pT1, and pTis, or as muscle-invasive BCa (MIBC), including all tumors with an expected tumor stage of ≥pT2a. The stratification of tumor grades into G1, G2, and G3 was done in accordance with the WHO classification from 1973 and into low-grade and high-grade tumors according to the WHO classification from 2004 [64]. As a reference method for the non-invasive detection of BCa, VUC specimens were prepared from urine samples from all BCa patients and control subjects. One experienced examiner (U.H.) evaluated these VUC specimens according to the ICUD/WHO classification [65].

4.2. Processing of Urine Samples, RNA Isolation, and cDNA Synthesis

Spontaneous urine samples (20–100 mL) were collected before therapeutic intervention from all BCa patients and control subjects. Urine collection was standardized in daily clinical practice (no morning urine, 2nd or 3rd urine of the day, clean catch in a sterile cup). The presence of erythrocytes, leucocytes, and bacteria was assessed by microscopic analysis of the sediment from 5–10 mL urine. Additionally, a VUC specimen was prepared from 5–10 mL urine. It was prefixed with *Esposti's fixative* overnight, centrifuged on glass slides, fixed with *Cytofix N* (Niepötter Labortechnik, Bürstadt, Germany), and stained by the Papanicolaou procedure [66].

The remaining urine was centrifuged at 1500× *g* for 10 min at 4 °C. After removal of the supernatant, the cellular pellet was washed twice with ice-cold phosphate-buffered saline (PBS) by centrifugation at 870× *g* for 5 min at 4 °C and resuspended in 700 µL *QIAzol Lysis Reagent* (Qiagen, Hilden, Germany). The lysates were frozen and stored at −80 °C until further processing. After thawing, total RNA was isolated using the *Direct-zol RNA MiniPrep kit* (Zymo Research, Freiburg, Germany) according to the manufacturer's recommendations. The RNA was eluted from the *Zymo-Spin IIC Column* with 40 μL nuclease-free water and quantified using the *NanoDrop 2000c* spectrophotometer (PEQLAB, Erlangen, Germany) and the *Agilent RNA 6000 Pico Kit* on an *Agilent 2100 Bioanalyzer* (Agilent Technologies, Ratingen, Germany).

If available, one-hundred nanograms total RNA (at least 50 ng) were employed for reverse transcription (RT) of the miRNAs using specific *TaqMan microRNA Assays* (Thermo Fisher Scientific, Darmstadt, Germany).

A multiplex RT was performed for the nine selected target miRNAs (Table 6: miR-21, -96, -125b, -126, -145, -183, -205, -210, and -221) and two reference RNAs (RNU44 andRNU48) in a final reaction volume of 30 μL comprised of 8 μL of the diluted RNA and 22 μL of the RT master mix. The latter consisted of dNTPs (each in a final concentration of 2 mM), *MultiScribe Reverse Transcriptase* (300 U), RT buffer, RNase inhibitor (7.6 U), and the respective RT primers (each 0.6×). The following temperature program was applied for the RT reaction: 30 min at 16 °C, 30 min at 42 °C, 5 min at 85 °C, followed by cooling down to 4 °C.

Table 6. The TaqMan microRNA assays used (Thermo Fisher Scientific, Darmstadt, Germany).

miRNA	Assay Name	Assay ID
miR-21-5p	hsa-miR-21	000397
miR-96-5p	mmu-miR-96 (for hsa-miR-96-5p)	000186
miR-125b-5p	hsa-miR-125b	000449
miR-126-3p	hsa-miR-126	002228
miR-145-5p	hsa-miR-145	002278
miR-183-5p	hsa-miR-183	002269
miR-205-5p	hsa-miR-205	000509
miR-210-3p	hsa-miR-210	000512
miR-221-3p	hsa-miR-221	000524
RNU44 (NR_002750) *	RNU44	001094
RNU48 (NR_002745) *	RNU48	001006

* TaqMan microRNA control assays.

4.3. Transcript Quantitation by Quantitative PCR

The individual mature miRNAs and reference RNAs were quantified separately on the *LightCycler 480 Real-Time PCR System* (Roche Diagnostics, Mannheim, Germany). Each qPCR with a final volume of 10 μL consisted of 1 μL of the undiluted cDNA product, the respective *TaqMan MicroRNA Assay* (Table 6), *GoTaq Probe qPCR Master Mix* (Promega, Mannheim, Germany), and nuclease-free water. The qPCR temperature program comprised the following steps: 10 min initial denaturation at 95 °C, 45 cycles of 15 s denaturation at 95 °C, and 1 min annealing/extension at 60 °C. The transcript quantitation was carried out in two independent reactions, and threshold cycles (C_T) determined by the second derivative method were averaged for each transcript per sample. In cases of a mean deviation >0.25 C_T-value, the measurements were repeated. Subsequently, the delta-delta-C_T method was used for the calculation of the relative miRNA levels normalized to the reference RNAs. For this, the geometric means of the C_T-values of RNU44 and RNU48 were utilized.

4.4. Statistical Analysis

For the assessment of potential differences in the relative miRNA levels between BCa patients and control subjects, the nonparametric two-tailed Mann–Whitney U test was applied. Bonferroni's correction for multiple comparisons was performed by multiplying the uncorrected *p*-values by a factor of 9 for nine miRNAs. Spearman's rank correlation coefficients (r_s) were calculated to reveal possible correlations among the relative expression levels of the different miRNAs and with tumor stage or grade. The distribution of the relative miRNA expression levels is depicted in box plots, where the bottom and top of the boxes represent the first and third quartiles, respectively. The median is shown as a solid line within the box, and the ends of the whiskers are depicted according to the Tukey method. Data outside the whiskers represent outliers and are marked as single circle symbols.

Differences in the relative miRNA levels between patients with different tumor stages and grades were assessed by the nonparametric two-tailed Mann–Whitney U test.

The diagnostic performance of the individual miRNAs was assessed by ROC curve analyses, followed by the above-mentioned Bonferroni's correction for multiple comparisons and the corresponding AUC values. The Youden index was calculated to determine optimal cutoff values, which were used to classify the relative expression levels of the different miRNAs into positive and negative indicators for tumor detection. Subsequently, the sensitivity (SNS), specificity (SPC), positive predictive value (PPV), negative predictive value (NPV), positive likelihood ratio (pLR), negative likelihood ratio (nLR), and accuracy (ACC) were calculated for each miRNA marker and for marker combinations according to standard statistical methods. The same was done for VUC alone or in combination with different miRNAs. For all analyses, two-sided p-values < 0.05 were considered statistically significant. All analyses were performed using *IBM SPSS Statistics Version 24.0.0.2* (IBM, Ehningen, Germany) and *GraphPad Prism Version 6.05 for Windows* (GraphPad Software, Inc, San Diego, CA, USA).

In addition, the diagnostic performance was assessed using penalized linear regression with miRNAs as predictor variables and tumor status as the outcome. The analysis was performed using the *R statistical environment* [67]. The predictive strength of the miRNAs for tumor status was investigated using the elastic net method [68] implemented in the R package *glmnet*. The importance of the miRNAs in predicting the tumor status and prediction accuracy were also assessed using the random forest method [69] implemented in the R package *randomForest* [70].

5. Conclusions

The literature-based selection of promising miRNAs as potential markers for the non-invasive detection of BCa in urine as alternative or adjunct markers to VUC revealed four suitable candidates (miR-125b/-145/-183/-221). In combination with VUC, an adequate performance was obtained, and the previously reported value as BCa-associated biomarkers could be confirmed for these four miRNAs. Prospective studies are required in order to reveal the real value of miRNAs in urine-based BCa diagnosis as a potential tool for the reduction of invasive and expensive diagnostic procedures like cystoscopies.

Supplementary Materials: Supplementary materials can be found at http://www.mdpi.com/1422-0067/21/11/3814/s1.

Author Contributions: Conceptualization: K.S. and S.F.; methodology: K.E., K.S., and S.F.; validation: K.E. and K.S.; formal analysis: K.E., K.S., and S.F.; investigation: U.H., A.L.-F., and R.F.; resources: M.F. and M.P.W.; data curation: K.S., A.K., I.R., and S.F.; writing, original draft preparation: S.F.; writing, review and editing: K.E., A.K., C.T., and S.F.; supervision: C.T. and M.P.W.; project administration: M.P.W. and S.F. All authors have read and agreed to the published version of the manuscript.

Funding: This research received no external funding.

Acknowledgments: We thank the individuals who consented to be included in the cohorts of this project.

Conflicts of Interest: The authors declare no conflict of interest.

Abbreviations

ACC	accuracy
AUC	area under the curve
BCa	bladder cancer
G	tumor grade
MIBC	muscle-invasive bladder cancer
miRNA or miR	microRNA
NGS	next-generation sequencing

nLR	negative likelihood ratio
NMIBC	non-muscle-invasive bladder cancer
ns	not significant
NPV	negative predictive value
pLR	positive likelihood ratio
PPV	positive predictive value
pT	pathological tumor stage
PUNLMP	papillary urothelial neoplasm of low malignant potential
qPCR	quantitative polymerase chain reaction
ROC	receiver operating characteristic
RT	reverse transcription
SNS	sensitivity
SPC	specificity
TUR-B	transurethral resection of the bladder
VUC	voided urine cytology

References

1. Richters, A.; Aben, K.K.H.; Kiemeney, L. The global burden of urinary bladder cancer: An update. *World J. Urol.* **2019**. [CrossRef] [PubMed]

2. Saginala, K.; Barsouk, A.; Aluru, J.S.; Rawla, P.; Padala, S.A.; Barsouk, A. Epidemiology of Bladder Cancer. *Med. Sci. (Basel)* **2020**, *8*, 15. [CrossRef] [PubMed]

3. Babjuk, M.; Bohle, A.; Burger, M.; Capoun, O.; Cohen, D.; Comperat, E.M.; Hernandez, V.; Kaasinen, E.; Palou, J.; Roupret, M.; et al. EAU Guidelines on Non-Muscle-invasive Urothelial Carcinoma of the Bladder: Update 2016. *Eur. Urol.* **2017**, *71*, 447–461. [CrossRef]

4. Sievert, K.D.; Amend, B.; Nagele, U.; Schilling, D.; Bedke, J.; Horstmann, M.; Hennenlotter, J.; Kruck, S.; Stenzl, A. Economic aspects of bladder cancer: What are the benefits and costs? *World J. Urol.* **2009**, *27*, 295–300. [CrossRef] [PubMed]

5. Svatek, R.S.; Hollenbeck, B.K.; Holmang, S.; Lee, R.; Kim, S.P.; Stenzl, A.; Lotan, Y. The economics of bladder cancer: Costs and considerations of caring for this disease. *Eur. Urol.* **2014**, *66*, 253–262. [CrossRef]

6. Maas, M.; Bedke, J.; Stenzl, A.; Todenhofer, T. Can urinary biomarkers replace cystoscopy? *World J. Urol.* **2019**, *37*, 1741–1749. [CrossRef]

7. Woldu, S.L.; Bagrodia, A.; Lotan, Y. Guideline of guidelines: Non-muscle-invasive bladder cancer. *BJU Int.* **2017**, *119*, 371–380. [CrossRef]

8. Chou, R.; Gore, J.L.; Buckley, D.; Fu, R.; Gustafson, K.; Griffin, J.C.; Grusing, S.; Selph, S. Urinary Biomarkers for Diagnosis of Bladder Cancer: A Systematic Review and Meta-analysis. *Ann. Intern. Med.* **2015**, *163*, 922–931. [CrossRef]

9. D'Costa, J.J.; Goldsmith, J.C.; Wilson, J.S.; Bryan, R.T.; Ward, D.G. A Systematic Review of the Diagnostic and Prognostic Value of Urinary Protein Biomarkers in Urothelial Bladder Cancer. *Bladder Cancer* **2016**, *2*, 301–317. [CrossRef]

10. Mengual, L.; Ribal, M.J.; Lozano, J.J.; Ingelmo-Torres, M.; Burset, M.; Fernandez, P.L.; Alcaraz, A. Validation study of a noninvasive urine test for diagnosis and prognosis assessment of bladder cancer: Evidence for improved models. *J. Urol.* **2014**, *191*, 261–269. [CrossRef]

11. Ribal, M.J.; Mengual, L.; Lozano, J.J.; Ingelmo-Torres, M.; Palou, J.; Rodriguez-Faba, O.; Witjes, J.A.; Van der Heijden, A.G.; Medina, R.; Conde, J.M.; et al. Gene expression test for the non-invasive diagnosis of bladder cancer: A prospective, blinded, international and multicenter validation study. *Eur. J. Cancer* **2016**, *54*, 131–138. [CrossRef] [PubMed]

12. Urquidi, V.; Netherton, M.; Gomes-Giacoia, E.; Serie, D.; Eckel-Passow, J.; Rosser, C.J.; Goodison, S. Urinary mRNA biomarker panel for the detection of urothelial carcinoma. *Oncotarget* **2016**, *7*, 38731–38740. [CrossRef]

13. Esquela-Kerscher, A.; Slack, F.J. Oncomirs—microRNAs with a role in cancer. *Nat. Rev. Cancer* **2006**, *6*, 259–269. [CrossRef] [PubMed]

14. Iorio, M.V.; Croce, C.M. microRNA involvement in human cancer. *Carcinogenesis* **2012**, *33*, 1126–1133. [CrossRef] [PubMed]

15. Frixa, T.; Donzelli, S.; Blandino, G. Oncogenic MicroRNAs: Key Players in Malignant Transformation. *Cancers* **2015**, *7*, 2466–2485. [CrossRef]

16. Dong, F.; Xu, T.; Shen, Y.; Zhong, S.; Chen, S.; Ding, Q.; Shen, Z. Dysregulation of miRNAs in bladder cancer: Altered expression with aberrant biogenesis procedure. *Oncotarget* **2017**, *8*, 27547–27568. [CrossRef]

17. Liu, X.; Liu, X.; Wu, Y.; Wu, Q.; Wang, Q.; Yang, Z.; Li, L. MicroRNAs in biofluids are novel tools for bladder cancer screening. *Oncotarget* **2017**, *8*, 32370–32379. [CrossRef]

18. Matullo, G.; Naccarati, A.; Pardini, B. MicroRNA expression profiling in bladder cancer: The challenge of next-generation sequencing in tissues and biofluids. *Int. J. Cancer* **2016**, *138*, 2334–2345. [CrossRef]

19. Ouyang, H.; Zhou, Y.; Zhang, L.; Shen, G. Diagnostic Value of MicroRNAs for Urologic Cancers: A Systematic Review and Meta-Analysis. *Medicine (Baltimore)* **2015**, *94*, e1272. [CrossRef]

20. Schubert, M.; Junker, K.; Heinzelmann, J. Prognostic and predictive miRNA biomarkers in bladder, kidney and prostate cancer: Where do we stand in biomarker development? *J. Cancer Res. Clin. Oncol.* **2016**, *142*, 1673–1695. [CrossRef]

21. Enokida, H.; Yoshino, H.; Matsushita, R.; Nakagawa, M. The role of microRNAs in bladder cancer. *Investig. Clin. Urol.* **2016**, *57*, 60–76. [CrossRef] [PubMed]

22. Canturk, K.M.; Ozdemir, M.; Can, C.; Oner, S.; Emre, R.; Aslan, H.; Cilingir, O.; Ciftci, E.; Celayir, F.M.; Aldemir, O.; et al. Investigation of key miRNAs and target genes in bladder cancer using miRNA profiling and bioinformatic tools. *Mol. Biol. Rep.* **2014**, *41*, 8127–8135. [CrossRef] [PubMed]

23. Catto, J.W.; Miah, S.; Owen, H.C.; Bryant, H.; Myers, K.; Dudziec, E.; Larre, S.; Milo, M.; Rehman, I.; Rosario, D.J.; et al. Distinct microRNA alterations characterize high- and low-grade bladder cancer. *Cancer Res.* **2009**, *69*, 8472–8481. [CrossRef] [PubMed]

24. Cheng, Y.; Deng, X.; Yang, X.; Li, P.; Zhang, X.; Li, P.; Tao, J.; Lu, Q.; Wang, Z. Urine microRNAs as biomarkers for bladder cancer: A diagnostic meta-analysis. *Onco Targets Ther.* **2015**, *8*, 2089–2096. [CrossRef]

25. Ding, M.; Li, Y.; Wang, H.; Lv, Y.; Liang, J.; Wang, J.; Li, C. Diagnostic value of urinary microRNAs as non-invasive biomarkers for bladder cancer: A meta-analysis. *Int. J. Clin. Exp. Med.* **2015**, *8*, 15432–15440.

26. Dyrskjot, L.; Ostenfeld, M.S.; Bramsen, J.B.; Silahtaroglu, A.N.; Lamy, P.; Ramanathan, R.; Fristrup, N.; Jensen, J.L.; Andersen, C.L.; Zieger, K.; et al. Genomic profiling of microRNAs in bladder cancer: miR-129 is associated with poor outcome and promotes cell death in vitro. *Cancer Res.* **2009**, *69*, 4851–4860. [CrossRef]

27. Han, Y.; Chen, J.; Zhao, X.; Liang, C.; Wang, Y.; Sun, L.; Jiang, Z.; Zhang, Z.; Yang, R.; Chen, J.; et al. MicroRNA expression signatures of bladder cancer revealed by deep sequencing. *PLoS ONE* **2011**, *6*, e18286. [CrossRef]

28. Itesako, T.; Seki, N.; Yoshino, H.; Chiyomaru, T.; Yamasaki, T.; Hidaka, H.; Yonezawa, T.; Nohata, N.; Kinoshita, T.; Nakagawa, M.; et al. The microRNA expression signature of bladder cancer by deep sequencing: The functional significance of the miR-195/497 cluster. *PLoS ONE* **2014**, *9*, e84311. [CrossRef]

29. Mengual, L.; Lozano, J.J.; Ingelmo-Torres, M.; Gazquez, C.; Ribal, M.J.; Alcaraz, A. Using microRNA profiling in urine samples to develop a non-invasive test for bladder cancer. *Int. J. Cancer* **2013**, *133*, 2631–2641. [CrossRef]

30. Sapre, N.; Macintyre, G.; Clarkson, M.; Naeem, H.; Cmero, M.; Kowalczyk, A.; Anderson, P.D.; Costello, A.J.; Corcoran, N.M.; Hovens, C.M. A urinary microRNA signature can predict the presence of bladder urothelial carcinoma in patients undergoing surveillance. *Br. J. Cancer* **2016**, *114*, 454–462. [CrossRef]

31. Zaravinos, A.; Radojicic, J.; Lambrou, G.I.; Volanis, D.; Delakas, D.; Stathopoulos, E.N.; Spandidos, D.A. Expression of miRNAs involved in angiogenesis, tumor cell proliferation, tumor suppressor inhibition, epithelial-mesenchymal transition and activation of metastasis in bladder cancer. *J. Urol.* **2012**, *188*, 615–623. [CrossRef] [PubMed]

32. Zhang, D.Z.; Lau, K.M.; Chan, E.S.; Wang, G.; Szeto, C.C.; Wong, K.; Choy, R.K.; Ng, C.F. Cell-free urinary microRNA-99a and microRNA-125b are diagnostic markers for the non-invasive screening of bladder cancer. *PLoS ONE* **2014**, *9*, e100793. [CrossRef]

33. Snowdon, J.; Boag, S.; Feilotter, H.; Izard, J.; Siemens, D.R. A pilot study of urinary microRNA as a biomarker for urothelial cancer. *Can. Urol. Assoc. J.* **2013**, *7*, 28–32. [CrossRef] [PubMed]

34. Pospisilova, S.; Pazourkova, E.; Horinek, A.; Brisuda, A.; Svobodova, I.; Soukup, V.; Hrbacek, J.; Capoun, O.; Hanus, T.; Mares, J.; et al. MicroRNAs in urine supernatant as potential non-invasive markers for bladder cancer detection. *Neoplasma* **2016**, *63*, 799–808. [CrossRef] [PubMed]

35. Dip, N.; Reis, S.T.; Srougi, M.; Dall'Oglio, M.F.; Leite, K.R. Expression profile of microrna-145 in urothelial bladder cancer. *Int. Braz. J. Urol.* **2013**, *39*, 95–101. [CrossRef] [PubMed]

36. Yun, S.J.; Jeong, P.; Kim, W.T.; Kim, T.H.; Lee, Y.S.; Song, P.H.; Choi, Y.H.; Kim, I.Y.; Moon, S.K.; Kim, W.J. Cell-free microRNAs in urine as diagnostic and prognostic biomarkers of bladder cancer. *Int. J. Oncol.* **2012**, *41*, 1871–1878. [CrossRef]

37. Mearini, E.; Poli, G.; Cochetti, G.; Boni, A.; Egidi, M.G.; Brancorsini, S. Expression of urinary miRNAs targeting NLRs inflammasomes in bladder cancer. *Onco Targets Ther.* **2017**, *10*, 2665–2673. [CrossRef]

38. Dambal, S.; Shah, M.; Mihelich, B.; Nonn, L. The microRNA-183 cluster: The family that plays together stays together. *Nucleic Acids Res.* **2015**, *43*, 7173–7188. [CrossRef]

39. Ma, Y.; Liang, A.J.; Fan, Y.P.; Huang, Y.R.; Zhao, X.M.; Sun, Y.; Chen, X.F. Dysregulation and functional roles of miR-183-96-182 cluster in cancer cell proliferation, invasion and metastasis. *Oncotarget* **2016**, *7*, 42805–42825. [CrossRef]

40. Zhang, Q.H.; Sun, H.M.; Zheng, R.Z.; Li, Y.C.; Zhang, Q.; Cheng, P.; Tang, Z.H.; Huang, F. Meta-analysis of microRNA-183 family expression in human cancer studies comparing cancer tissues with noncancerous tissues. *Gene* **2013**, *527*, 26–32. [CrossRef]

41. Yamada, Y.; Enokida, H.; Kojima, S.; Kawakami, K.; Chiyomaru, T.; Tatarano, S.; Yoshino, H.; Kawahara, K.; Nishiyama, K.; Seki, N.; et al. MiR-96 and miR-183 detection in urine serve as potential tumor markers of urothelial carcinoma: Correlation with stage and grade, and comparison with urinary cytology. *Cancer Sci.* **2011**, *102*, 522–529. [CrossRef] [PubMed]

42. Eissa, S.; Habib, H.; Ali, E.; Kotb, Y. Evaluation of urinary miRNA-96 as a potential biomarker for bladder cancer diagnosis. *Med. Oncol.* **2015**, *32*, 413. [CrossRef] [PubMed]

43. Eissa, S.; Matboli, M.; Essawy, N.O.; Kotb, Y.M. Integrative functional genetic-epigenetic approach for selecting genes as urine biomarkers for bladder cancer diagnosis. *Tumour Biol.* **2015**, *36*, 9545–9552. [CrossRef]

44. Urquidi, V.; Netherton, M.; Gomes-Giacoia, E.; Serie, D.J.; Eckel-Passow, J.; Rosser, C.J.; Goodison, S. A microRNA biomarker panel for the non-invasive detection of bladder cancer. *Oncotarget* **2016**, *7*, 86290–86299. [CrossRef]

45. Pardini, B.; Cordero, F.; Naccarati, A.; Viberti, C.; Birolo, G.; Oderda, M.; Di Gaetano, C.; Arigoni, M.; Martina, F.; Calogero, R.A.; et al. microRNA profiles in urine by next-generation sequencing can stratify bladder cancer subtypes. *Oncotarget* **2018**, *9*, 20658–20669. [CrossRef] [PubMed]

46. Hanke, M.; Hoefig, K.; Merz, H.; Feller, A.C.; Kausch, I.; Jocham, D.; Warnecke, J.M.; Sczakiel, G. A robust methodology to study urine microRNA as tumor marker: microRNA-126 and microRNA-182 are related to urinary bladder cancer. *Urol. Oncol.* **2010**, *28*, 655–661. [CrossRef] [PubMed]

47. Eissa, S.; Matboli, M.; Hegazy, M.G.; Kotb, Y.M.; Essawy, N.O. Evaluation of urinary microRNA panel in bladder cancer diagnosis: Relation to bilharziasis. *Transl. Res.* **2015**, *165*, 731–739. [CrossRef] [PubMed]

48. Long, J.D.; Sullivan, T.B.; Humphrey, J.; Logvinenko, T.; Summerhayes, K.A.; Kozinn, S.; Harty, N.; Summerhayes, I.C.; Libertino, J.A.; Holway, A.H.; et al. A non-invasive miRNA based assay to detect bladder cancer in cell-free urine. *Am. J. Transl. Res.* **2015**, *7*, 2500–2509.

49. Matsuzaki, K.; Fujita, K.; Jingushi, K.; Kawashima, A.; Ujike, T.; Nagahara, A.; Ueda, Y.; Tanigawa, G.; Yoshioka, I.; Ueda, K.; et al. MiR-21-5p in urinary extracellular vesicles is a novel biomarker of urothelial carcinoma. *Oncotarget* **2017**, *8*, 24668–24678. [CrossRef]

50. Michailidi, C.; Hayashi, M.; Datta, S.; Sen, T.; Zenner, K.; Oladeru, O.; Brait, M.; Izumchenko, E.; Baras, A.; VandenBussche, C.; et al. Involvement of epigenetics and EMT-related miRNA in arsenic-induced neoplastic transformation and their potential clinical use. *Cancer Prev. Res. (Phila)* **2015**, *8*, 208–221. [CrossRef]

51. Wang, G.; Chan, E.S.; Kwan, B.C.; Li, P.K.; Yip, S.K.; Szeto, C.C.; Ng, C.F. Expression of microRNAs in the urine of patients with bladder cancer. *Clin. Genitourin. Cancer* **2012**, *10*, 106–113. [CrossRef] [PubMed]

52. Kim, S.S.; Choi, C.; Kwon, D.D. Urinary microRNAs as potential biomarkers for differentiating the "atypical urothelial cells" category of the Paris system for reporting urine cytology. *Int. J. Clin. Exp. Pathol.* **2017**, *10*, 8303–8313. [PubMed]

53. Fendler, A.; Stephan, C.; Yousef, G.M.; Jung, K. MicroRNAs as regulators of signal transduction in urological tumors. *Clin. Chem.* **2011**, *57*, 954–968. [CrossRef] [PubMed]

54. Gulia, C.; Baldassarra, S.; Signore, F.; Rigon, G.; Pizzuti, V.; Gaffi, M.; Briganti, V.; Porrello, A.; Piergentili, R. Role of Non-Coding RNAs in the Etiology of Bladder Cancer. *Genes (Basel)* **2017**, *8*, 339. [CrossRef] [PubMed]

55. Batista, R.; Vinagre, N.; Meireles, S.; Vinagre, J.; Prazeres, H.; Leao, R.; Maximo, V.; Soares, P. Biomarkers for Bladder Cancer Diagnosis and Surveillance: A Comprehensive Review. *Diagnostics (Basel)* **2020**, *10*, 39. [CrossRef] [PubMed]

56. Valenberg, F.; Hiar, A.M.; Wallace, E.; Bridge, J.A.; Mayne, D.J.; Beqaj, S.; Sexton, W.J.; Lotan, Y.; Weizer, A.Z.; Jansz, G.K.; et al. Prospective Validation of an mRNA-based Urine Test for Surveillance of Patients with Bladder Cancer. *Eur. Urol.* **2019**, *75*, 853–860. [CrossRef] [PubMed]

57. Witjes, J.A.; Morote, J.; Cornel, E.B.; Gakis, G.; van Valenberg, F.J.P.; Lozano, F.; Sternberg, I.A.; Willemsen, E.; Hegemann, M.L.; Paitan, Y.; et al. Performance of the Bladder EpiCheck Methylation Test for Patients Under Surveillance for Non-muscle-invasive Bladder Cancer: Results of a Multicenter, Prospective, Blinded Clinical Trial. *Eur. Urol. Oncol.* **2018**, *1*, 307–313. [CrossRef]

58. Trenti, E.; Pycha, S.; Mian, C.; Schwienbacher, C.; Hanspeter, E.; Kafka, M.; Spedicato, G.A.; Vjaters, E.; Degener, S.; Pycha, A.; et al. Comparison of 2 new real-time polymerase chain reaction-based urinary markers in the follow-up of patients with non-muscle-invasive bladder cancer. *Cancer Cytopathol.* **2020**, *128*, 341–347. [CrossRef]

59. Sathianathen, N.J.; Butaney, M.; Weight, C.J.; Kumar, R.; Konety, B.R. Urinary Biomarkers in the Evaluation of Primary Hematuria: A Systematic Review and Meta-Analysis. *Bladder Cancer* **2018**, *4*, 353–363. [CrossRef]

60. Van Kessel, K.E.; Beukers, W.; Lurkin, I.; Ziel-van der Made, A.; van der Keur, K.A.; Boormans, J.L.; Dyrskjot, L.; Marquez, M.; Orntoft, T.F.; Real, F.X.; et al. Validation of a DNA Methylation-Mutation Urine Assay to Select Patients with Hematuria for Cystoscopy. *J. Urol.* **2017**, *197*, 590–595. [CrossRef]

61. Sasaki, H.; Yoshiike, M.; Nozawa, S.; Usuba, W.; Katsuoka, Y.; Aida, K.; Kitajima, K.; Kudo, H.; Hoshikawa, M.; Yoshioka, Y.; et al. Expression Level of Urinary MicroRNA-146a-5p Is Increased in Patients With Bladder Cancer and Decreased in Those After Transurethral Resection. *Clin. Genitourin. Cancer* **2016**, *14*, e493–e499. [CrossRef] [PubMed]

62. Zhang, X.; Zhang, Y.; Liu, X.; Fang, A.; Wang, J.; Yang, Y.; Wang, L.; Du, L.; Wang, C. Direct quantitative detection for cell-free miR-155 in urine: A potential role in diagnosis and prognosis for non-muscle invasive bladder cancer. *Oncotarget* **2016**, *7*, 3255–3266. [CrossRef] [PubMed]

63. *TNM Classification of Malignant Tumours*; Sobin, L.H.; Gospodarowicz, M.K.; Wittekind, C.E. (Eds.) Wiley-Blackwell: Hoboken, NJ, USA, 2011.

64. Humphrey, P.A.; Moch, H.; Cubilla, A.L.; Ulbright, T.M.; Reuter, V.E. The 2016 WHO Classification of Tumours of the Urinary System and Male Genital Organs-Part B: Prostate and Bladder Tumours. *Eur. Urol.* **2016**, *70*, 106–119. [CrossRef] [PubMed]

65. Amin, M.B.; Smith, S.C.; Reuter, V.E.; Epstein, J.I.; Grignon, D.J.; Hansel, D.E.; Lin, O.; McKenney, J.K.; Montironi, R.; Paner, G.P.; et al. Update for the practicing pathologist: The International Consultation On Urologic Disease-European association of urology consultation on bladder cancer. *Mod. Pathol.* **2015**, *28*, 612–630. [CrossRef]

66. Papanicolaou, G.N.; Marshall, V.F. URINE SEDIMENT SMEARS AS A DIAGNOSTIC PROCEDURE IN CANCERS OF THE URINARY TRACT. *Science* **1945**, *101*, 519–520. [CrossRef]

67. Marano, G.; Boracchi, P.; Biganzoli, E.M.; R Core Team. R: A language and environment for statistical computing. R Foundation for Statistical Computing, Vienna. *Open J. Stat.* **2016**, *6*, 3.

68. Friedman, J.; Hastie, T.; Tibshirani, R. Regularization Paths for Generalized Linear Models via Coordinate Descent. *J. Stat. Softw.* **2010**, *33*, 1–22. [CrossRef]

69. Breiman, L. Random Forests. *Mach. Learn.* **2001**, *45*, 5–32. [CrossRef]

70. Liaw, A.; Wienertitle, M. Classification and Regression by randomForest. *R News* **2002**, *2*, 18–22.

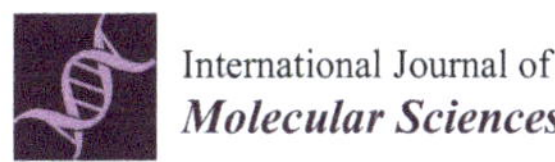

International Journal of
Molecular Sciences

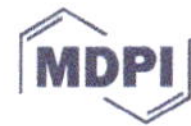

Article

Inhibition of Heparanase Expression Results in Suppression of Invasion, Migration and Adhesion Abilities of Bladder Cancer Cells

Yoshihiro Tatsumi [1,2], Makito Miyake [1], Keiji Shimada [2], Tomomi Fujii [2], Shunta Hori [1], Yosuke Morizawa [1], Yasushi Nakai [1], Satoshi Anai [1], Nobumichi Tanaka [1], Noboru Konishi [2] and Kiyohide Fujimoto [1,*]

1   Department of Urology, Nara Medical University, 840 Shijo-cho, Nara 634-8522, Japan;
    takuro.birds.nest@gmail.com (Y.T.); makitomiyake@yahoo.co.jp (M.M.); horimaus@gmail.com (S.H.);
    tigers.yosuke@gmail.com (Y.M.); nakaiyasusiuro@live.jp (Y.N.); sanai@naramed-u.ac.jp (S.A.);
    sendo@naramed-u.ac.jp (N.T.)
2   Department of Pathology, Nara Medical University, 840 Shijo-cho, Nara 634-8522, Japan;
    k-shimada@nara-jadecom.jp (K.S.); fujiit@naramed-u.ac.jp (T.F.); n-konishi@takai-hp.com (N.K.)
*   Correspondence: kiyokun@naramed-u.ac.jp; Tel.: +81-744-22-3051 (ext. 2338)

Received: 28 April 2020; Accepted: 26 May 2020; Published: 27 May 2020

Abstract: Heparan sulfate proteoglycan syndecan-1, CD138, is known to be associated with cell proliferation, adhesion, and migration in malignancies. We previously reported that syndecan-1 (CD138) may contribute to urothelial carcinoma cell survival and progression. We investigated the role of heparanase, an enzyme activated by syndecan-1 in human urothelial carcinoma. Using human urothelial cancer cell lines, MGH-U3 and T24, heparanase expression was reduced with siRNA and RK-682, a heparanase inhibitor, to examine changes in cell proliferation activity, induction of apoptosis, invasion ability of cells, and its relationship to autophagy. A bladder cancer development mouse model was treated with RK-682 and the bladder tissues were examined using immunohistochemical analysis for Ki-67, E-cadherin, LC3, and CD31 expressions. Heparanase inhibition suppressed cellular growth by approximately 40% and induced apoptosis. The heparanase inhibitor decreased cell activity in a concentration-dependent manner and suppressed invasion ability by 40%. Inhibition of heparanase was found to suppress autophagy. In N-butyl-N-(4-hydroxybutyl) nitrosamine (BBN)-induced bladder cancer mice, treatment with heparanase inhibitor suppressed the progression of cancer by 40%, compared to controls. Immunohistochemistry analysis showed that heparanase inhibitor suppressed cell growth, and autophagy. In conclusion, heparanase suppresses apoptosis and promotes invasion and autophagy in urothelial cancer.

Keywords: heparanase; syndecan-1; heparan sulfate proteoglycans (HSPGs); urothelial carcinoma

1. Introduction

Heparan sulfate proteoglycans (HSPGs) are glycoproteins containing heparan sulfate (HS) groups that are covalently attached [1]. They are widely expressed and play critical roles in numerous cellular processes, including endocytosis, migration, and adhesion. Their actions are mediated through interactions with ligands such as growth factors, cytokines, extracellular matrix proteins, and enzymes. HSPGs are also involved in the malignant transformation of cells. Growth factors are released through cellular degradation, which promote the invasion and proliferation of cancer cells [2,3]. Syndecan-1 (SDC1) is an HSPG that is overexpressed in both normal and malignant cells, contributing to the development of hematopoietic and carcinoma development [4–9]. Syndecan-1 regulates substance permeation and constitutes a reservoir for various growth factors and cytokines in the basement membrane of cells. It plays a critical role in the progression and invasion of urothelial cancer through enhanced angiogenesis.

We have previously reported that syndecan-1 (CD138) suppresses apoptosis and increases the capacity for cell proliferation via junB-FLIP long signal in urothelial cancer [10]. Urothelial cancers can be broadly classified into low-grade, non-invasive, and high-grade invasive cancers [11]. Invasive urothelial cancers exhibit significantly higher syndecan-1 expression. In vitro experiments showed that knocking down syndecan-1 using siRNA induces cellular apoptosis and decreases the capacity for cellular proliferation. The enzyme heparanase controls the activation of syndecan-1.

Heparanase is an endoglycosidase enzyme that targets HSPG proteins expressed in the extracellular matrix (ECM) and basement membrane (BM) for degradation [12]. Heparanase activation expedites the movement of tumor cells through the ECM and BM, facilitating metastasis. Heparanase is also known to be expressed in many types of malignant tumors, and is associated with metastasis and angiogenesis [13,14]. Heparinase cleavage of HSPGs produces soluble proteins that infiltrate into the tumor microenvironment, where they interact with ligands such as growth factors, modifying signaling pathways [15]. SDC1 in the stroma promotes breast carcinoma growth by enhancing FGF2 signaling [16]. Heparanase-neutralizing antibodies have been suggested for the treatment of diffuse non-Hodgkin's B-cell and follicular lymphomas [17] through the inhibition of cell invasion and tumor metastasis processes [17–19]. Recently, a small molecule inhibitor of heparanase was shown to reduce metastatic characteristics in a hepatocellular carcinoma model [20]. In vivo studies using heparanase inhibitors in animal tumor models have also demonstrated reductions in tumor metastasis [21–23]. As heparinase is absent or expressed at low levels in normal tissue [24,25], it may be a potential target candidate for therapeutic interventions. Various studies have investigated the underlying mechanism for heparanase activity in cancer, including enhancement of angiogenesis and promotion of apoptosis and autophagy [14,26–30]. Reports indicate that autophagy contributes to chemotherapy resistance development, making this an important research focus area.

In this study, we analyzed the function of heparanase, an activator of syndecan-1, in angiogenesis, apoptosis, and autophagy. The aim was to establish heparanase as a target for molecular therapy in urothelial carcinoma.

2. Results

2.1. Heparanase Is Overexpressed in Human Urothelial Carcinoma of the Urinary Bladder, and Heparanase Expression Levels Are Associated with Intravesical Recurrence

The patterns of heparanase expression in resected bladder cancer tissue samples were analyzed using immunohistochemical (IHC) staining. The relationship between heparanase expression and recurrence, metastasis, and prognosis of urothelial cancer was examined. Tissue specimens ($n = 57$) were resected from the renal pelvis, ureter, and bladder of patients with multifocal onset, relapse, metastasis, and prognosis cases of urothelial cancer. Table 1 summarizes patient clinicopathological data using the 2009 World Health Organization (WHO) grading and staging of tumors classification [31]. The total number of Ta cases was 20 and the grade was low grade:high grade, 13:7. Among the 17 cases of T1, low grade:high grade, 3:14, and all 10 cases of Tis were high grade.

Table 1. Characterization of urothelial carcinomas.

	*p*Ta (*n* = 20)	*p*T1 (*n* = 17)	*p*Tis (*n* = 10)
Age	71.3 (61–82)	72.9 (5–80)	72.4 (62–86)
Gender (M:F)	16:4	14:3	8:2
Grade			
Low grade	13	3	0
High grade	7	14	10

*p*Ta = low-grade non-muscle invasive bladder cancer; *p*T1 = intermediate risk non-muscle invasive bladder cancer; *p*Tis = in situ neoplasia.

The expression of heparanase is diffusely expressed in both the cell membrane and cytoplasm. The expression of heparanase protein was approximately 10% in normal urothelium but increased to approximately 30% in urothelial carcinoma samples ($p < 0.05$). Heparanase expression was elevated in high-grade compared to low-grade carcinoma samples (34.7% vs. 23.4%, respectively) (Figure 1a,b). The immunohistochemical staining of surgically resected specimens from 47 bladder cancer patients showed that positive heparanase expression was observed predominantly in cases exhibiting intravesical relapse ($p < 0.05$) (Figure 1c).

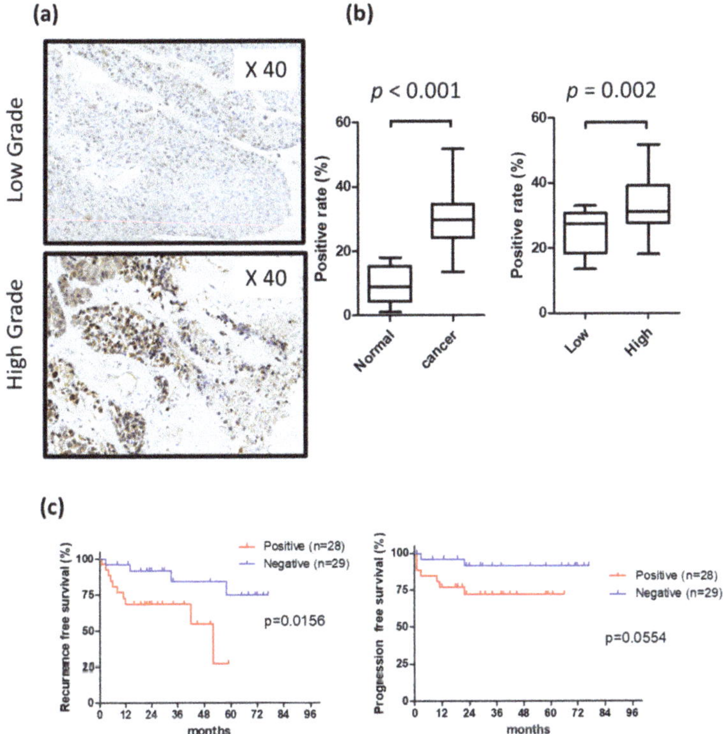

Figure 1. Immunohistological examination of expression of heparanase in bladder tissue; (**a**) positive ratio in low grade bladder cancer and high grade bladder cancer; (**b**) heparanase expression rate; (**c**) Kaplan–Meier curve of intravesical recurrence and invasion.

2.2. *Knockdown of Heparanase-Induced Apoptosis in Urothelial Carcinoma Cells*

Heparanase expression was studied in the human urothelial cancer cell lines MGH-U3 and T24 and found to increase compared to the normal urothelial cell line (UROtsa). The expression levels of heparanase were similar in MGH-U3 and T24 (Supplementary Figure S1). We first examined the suppression of heparanase protein expression and mRNA expression by knockdown with Si RNA (Supplementary Figure S2). MGH-U3 showed a significant decrease in cell activity due to heparanase knockdown compared to T24. There is a difference that MGH-U3 cells are suppressed by about 15% and T24 cells are suppressed by about 25% by knockdown by Si RNA. Inhibiting the expression of heparanase by siRNA suppressed the proliferative activity of cancer cells strongly, and cytotoxicity was observed (Figure 2a). In the MGH-U3 cell line, proliferation activity was suppressed by approximately 80% compared to approximately 40% in T24 cells. In the UROtsa cell line, heparanase knockdown suppressed growth activity by 15%. Further, heparanase knock-down by siRNA induced apoptosis (Figure 2b).

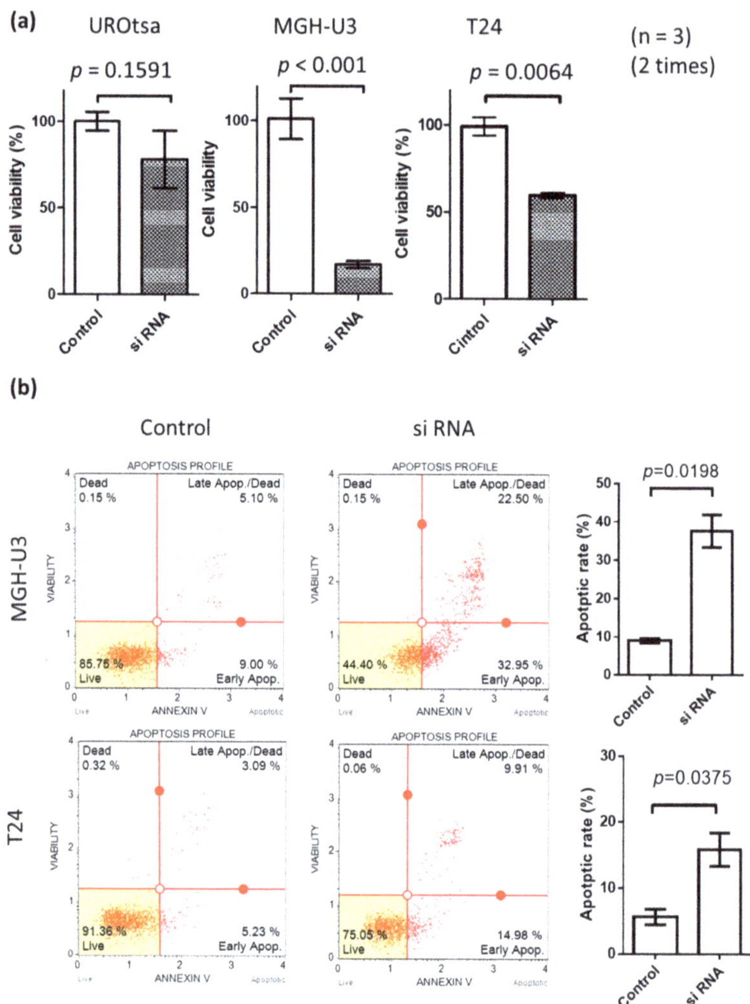

Figure 2. (**a**) Effect of heparanase knockdown on cell survival in urothelial carcinoma cells. Cell viability was assessed by an MTS assay 72 h following transfection; (**b**) 48 h following transfection, cells stained with Annexin V and propidium iodide were analyzed by flow cytometry (upper panels) and the percentages of apoptotic cells (AV[+]/PI[]) calculated (lower panels). Inset photograph is an immunofluorescence microscopy image showing cells positive for FITC-conjugated Annexin V (AV). Each value is the mean ± standard error. C, control RNA (non-specific siRNA); Si RNA, heparanase siRNA.

2.3. The Multi Enzyme Inhibitor RK-682, Which Is Also a Heparanase Inhibitor, Suppresses Cell Proliferation and Autophagy in Human Urothelial Cancer Cell Lines

RK-682 is an inhibitor of various enzymes including heparanase, phospholipase A_2, HIV-1 protease, some dual-specificity phosphatases (DSP), and a protein tyrosine phosphatase (PTP), CD45. The inhibition of heparanase by RK-682 was examined using MGH-U3 and T24 cell lines. Treatment with RK-682 suppressed heparanase protein expression and mRNA expression in these cells (Supplementary Figure S3). MGH-U3 and T24 cell lines were treated with RK-682 and examined in a cell viability assay to determine cytotoxicity. RK-682-treated MGH-U3 and T24 cells showed a concentration-dependent cytotoxicity (Figure 3a). The half-maximal inhibitory concentration (IC50) of RK-682 was 78.2 nM in

MGH-U3 cells, 43.2 nM in T24 cells, and 145 nM in UROtsa. The cytotoxicity was 2–3 times higher than that of the cancer cell line. UROtsa, which has low expression of heparanae, has an IC50 of RK-682 about 2–3 times higher than that of urothelial carcinoma cell line, MGH-U3 cell line and T24 cell line which has high expression of heparanase. In the heparanse knockdown experiment with Si RNA, the UROtsa cell line showed almost no inhibition of the cell activity, whereas RK-682 inhibited the cell activity of the UROtsa cell line at a high concentration. From this fact, it is considered that RK-682 has an action other than the inhibition of heparanase. The effect of RK-682 treatment was also examined in an invasion migration assay. In MGH-U3 and T24 cell lines, migratory ability decreased by approximately 20% following treatment with RK-682. In RK-682-treated MGH-U3 and T24 cells, invasion ability reduced by 55% and 40%, respectively (Figure 3b). MGH-U3 and T24 cells treated with RK-682 were also tested in an autophagy assay. The expression of autophagy decreased following the treatment with RK-682 (Figure 3c).

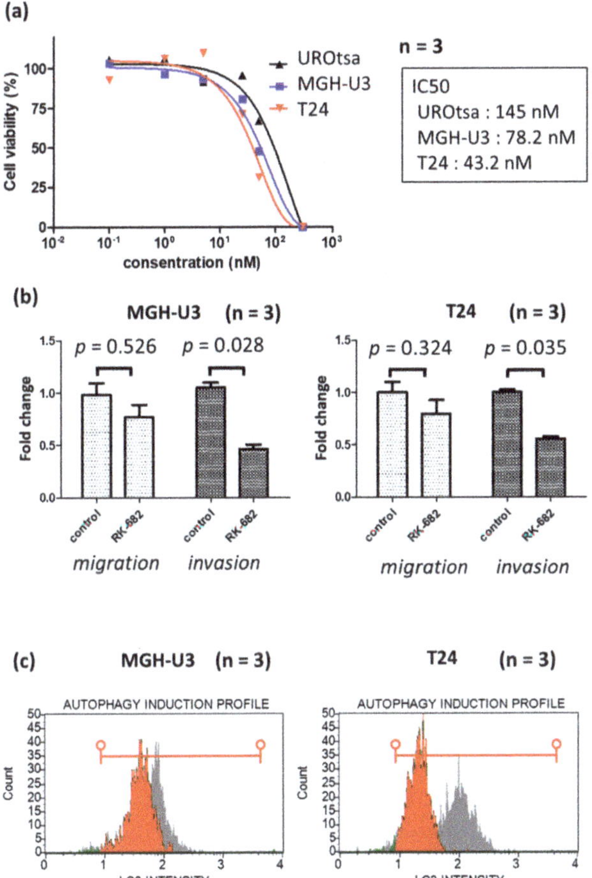

Figure 3. (**a**) Treatment with the multi enzyme inhibitor RK-682 inhibited cell proliferation in MGH-U3, T24 cells and UROtsa. Cells were incubated in serum-free media for 24 h and treated with different concentrations of RK-682 for a further 48 h. The number of viable cells was measured by an MTS assay and expressed as a percentage of viable cells; (**b**) effect of RK-682 on MGH-U3 and T24 cells. RK-682 treatment resulted in a significant inhibition of MGH-U3 and T24 cell invasion ($p < 0.05$); (**c**) 48 h treatment with heparanase inhibitor RK-682 inhibited cell autophagy in MGH-U3 and T24 cells. The red horizontal line shows the range of LC3 intensity after KR-682 treatment.

2.4. In Vivo Growth of Urothelial Carcinoma Is Suppressed by RK-682 in the BBN-Induced Mouse Bladder Cancer Model

The effects of the multi enzyme inhibitor RK-682 were tested using an in vivo model of bladder cancer treated with BBN (Figure 4a). Figure 4a briefly illustrates the experimental protocol for the present study. Six-week-old C57BL/6J mice were orally administered with 0.05% BBN. Bladder cancer-induced mice were prepared in approximately 22 weeks. The animals were divided into two groups, the treatment group (*n* = 7), and the non-treatment group (*n* = 5), totaling *n* = 14 animals. The heparanase inhibitor RK-682 was administered at 2.5 mg/100 μL, into the bladder four times a week through a catheter inserted into the bladder.

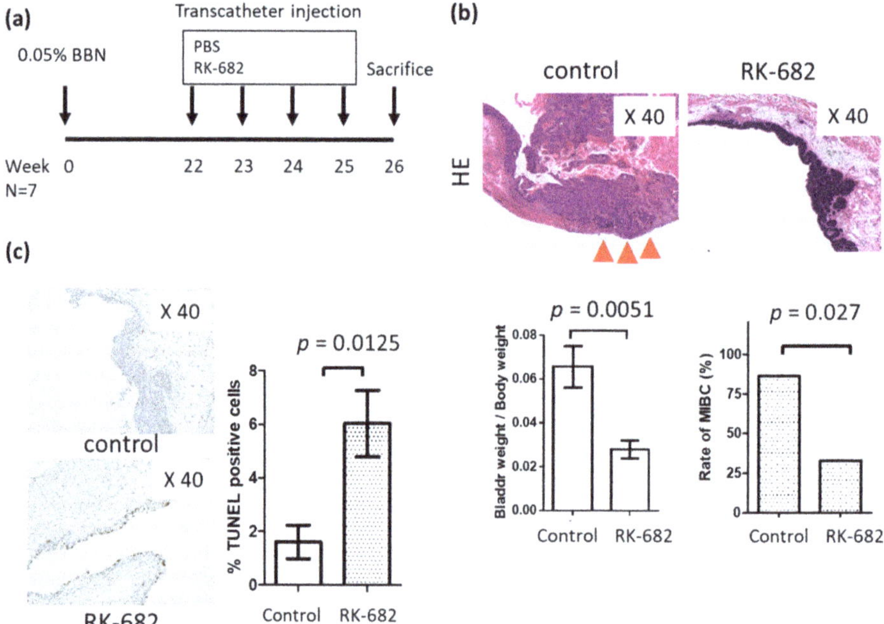

Figure 4. Intravesical injection of RK-682 inhibits in vivo tumor growth in the mouse N-butyl-N-(4-hydroxybutyl) nitrosamine (BBN)-induced bladder cancer implant model. (**a**) Diagrammatic experimental procedure; (**b**) RK-682 or control was transurethrally instilled into the bladder lumen. Bladders were resected post-instillation. Hematoxylin Eosin (HE) staining of bladder, comparison of bladder weight, ratio of muscle layer infiltration. Red triangle indicate images of muscle invasive bladder cancer.; (**c**) the percentage of cells in resected bladder specimens immunoreactive with TUNEL reagent, calculated per 1000 cells/in a high-power field. Each value is the mean ± standard error.

There was no significant difference in body weight between the RK-682-treated group and the control group after the end of treatment. (RK-682 group vs. control group; 24.5 g vs. 25.6 g *p* = 0.765). There was a significant decrease in the bladder weight/body wight, (RK-682 group vs. control group; 0.028 vs. 0.056 *p* = 0.0051) and ratio of infiltrative bladder cancer (RK-682 group vs. control group; 28.6% vs. 85.7% *p* = 0.027) in the RK-682 treatment group compared to the control group (Figure 4b). A TUNEL assay showed that apoptosis was more frequent in the RK-682 treatment group (Figure 4c). IHC studies of the mouse tissue showed decreased expression of Ki67, LC3, and CD31 markers in the specimens from animals treated with RK-682. In contrast, E-cadherin expression level increased after treatment with the inhibitor (Figure 5).

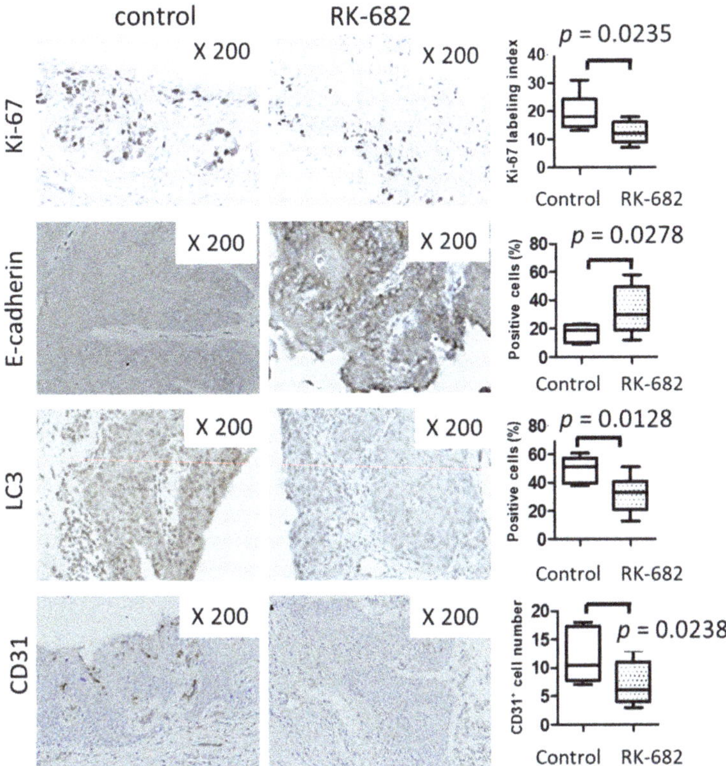

Figure 5. Immunohistochemical analysis of the mouse BBN-induced bladder cancer implant model. Immunohistochemistry for Ki-67, E-cadherin, LC3 and CD31 expression. The percentage of immunopositive cells was determined per 1000 cells in a high-power field.

3. Discussion

Heparanase expression is elevated in many types of tumors and is associated with more aggressive cancer and a poor prognosis [3,13,14,26]. We have previously reported that syndecan-1 is involved in urothelial cancer development through the promotion of angiogenesis [10]. In this study, we investigated heparanase, an activator of syndecan-1, and analyzed its function in urothelial cancer. We have demonstrated that inhibition of heparanase suppresses cell proliferation, epithelial-mesenchymal transition (EMT), autophagy and angiogenesis.

In other cancer types, heparanase activation has been indicated in promoting metastasis and tumor progression. In bladder cancer, Gohji et al. [32] reported that cancer-specific survival rates are significantly lower when heparanase expression is elevated in bladder cancer patients. In our study, increased expression of heparanase in bladder cancer tissue samples correlated with higher recurrence rates within the bladder and progression to muscle-invasive cancer.

Chen et al. [30] suggested an association between heparanase expression and cell adhesion, and metastasis in hepatocellular carcinoma cell lines. Heparanase plays a proadhesive role in cell adhesion and tumor microembolus in hepatocellular carcinoma. In this study, inhibition of heparanase activity significantly reduced the ability of cancer cells to migrate and infiltrate. Furthermore, it was confirmed that the inhibition of autophagy resulted from heparanase inhibition.

Shteingauz et al. [33] reported the regulation of autophagy in normal and malignant cells by heparanse, conferring survival advantages and the development of resistance to chemotherapy. In the spontaneous bladder cancer mouse model, heparanase inhibition significantly suppressed bladder cancer invasion. This study confirmed that the suppression of heparanase induces apoptosis, suppresses cell proliferation and inhibits autophagy.

This report is the first to investigate heparanase inhibition and its effects on the suppression of cancer invasion, autophagy and apoptosis in bladder cancer. Intravesical treatment with a heparanase inhibitor did not result in serious side effects in the in vivo mouse model used here and hence this study was conducted as planned. As a treatment option for bladder cancer, intravesical infusion therapy allows the penetration of a drug directly into cancer cells and has mild side effects. In combination, these observations indicate that heparanase is a potential candidate for targeted therapy in bladder cancer.

This study has limitations. RK-682 is a multi-enzyme inhibitory locus targeting several enzymes including heparanase, protein tyrosine phosphatase (PTP), phospholipase A_2 and other enzymes. The T24 cell line is found to be less sensitive to siRNA inhibition compared with the MGH-U3 cell line, but is more sensitive to RK-682 inhibition. This may explain other effects of RK-682-mediated inhibition observed in this study. In UROtsa cells, the cell activity induced by siRNA was reduced by approximately 20%. However, RK-682 treatment showed cytotoxicity in a dose-dependent manner. The cytotoxicity observed was 2–3 times higher compared to the cancer cell line. Expression analysis shows that RK-682 does have a heparanase inhibitory effect (Supplementary Figure S3). However, heparanase activity alone does explain changes in migration, invasion, and autophagy in bladder cancer cells. Further experiments are required to investigate the molecular function of heparanase.

4. Materials and Methods

4.1. Cell Culture, Plasmids and Chemicals

Human urothelial carcinoma cell lines MGH-U3, T24, and human urothelial cell line (UROtsa) were supplied by American Type Culture Collection (Manassas, VA, USA). MGH-U3 and T24 cells originated from human papillary bladder cancer [34]. T24 cells were cultured in RPMI1640 media supplemented with 10% fetal bovine serum and 50 units/mL penicillin-streptomycin at 37 °C in 5% CO_2.

The antibodies, anti-Ki67, LC3, and CD31, and E-cadherin, were purchased from Abcam (Cambridge, UK). The heparanase inhibitor RK-682 was purchased from Cayman Chemical Company (Ann Arbor, MI, USA). siRNA molecules were purchased from Thermo Fisher Scientific (K.K. Japan).

4.2. siRNA Transfection of Heparanase

For transfection analyses, 10^6 cells from each cell line were seeded into 6-cm dishes. They were transfected with either 100 nM of control RNA (Santa Cruz Biotechnology, Dallas, TX, USA) or with the heparanase siRNA. Transfections were performed with the Lipofectamine system (Invitrogen Japan, Tokyo, Japan) following the manufacturer's protocol.

The primers used were: HPSE sense 5′-AGUACUUGCGGUUACCCUATT-3′; HPSE antisense 5′-UAGGGUAACCGCAAGUACUTG-3′.

Actin sense 5′-CTCTTCCAGCCTTCCTTCCT-3′; Actin antisense 5′-AGCACTGTGTTGGCGTACAG-3′.

Gene expression analysis of cell cycle-related genes was performed by qPCR using the PrimerArray Cell Cycle (Takara, Otsu, Japan).

4.3. Tissue Samples and Immunohistochemistry (IHC)

This study was approved by the Medical Ethics Committee of Nara Medical University. The requirement for informed patient consent was waived due to the retrospective nature of the study (Study ID: NMU 900, July 23, 2013). A total of 57 patients diagnosed with organ-confined urothelial cancer between April 2007 and June 2010 at the Nara Medical University hospital were included in this study. The clinicopathological data and follow-up data were collected via a retrospective chart review. All pathological examinations were performed under the guidance of two pathologists (K.S. and N.K.) according to the 2009 TNM classification system [32]. All patients had bladder cancer and underwent transurethral resection of the bladder tumor (TURBT). IHC staining of 57 TURBT specimens using paraffin-embedded, formalin-fixed tissue blocks was performed as previously described [10,33]. Antibodies against heparinase were used as the primary antibodies at a dilution of 1:500. Staining was scored based on the positive cell ratio using standard light microscopy. Staining outcomes were evaluated by two independent observers (Y.T. and K.S), who were blinded to patient clinicopathological data.

4.4. Cell Proliferation Assay

The CellTiter 96 AQueous One Solution Cell Proliferation Assay (Promega, Madison, WI, USA) was used to measure cell proliferation by MTS assay as previously described [11]. Data were collected from triplicate experiments.

4.5. Apoptosis Detection Assay

Following the transfection with siRNA, cells were stained with propidium iodide (PI) and Fluorescein-5-isothiocyanate (FITC)-conjugated Annexin V (AV) following the manufacturer's protocol (TACS Annexin V-FITC kit; R&D Systems). Apoptotic cells were quantified by calculating the number of cells positive for AV and negative for PI. Experiments were performed a minimum three times of duplicate.

4.6. TdT-Mediated dUTP Nick End Labeling (TUNEL) Assay

Formalin-fixed and paraffin-embedded 5-l-m thick sections of tumor specimens were stained using a TUNEL assay: Tumor TACS in situ apoptosis detection kit (R&D Systems, Minneapolis, MN, USA). The apoptotic index (the number of apoptotic cells per total number of cells) was calculated as per 400 microscopic fields per sample.

4.7. Cell Viability Assay

UROtsa, MGH-U3 and T24 cells were seeded into 96-well plates at 2×10^3 cells/well and incubated overnight. The growth medium was removed, and the cells were washed once with phosphate-buffered saline (PBS). Fresh serum-free medium with or without heparinase inhibitor (RK-682) was applied. Cells were then treated with RK-682 (between 1–1000 nM) for 72 h to evaluate cell viability. The IC50 was determined based on the concentration-effect relationship using PRISM software version 5.00 (GraphPad Software, San Diego, CA, USA). Cell viability was measured using a Cell Counting Kit-8 (Dojindo, Kumamoto, Japan) according to the manufacturer's protocol. Absorbance was measured at 490 nm with a reference at 630 nm using an Infinite 200M PRO microplate autoreader (Tecan, Männedorf, Switzerland).

4.8. Migration Assay

A migration assay was performed using the BD Falcon FluoroBlok Insert System (Becton Dickinson, Franklin Lakes, NJ, USA) according to the manufacturer's instructions. Cells were starved in serum-free media for 24 h, then seeded at a density of 2.5×10^4 cells/well in serum-free media plus RK-682 inhibitor. RPMI1640 media with 10% FBS chemoattractant was contained within the lower wells. The cells were incubated in a humidified environment at 37 °C with 5% CO_2 for 48 h. Cells that were attached to the membrane were stained with the cell viability indicator Calcein AM Fluorescent Dye for 30 min (Promo Kine, Heidelberg, Germany) and quantified with an Infinite 200M PRO microplate spectrophotometer (Tecan, Männedorf, Switzerland) at 495 mm excitation and 515 nm emission. Cells were inspected via fluorescent microscopy.

4.9. Autophagy Assay

Autophagy assays were performed using Muse™ Cell Analyzer from Millipore (Hayward, CA, USA) following the manufacturer's instructions. Following treatment of MGH-U3 and T24 cells with heparinase inhibiter RK-682 (Cayman Chemical Company, Ann Arbor, MI, USA), the treated cells were washed with PBS buffer. The autophagy assays were analyzed using the Muse™ Autophagy LC3-antibody based kit (Millipore) according to the manufacturer's protocol.

4.10. BBN-Induced Mouse Bladder Cancer Model

An in vivo mouse model of bladder cancer was treated with BBN. Fourteen 6-week-old C57BL/6J female mice were obtained from Oriental Bio Service (Kyoto, Japan). All animal studies were approved by Nara Medical University affiliated Frist People's Hospital Committee on Use and Care of Animals and conducted in accordance with local humane animal care standard (Reference Number: 11389). BBN B0938 (Tokyo Chemical Industry, Tokyo, Japan) treated bladder cancer model mice were treated with the heparanase inhibitor RK-682 in the bladder once a week for four weeks by injection. Mice were randomized into a control group (control PBS, $n = 7$) or heparanase inhibitor (RK-682, $n = 7$) treatment group and received a single intravesical treatment instillation that was retained for 1 h with a purse-string suture. Mice were sacrificed (at week 25) after four treatments. Bladders were removed, placed open on filter paper, and fixed in 10% neutral buffered formalin. Bladders were then embedded in paraffin, step-sectioned, and stained with hematoxylin-eosin (H&E) and IHC staining for E-cadherin, Ki67, CD31 and LC3 (Abcam, Tokyo, Japan).

4.11. Statistical Analysis

Differences in cell migration were evaluated with the Student's *t*-test. The correlation of IHC staining intensity was assessed with the Man–Whitney U test. IBM SPSS Version 21 (SPSS Inc., Chicago, IL, USA) and PRISM software version 5.00 (San Diego, CA, USA) were used for statistical analyses and data plotting, respectively. Statistical significance was set at $p < 0.05$, and all reported p values were two-sided.

5. Conclusions

Heparanase induces invasion and autophagy in urothelial carcinoma. Downregulation of heparanase induces apoptosis. Heparanase may contribute to urothelial carcinoma cell survival and invasion.

Supplementary Materials: The following are available online at http://www.mdpi.com/1422-0067/21/11/3789/s1, Figure S1: Heparanse protein expression levels and mRNA expression levels in MGH-U3, T24 and U Rotsa cell lines, Figure S2: The suppression of heparanase protein expression and mRNA expression by knockdown with Si RNA MGH-U3, T24 and U Rotsa cell lines, Figure S3: The suppression of heparanase protein expression and mRNA expression by treated with the multi enzyme inhibitor RK-682 in MGH-U3, T24 and U Rotsa cell lines.

Author Contributions: Conceptualization, Y.T. and K.F.; Methodology, Y.T.; Software, Y.T. and T.F.; Validation, Y.T., K.S. and N.K.; Formal analysis, Y.T.; Investigation, Y.T., S.H., Y.M., Y.N., N.K. and K.F.; Resources, Y.T.; Data curation, Y.T., S.H. and Y.M.; Writing—Original draft preparation, Y.T.; Writing—Review and editing, M.M.; Visualization, Y.T.; Supervision, K.S., M.M., S.A., N.T., N.K. and K.F.; Project administration, Y.T., K.S. and M.M.; Funding acquisition, Y.T., N.K. and K.F. All authors have read and agreed to the published version of the manuscript.

Funding: This research received no external funding.

Acknowledgments: Editorial support, in the form of medical writing, assembling tables and creating high-resolution images based on authors' detailed directions, collating author comments, copyediting, fact-checking, and referencing, was provided by Editage, Cactus Communications.

Conflicts of Interest: The authors declare no conflict of interest.

Abbreviations

AV	Annexin V
FITC	Fluorescein-5-isothiocyanate
IC50	half-maximal inhibitory concentration
IHC	Immunohistochemistry
PBS	phosphate-buffered saline

PI	propidium iodide
siRNA	Small Interfering Ribonucleic Acid
qPCR	Quantitative Polymerase Chain Reaction
TUNEL	TdT-mediated dUTP nick end labeling
TURBT	Transurethral resection of the bladder tumor

References

1. Sarrazin, S.; Lamanna, W.C.; Esko, J.D. Heparan sulfate proteoglycans. *Cold Spring Harb. Perspect. Biol.* **2011**, *3*, a004952. [CrossRef] [PubMed]
2. Hammond, E.; Khurana, A.; Shridhar, V.; Dredge, K. The Role of heparanase and sulfatases in the modification of heparan sulfate proteoglycans within the tumor microenvironment and opportunities for novel cancer therapeutics. *Front. Oncol.* **2014**, *4*, 195. [CrossRef] [PubMed]
3. Barash, U.; Cohen-Kaplan, V.; Dowek, I.; Sanderson, R.D.; Ilan, N.; Vlodavsky, I. Proteoglycans in health and disease: New concepts for heparanase function in tumor progression and metastasis. *FEBS J.* **2010**, *277*, 3890–3903. [CrossRef]
4. Dhodapkar, M.V.; Abe, E.; Theus, A.; Lacy, M.; Langford, J.K.; Barlogie, B.; Sanderson, R.D. Syndecan-1 is a multifunctional regulator of myeloma pathobiology: Control of tumor cell survival, growth, and bone cell differentiation. *Blood* **1998**, *91*, 2679–2688. [CrossRef]
5. Mahtouk, K.; Cremer, F.W.; Rème, T.; Jourdan, M.; Baudard, M.; Moreaux, J.; Requirand, G.; Fiol, G.; De Vos, J.; Moos, M.; et al. Heparan sulphate proteoglycans are essential for the myeloma cell growth activity of EGF-family ligands in multiple myeloma. *Oncogene* **2006**, *25*, 7180–7191. [CrossRef]
6. Derksen, P.W.; Keehnen, R.M.; Evers, L.M.; Van Oers, M.H.; Spaargaren, M.; Pals, S.T. Cell surface proteoglycan syndecan-1 mediates hepatocyte growth factor binding and promotes Met signaling in multiple myeloma. *Blood* **2002**, *99*, 1405–1410. [CrossRef]
7. Yang, Y.; MacLeod, V.; Dai, Y.; Khotskaya-Sample, Y.; Shriver, Z.; Venkataraman, G.; Sasisekharan, R.; Naggi, A.; Torri, G.; Casu, B.; et al. The syndecan-1 heparan sulfate proteoglycan is a viable target for myeloma therapy. *Blood* **2007**, *110*, 2041–2048. [CrossRef] [PubMed]
8. Nikolova, V.; Koo, C.Y.; Ibrahim, S.A.; Wang, Z.; Spillmann, D.; Dreier, R.; Kelsch, R.; Fischgrabe, J.; Smollich, M.; Rossi, L.H.; et al. Differential roles for membrane-bound and soluble syndecan-1 (CD138) in breast cancer progression. *Carcinogenesis* **2009**, *30*, 397–407. [CrossRef] [PubMed]
9. Shimada, K.; Nakamura, M.; Anai, S.; De Velasco, M.; Tanaka, M.; Tsujikawa, K.; Ouji, Y.; Konishi, N. A novel human AlkB homologue, ALKBH8, contributes to human bladder cancer progression. *Cancer Res.* **2009**, *69*, 3157–3164. [CrossRef]
10. Shimada, K.; Matsuyoshi, S.; Nakamura, M.; Ishida, E.; Konishi, N. Phosphorylation status of Fas-associated death domain-containing protein (FADD) is associated with prostate cancer progression. *J. Pathol.* **2005**, *206*, 423–432. [CrossRef] [PubMed]
11. Shimada, K.; Nakamura, M.; De Velasco, M.A.; Tanaka, M.; Ouji, Y.; Konishi, N. Syndecan-1, a new target molecule involved in progression of androgen-independent prostate cancer. *Cancer Sci.* **2009**, *100*, 1248–1254. [CrossRef] [PubMed]
12. Vlodavsky, I.; Ilan, N.; Naggi, A.; Casu, B. Heparanase: Structure, biological functions, and inhibition by heparin-derived mimetics of heparan sulfate. *Curr. Pharm. Des.* **2007**, *13*, 2057–2073. [CrossRef] [PubMed]
13. Vlodavsky, I.; Elkin, M.; Abboud-Jarrous, G.; Levi-Adam, F.; Fuks, L.; Shafat, I.; Ilan, N. Heparanase: One molecule with multiple functions in cancer progression. *Connect. Tissue Res.* **2008**, *49*, 207–210. [CrossRef]
14. Ilan, N.; Elkin, M.; Vlodavsky, I. Regulation, function and clinical significance of heparanase in cancer metastasis and angiogenesis. *Int. J. Biochem. Cell Biol.* **2006**, *38*, 2018–2039. [CrossRef]
15. Whitelock, J.M.; Iozzo, R.V. Heparan sulfate: A complex polymer charged with biological activity. *Chem. Rev.* **2005**, *105*, 2745–2764. [CrossRef]
16. Maeda, T.; Desouky, J.; Friedl, A. Syndecan-1 expression by stromal fibroblasts promotes breast carcinoma growth in vivo and stimulates tumor angiogenesis. *Oncogene* **2006**, *25*, 1408–1412. [CrossRef]
17. Weissmann, M.; Arvatz, G.; Horowitz, N.; Feld, S.; Naroditsky, I.; Zhang, Y.; Ng, M.; Hammond, E.; Nevo, E.; Vlodavsky, I.; et al. Heparanase-neutralizing antibodies attenuate lymphoma tumor growth and metastasis. *Proc. Natl. Acad. Sci. USA* **2016**, *113*, 704–709. [CrossRef] [PubMed]

18. Zhang, Y.F.; Tang, X.D.; Gao, J.H.; Fang, D.C.; Yang, S.M. Heparanase: A universal immunotherapeutic target in human cancers. *Drug Discov. Today* **2011**, *16*, 412–417. [CrossRef] [PubMed]

19. Chen, T.; Tang, X.D.; Wan, Y.; Chen, L.; Yu, S.T.; Xiong, Z.; Fang, D.C.; Liang, G.P.; Yang, S.M. HLA-A2-restricted cytotoxic T lymphocyte epitopes from human heparanase as novel targets for broad-spectrum tumor immunotherapy. *Neoplasia (N. Y. NY)* **2008**, *10*, 977–986. [CrossRef] [PubMed]

20. Baburajeev, C.P.; Mohan, C.D.; Rangappa, S.; Mason, D.J.; Fuchs, J.E.; Bender, A.; Barash, U.; Vlodavsky, I.; Basappa; Rangappa, K.S. Identification of novel class of triazolo-thiadiazoles as potent inhibitors of human heparanase and their anticancer activity. *BMC Cancer* **2017**, *17*, 235. [CrossRef]

21. Miao, H.Q.; Liu, H.; Navarro, E.; Kussie, P.; Zhu, Z. Development of heparanase inhibitors for anti-cancer therapy. *Curr. Med. Chem.* **2006**, *13*, 2101–2111. [CrossRef] [PubMed]

22. Parish, C.R.; Freeman, C.; Brown, K.J.; Francis, D.J.; Cowden, W.B. Identification of sulfated oligosaccharide-based inhibitors of tumor growth and metastasis using novel in vitro assays for angiogenesis and heparanase activity. *Cancer Res.* **1999**, *59*, 3433–3441. [PubMed]

23. Borsig, L. Antimetastatic activities of modified heparins: Selectin inhibition by heparin attenuates metastasis. *Semin. Thromb. Hemost.* **2007**, *33*, 540–546. [CrossRef] [PubMed]

24. Vlodavsky, I.; Friedmann, Y.; Elkin, M.; Aingorn, H.; Atzmon, R.; Ishai-Michaeli, R.; Bitan, M.; Pappo, O.; Peretz, T.; Michal, I.; et al. Mammalian heparanase: Gene cloning, expression and function in tumor progression and metastasis. *Nat. Med.* **1999**, *5*, 793–802. [CrossRef]

25. Hulett, M.D.; Freeman, C.; Hamdorf, B.J.; Baker, R.T.; Harris, M.J.; Parish, C.R. Cloning of mammalian heparanase, an important enzyme in tumor invasion and metastasis. *Nat. Med.* **1999**, *5*, 803–809. [CrossRef]

26. Parish, C.R.; Freeman, C.; Hulett, M.D. Heparanase: A key enzyme involved in cell invasion. *Biochim. Biophys. Acta* **2001**, *1471*, M99–M108. [CrossRef]

27. Vlodavsky, I.; Friedmann, Y. Molecular properties and involvement of heparanase in cancer metastasis and angiogenesis. *J. Clin. Investig.* **2001**, *108*, 341–347. [CrossRef]

28. Vlodavsky, I.; Beckhove, P.; Lerner, I.; Pisano, C.; Meirovitz, A.; Ilan, N.; Elkin, M. Significance of heparanase in cancer and inflammation. *Cancer Microenviron.* **2012**, *5*, 115–132. [CrossRef]

29. Jung, O.; Trapp-Stamborski, V.; Purushothaman, A.; Jin, H.; Wang, H.; Sanderson, R.D.; Rapraeger, A.C. Heparanase-induced shedding of syndecan-1/CD138 in myeloma and endothelial cells activates VEGFR2 and an invasive phenotype: Prevention by novel synstatins. *Oncogenesis* **2016**, *5*, e202. [CrossRef]

30. Chen, X.-P.; Luo, J.-S.; Tian, Y.; Nie, C.-L.; Cui, W.; Zhang, W.-D. Downregulation of heparanase expression results in suppression of invasion, migration, and adhesion abilities of hepatocellular carcinoma cells. *BioMed Res. Int.* **2015**, *2015*, 241983. [CrossRef]

31. Comperat, E.M.; Burger, M.; Gontero, P.; Mostafid, A.H.; Palou, J.; Roupret, M.; van Rhijn, B.W.G.; Shariat, S.F.; Sylvester, R.J.; Zigeuner, R.; et al. Grading of urothelial carcinoma and the new "world health organisation classification of tumours of the urinary system and male genital organs 2016". *Eur. Urol. Focus* **2019**, *5*, 457–466. [CrossRef] [PubMed]

32. Gohji, K.; Okamoto, M.; Kitazawa, S.; Toyoshima, M.; Dong, J.; Katsuoka, Y.; Nakajima, M. Heparanase protein and gene expression in bladder cancer. *J. Urol.* **2001**, *166*, 1286–1290. [CrossRef]

33. Shteingauz, A.; Boyango, I.; Naroditsky, I.; Hammond, E.; Gruber, M.; Doweck, I.; Ilan, N.; Vlodavsky, I. Heparanase enhances tumor growth and chemoresistance by promoting autophagy. *Cancer Res.* **2015**, *75*, 3946–3957. [CrossRef] [PubMed]

34. Sabichi, A.; Keyhani, A.; Tanaka, N.; Delacerda, J.; Lee, I.L.; Zou, C.; Zhou, J.H.; Benedict, W.F.; Grossman, H.B. Characterization of a panel of cell lines derived from urothelial neoplasms: Genetic alterations, growth in vivo and the relationship of adenoviral mediated gene transfer to coxsackie adenovirus receptor expression. *J. Urol.* **2006**, *175*, 1133–1137. [CrossRef]

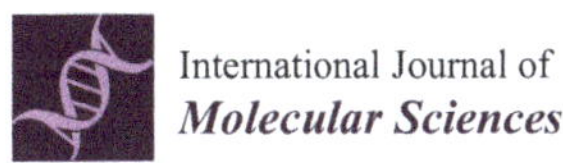 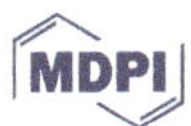

International Journal of
Molecular Sciences

Article

Malignancy Grade-Dependent Mapping of Metabolic Landscapes in Human Urothelial Bladder Cancer: Identification of Novel, Diagnostic, and Druggable Biomarkers

Aikaterini Iliou [1,†], Aristeidis Panagiotakis [1,†], Aikaterini F. Giannopoulou [2,†], Dimitra Benaki [1], Mariangela Kosmopoulou [1], Athanassios D. Velentzas [2], Ourania E. Tsitsilonis [3], Issidora S. Papassideri [2], Gerassimos E. Voutsinas [4], Eumorphia G. Konstantakou [5], Evagelos Gikas [1,*,‡], Emmanuel Mikros [1,*,‡] and Dimitrios J. Stravopodis [2,*,‡]

[1]   Section of Pharmaceutical Chemistry, Department of Pharmacy, School of Health Sciences, National and Kapodistrian University of Athens (NKUA), 15701 Athens, Greece; katerinail@pharm.uoa.gr (A.I.); arispan@pharm.uoa.gr (A.P.); dbenaki@pharm.uoa.gr (D.B.); mrgkosm@gmail.com (M.K.)

[2]   Section of Cell Biology and Biophysics, Department of Biology, School of Science, National and Kapodistrian University of Athens (NKUA), 15701 Athens, Greece; aigiann@biol.uoa.gr (A.F.G.); tveletz@biol.uoa.gr (A.D.V.); ipapasid@biol.uoa.gr (I.S.P.)

[3]   Section of Animal and Human Physiology, Department of Biology, School of Science, National and Kapodistrian University of Athens (NKUA), 15701 Athens, Greece; rtsitsil@biol.uoa.gr

[4]   Laboratory of Molecular Carcinogenesis and Rare Disease Genetics, Institute of Biosciences and Applications, National Center for Scientific Research (NCSR) "Demokritos", 15701 Athens, Greece; mvoutsin@bio.demokritos.gr

[5]   Harvard Medical School, Massachusetts General Hospital Cancer Center (MGHCC), Charlestown, MA 021004, USA; ekonstantakou@mgh.harvard.edu

*   Correspondence: vgikas@pharm.uoa.gr (E.G.); mikros@pharm.uoa.gr (E.M.); dstravop@biol.uoa.gr (D.J.S.)

†   These authors contributed equally to this work.

‡   These authors contributed equally to this work.

Received: 31 January 2020; Accepted: 8 March 2020; Published: 10 March 2020

Abstract: Background: Urothelial bladder cancer (UBC) is one of the cancers with the highest mortality rate and prevalence worldwide; however, the clinical management of the disease remains challenging. Metabolomics has emerged as a powerful tool with beneficial applications in cancer biology and thus can provide new insights on the underlying mechanisms of UBC progression and/or reveal novel diagnostic and therapeutic schemes. Methods: A collection of four human UBC cell lines that critically reflect the different malignancy grades of UBC was employed; RT4 (grade I), RT112 (grade II), T24 (grade III), and TCCSUP (grade IV). They were examined using Nuclear Magnetic Resonance, Mass Spectrometry, and advanced statistical approaches, with the goal of creating new metabolic profiles that are mechanistically associated with UBC progression toward metastasis. Results: Distinct metabolic profiles were observed for each cell line group, with T24 (grade III) cells exhibiting the most abundant metabolite contents. AMP and creatine phosphate were highly increased in the T24 cell line compared to the RT4 (grade I) cell line, indicating the major energetic transformation to which UBC cells are being subjected during metastasis. Thymosin $\beta4$ and $\beta10$ were also profiled with grade-specific patterns of expression, strongly suggesting the importance of actin-cytoskeleton dynamics for UBC advancement to metastatic and drug-tolerant forms. Conclusions: The present study unveils a novel and putatively druggable metabolic signature that holds strong promise for early diagnosis and the successful chemotherapy of UBC disease.

Keywords: biomarker; bladder; cancer; grade; metabolomics; MS; NMR

---

1. Introduction

Urothelial bladder cancer (UBC) exhibits the highest mortality rate worldwide, being categorized as the second most common genitourinary disease in the USA [1]. UBC still remains a major clinical challenge and its treatment mainly depends on early diagnosis [2]. It can be generally classified as a low-grade (I and II) non-muscle-invasive and a high-grade (III and IV) muscle-invasive disease that is prone to metastasis, based on histological differentiations from normal bladder cells [3]. One third of non-muscle-invasive UBCs progress to high(er) grades or stages of malignancy [4], which, along with the symptom-to-treatment delay for affected patients [5], compromise the therapeutic effectiveness and success of clinically applied regimens. UBC is characterized by high recurrence rates, with the continuous monitoring of patients being a medical practice of great importance [6]. Notably, despite their initial chemosensitivity, UBC patients will eventually develop chemoresistance due to tumors' mutational heterogeneity, leading to a median survival expectancy of 13–19 months [7,8]. Thereby, novel, early diagnosis, and druggable biomarkers for UBC need to be promptly discovered.

Metabolomics, according to Professor J. Nicolson's definition, is "the quantitative measurement of the dynamic and multi-parametric metabolic response of living systems to pathophysiological stimuli or genetic modifications" [9], with its great potential and promise in cancer research being continuously proved. The reprogramming of cellular metabolism seems to act as a strong force in tumorigenesis [10]. Malignant hallmarks, such as cell survival under stress conditions, as well as tumors' ability to utilize nutrients and successfully encounter high-energy demands, are tightly correlated with metabolic alterations, thus indicating the major roles of metabolic landscapes in Cancer Biology [11–14]. Metabolic activities may significantly differ among distinct subtypes or malignancy grades/stages of the same type of cancer, leading to different metabolic networks and metabolomes [15,16]. Metabolomics has gained great value, power, and importance for cancer research, not only as a multifaceted tool in early diagnosis, but also as a valuable platform for the discovery of novel mechanisms controlling tumorigenesis, thus paving the way to new treatment strategies and therapies. Research on several cancers has significantly profited from the engagement of metabolomics technology. However, its application to early detection, progression, and the chemotherapeutic management of human malignancies and especially UBC remains still limited, and it needs to be further expanded [15–20].

Most metabolomics studies in UBC cell lines have focused on differentiating between normal bladder and UBC cells, and they have shown the importance of several metabolites involved in pathways related to energy production, such as fatty acids, amino acids, and organic acids. [21,22]. The effect of the oncometabolome on progression of the disease has recently emerged as a new field in UBC research [23–26]. Few studies used two cell lines, for low and high-grade UBC, in order to find distinct metabolic profiles between the two grades [27,28]. They observed that pyruvate consumption, as well as alanine and lactate levels, might be related to UBC aggressiveness, and they also suggested the role of fatty acid biosynthesis and amino acid metabolism in disease progression.

To further expand these studies, we herein engaged a collection of four human UBC cell lines that critically reflect the distinct de-differentiation stage, malignancy grade (I, II, III, and IV), mutational signature, genetic heterogeneity, metastatic capacity, and chemotherapeutic tolerance of UBC to thoroughly investigate the metabolic alterations to which UBC cells are being subjected during disease progression. Our findings are expected to shed light into mechanisms regulating the transition of normal to the oncogenic and, finally, metastatic cell phase. Employment of the two state-of-the-art analytical platforms, Nuclear Magnetic Resonance (NMR) and Mass Spectrometry (MS), which are complementary, allows the more comprehensive metabolic profiling of UBC, with the grade-specific metabolic signatures revealed essentially contributing to the significant advancement in the success, efficacy, and safety of conducted research. High-scale UBC cell culturing enabled the high-resolution metabolic landscaping, while the high density of cells upon harvesting portrayed tumor architectural organization in vivo.

2. Results

In this study, a comparative NMR and LC-MS-mediated metabolic profiling was performed in four UBC human cell lines in order to thoroughly examine the effects of oncometabolome composition on progression of the disease.

2.1. NMR Analysis

The ^{1}H 1D NMR spectra of the four UBC cell lines with the respective standard deviations obtained from each group are shown in Figure 1. The observed within-group variability has proved to be very low, thus confirming the precision and high-technical value of the procedure being followed for sample preparation and the subsequent instrumental analysis. In total, 42 metabolites have been identified (Supplementary Table S1), with the annotated and grade-dependent metabolites being described in Figure 2 as boxplot-type graphs.

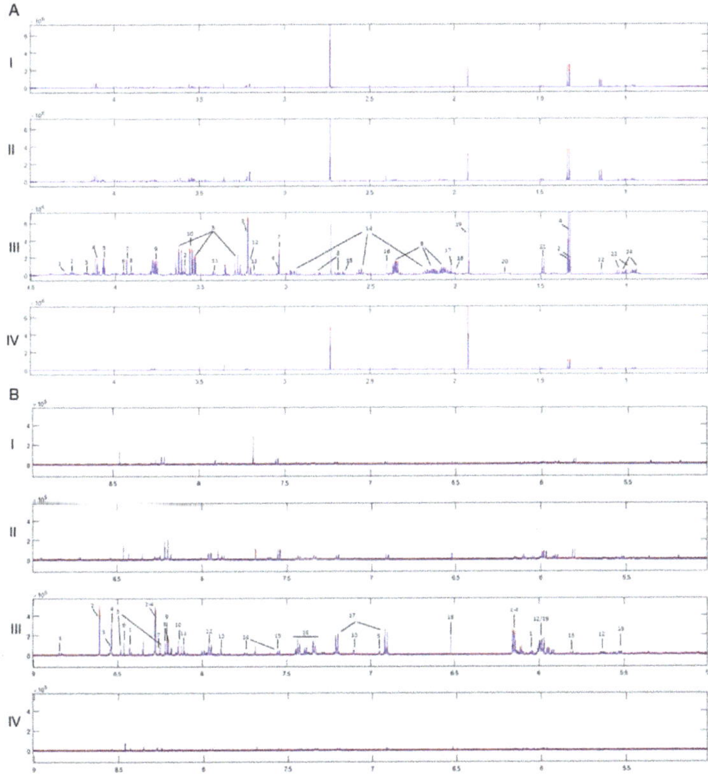

Figure 1. Average ^{1}H NMR spectra of the four groups and their standard deviation, where very low within-group variability is observed. Annotation is shown on the most abundant spectrum of the grade III group. (I. Grade I, II. Grade II, III. Grade III, IV. Grade IV). Red Line: Average + standard deviation, Blue Line: Average–standard deviation. (**A**) Aliphatic region: 1. UDPs, 2. Threonine, 3. Choline phosphate, 4. Lactate, 5. Myo-inositol, 6. Creatine phosphate, 7. Creatine, 8. Aspartate, 9. Glutamate, 10. Glycine, 11. Taurine, 12. Choline, 13. β-Alanine, 14. Glutathione, 15. Malate, 16. Succinate, 17. N-Acetylglutamine, 18. Proline, 19. Acetate, 20. Leucine, 21. Alanine, 22. Propylene glycol, 23. Valine, 24. Isoleucine. (**B**) Aromatic region: 1. NAD+, 2. AMP, 3. ATP, 4. ADP, 5. NADH, 6. Formate, 7. Adenine, 8. Hypoxanthine, 9. Oxypurinol, 10. GTP, 11. UMP, 12. UDPs, 13. Histidine, 14. Tryptophan, 15. Uracil, 16. Phenylalanine, 17. Tyrosine, 18. Fumarate, 19. UDP-GlcNAc.

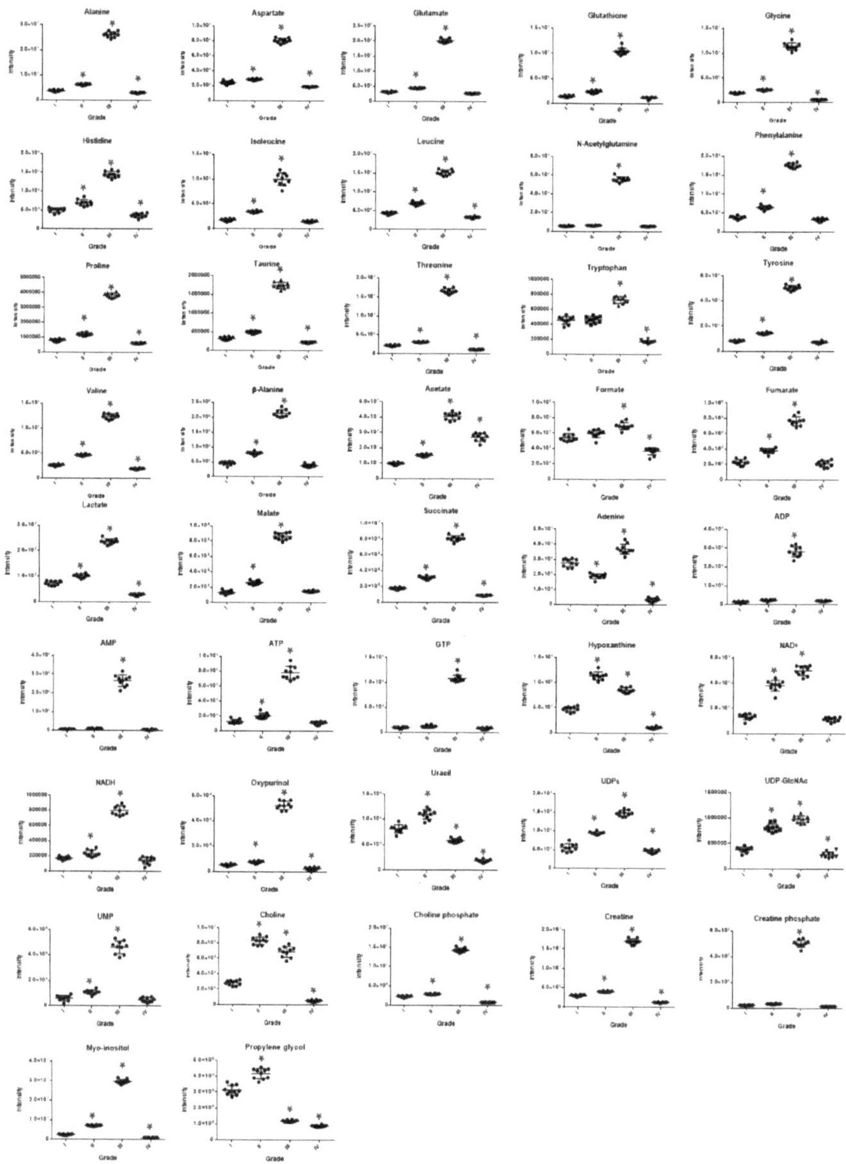

Figure 2. Boxplots of the 42 most significant metabolites, using ANOVA for the four-group urothelial bladder cancer (UBC) member comparisons. Myo-inositol, creatine phosphate, amino acids (e.g., histidine), organic acids (e.g., malate, succinate, and acetate), AXPs (AMP, ADP, and ATP), GTP, UMP, and oxypurinol follow the pattern of "metabolic inversion" that is being typified by their highly elevated contents in grade III (T24) group but reduced (restored) to the cell line-reference-like ones (RT4; grade I) in the grade IV (TCCSUP) UBC cell group. However, some metabolites are not subjected to the same pattern of grade-dependent deregulation (e.g., tryptophan, formate, uracil, adenine, propylene glycol, and choline). Remarkably, uracil and propylene glycol are presented with significant decreases during cellular transition from low to high grades (III and IV) of UBC malignancy.

For the multivariate analysis, Principal Component Analysis (PCA) was first conducted to search for outliers and trends of discrimination. No outliers were detected (Hotteling eclipse, 95% confidence level), and a clear separation of the four UBC groups was observed (Supplementary Figure S1). Partial Least Square-Discriminant Analysis (PLS-DA) confirmed the clear separation of the examined groups, with good quality parameters and prediction power [R2X(cum) = 0.982 and Q2(cum) = 0.977]. Orthogonal Partial Least Square-Discriminant Analysis (OPLS-DA) pairwise comparisons were also performed to search for discriminatory variables for each grade-specific UBC cell line. The S-plot between grade I (RT4) and grade III (T24) UBC cells revealed that the T24 cell line exhibits notably upregulated levels of most metabolites, including, among others, amino acids (glutamate, alanine, threonine), organic acids (acetate, lactate), myo-inositol, creatine, and choline phosphate, while decreased contents of few metabolites (uracil, histidine, and propylene glycol) were observed (Figure 3A). The S-plot between grade III (T24) and grade IV (TCCSUP) UBC cells unveiled that the grade IV-specific levels of most metabolites were significantly reduced and restored almost to the grade I (RT4) respective levels, indicating a "metabolic inversion" effect during the advanced (late stage) UBC development (Figure 3B). This is observed in the PLS-DA scores plot of UBC groups, with RT4 and TCCSUP showing an inability to be discriminated on the first PC, while grade III (T24) was being proved as the most distant UBC group on the same component (Figure 3C). Validation of the PLS-DA model using permutation testing is shown in Figure 3D. Table 1 summarizes the results of univariate analysis of the identified metabolites, considering grade I (RT4) as the UBC cell line of reference (control) in order to explore malignancy grade-specific metabolic changes occurring during disease progression. Grade-dependent metabolites were detected and shown to be implicated in diverse metabolic pathways, such as amino acid metabolism, the tricarboxylic acid (TCA) cycle, and energy metabolism, as well as purine and pyrimidine metabolism. In accordance to the multivariate analysis, elevated contents of most metabolites are observed in grade III (T24), whereas they are restored (reduced) to their respective levels of the reference grade I group (RT4) [Fold Change (x) close to 1], or even lower, in the grade IV (TCCSUP) cells. Since the majority of metabolites (40 out of 42) exhibited significant increase in the grade III (T24) group, further investigation was performed in order to take into account dilution effects and metabolic dependencies. For the identified metabolites, all pairwise ratios were examined, and the fold change (x) of each metabolic trait was calculated. A heat map of the fold change (x) values of metabolic ratios between grade III (T24) and grade I (RT4) UBC cell groups is presented in Supplementary Figure S2. Among the 42 metabolites that were found to be significant, the pairwise ratios analysis highlighted the importance of a sub-collection containing 14 of them. Remarkably, uracil, hypoxanthine, adenine, tryptophan, propylene glycol, formate, UDPs, and choline ratios exhibited the highest decrease in grade III (T24) compared to grade I (RT4), whereas ADP, AMP, GTP, oxypurinol, creatine phosphate, and myo-inositol ratios showed the most significant increase in grade III (T24) [compared to grade I (RT4) reference group] cells. Importantly, the reduced metabolite contents, except for the uracil and propylene glycol ones, were found to be elevated in the analysis of metabolite concentrations only (expressed as signals). On the contrary, most of these metabolite ratios were shown to be decreased, which suggests that the analysis of metabolite concentrations only may lead to erroneous results when such enormous biological differences between compared groups are observed.

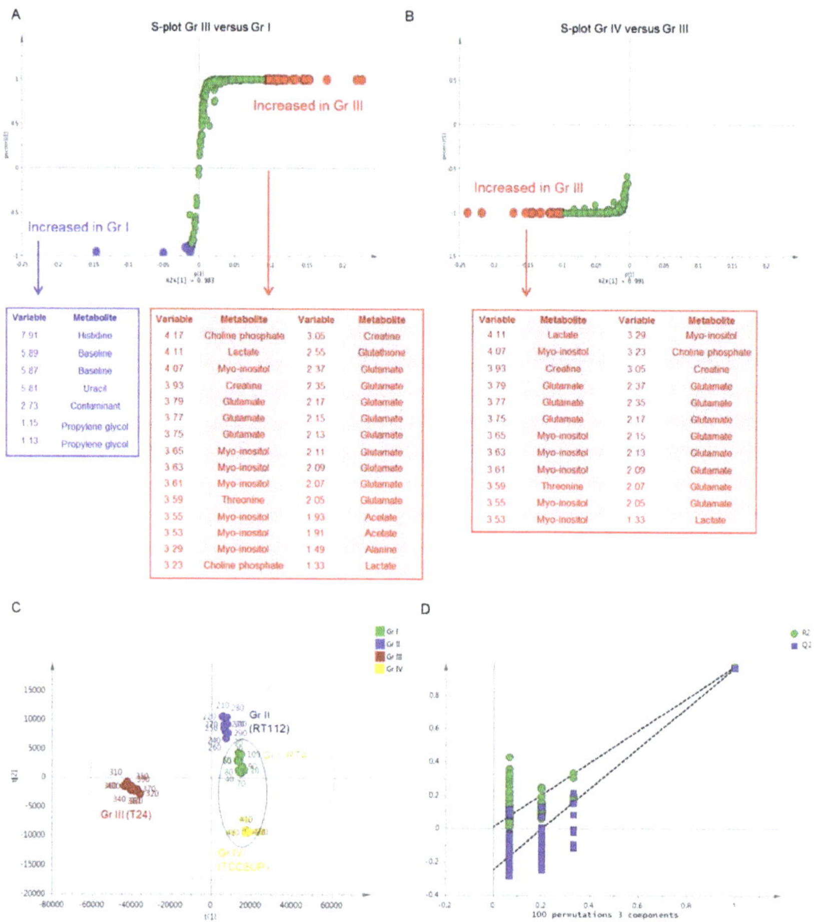

Figure 3. Multivariate analysis of ^{1}H NMR spectra of the four UBC cell lines. (**A**) S-plot of Orthogonal Partial Least Square-Discriminant Analysis (OPLS-DA) model of grade I (RT4) versus grade III (T24) cell line and the respective loadings. Red dots: increased in grade III (T24), Blue dots: increased in grade I (RT4). (**B**) S-plot of OPLS-DA model of grade III (T24) versus grade IV (TCCSUP) cell line and the respective loadings. Red dots: increased in grade III (T24). (**C**) Scores plot of Partial Least Square-Discriminant Analysis (PLS-DA) model of the four UBC cell lines. Grade I (RT4) and grade IV (TCCSUP) groups seem unable to be discriminated, among each other, on the first principal component, while the grade III (T24) group is the most distant from the initial conditions on the same component. (**D**) Permutation test of the PLS-DA model of the four UBC cell lines. Gr: (malignancy) grade.

In order to systemically map and integrate the metabolic hits into their related biological pathways, the statistically significant metabolites were imported into CytoScape 3.7.0, using MetScape for metabolomics data visualization. Extracted pathway and metabolic course analyses are illustrated in Figure 4A. Among others, it seems that purine and pyrimidine metabolism (including the one of uracil) can critically control (positively or negatively) UBC progression to late-malignancy stages (Figure 4B). Importantly, propylene glycol (Kyoto Encyclopedia of Genes and Genomes (KEGG): 1, 2 propanediol), which is implicated in lactaldehyde metabolism, as shown in the constructed network (Figure 4A), may also be notably downregulated during UBC advancement toward metastasis (e.g., T24; grade III).

Figure 4C describes the enzymatic reaction of aldo-keto reductase family 1 member B (AKR1B1), which is the enzyme that catalyzes the NADP-dependent conversion of propylene glycol to lactaldehyde in human (KEGG Reaction R02577, EC 1.1.1.21).

Table 1. The identified metabolites and the calculated fold change (×) during UBC progression, taking grade I (RT4) as the cell group of reference. A three-color gradient is applied, depending on the fold change (×) value. Red denotes the highest value(s). Gr: (malignancy) grade.

Metabolites	Gr II/Gr I	Gr III/Gr I	Gr IV/Gr I
Alanine	1.66	6.99	0.81
Aspartate	1.18	3.33	0.78
Glutamate	1.41	6.44	0.88
Glutathione	1.65	7.18	0.87
Glycine	1.33	5.71	0.32
Histidine	1.41	2.91	0.74
Isoleucine	1.96	5.62	0.86
Leucine	1.61	3.51	0.77
N-Acetylglutamine	1.14	10.17	0.99
Phenylalanine	1.82	5.92	0.86
Proline	1.5	4.77	0.75
Taurine	1.55	5.5	0.67
Threonine	1.42	5.38	0.74
Tryptophan	1.01	1.6	0.37
Tyrosine	1.77	6.25	0.88
Valine	1.79	4.81	0.74
β-Alanine	1.68	4.54	0.82
Acetate	1.56	4.17	2.78
Formate	1.13	1.28	0.68
Fumarate	1.65	3.34	0.92
Lactate	1.39	3.22	0.39
Malate	1.95	6.5	1.12
Succinate	1.79	4.65	0.51
Adenine	0.68	1.33	0.12
ADP	1.76	20.76	1.49
AMP	1.45	34.33	0.79
ATP	1.6	6.1	0.88
GTP	1.29	11.31	0.88
Hypoxanthine	2.41	1.81	0.21
NAD+	2.86	3.76	0.86
NADH	1.36	4.62	0.83
Oxypurinol	1.46	10.16	0.45
Uracil	1.36	0.72	0.23
UDPs	1.71	2.66	0.83
UDP-GlcNAc	2.43	3.25	0.75
UMP	1.82	7.77	0.82
Choline	2.96	2.44	0.19
Choline phosphate	1.27	6.26	0.37
Creatine	1.35	5.73	0.45
Creatine phosphate	1.51	22.99	0.66
Myo-inositol	2.89	12.06	0.37
Propylene glycol	1.34	0.38	0.29

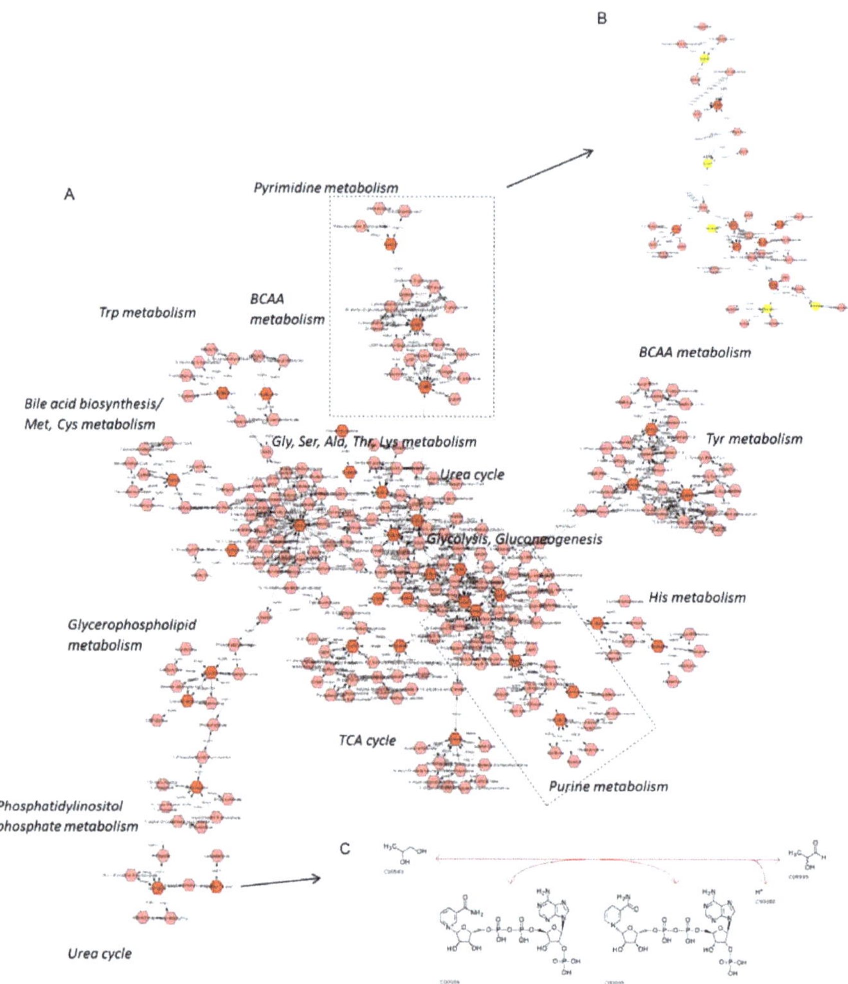

Figure 4. UBC metabolic network construction. (**A**) Hits (red) of the ^{1}H NMR metabolomic analysis inserted into Cytoscape and the related pathways assembled. Purine/pyrimidine metabolism seems to play a crucial role in UBC progression. (**B**) Hits of the purine/pyrimidine metabolism in grade III (T24) versus grade I (RT4) cell group comparison. Red: increased in grade III (T24), Yellow: decreased in grade III (T24). (**C**) Propylene glycol (or propane-1, 2-diol) has emerged as a novel, putative biomarker, with the EC 1.1.1.21 enzyme reaction for propylene glycol having been taken from KEGG.

2.2. MS Analysis

Representative LC-MS chromatograms of each one of the four UBC cell lines are shown in Supplementary Figure S3. PCA scores plots, before and after filtering of the features based on the % Relative Standard Deviation in Quality Control samples (QCs) and QC-based Signal-correction Method (QC-RLSC) correction (Supplementary Figure S4A,B, respectively), for instrument drift and signal attenuation, remarkably lead to more consistent clustering of QCs after normalization, therefore improving the repeatability and accuracy of the study.

In order to more deeply investigate for grade-specific variables among the four UBC cell groups that are able to uniquely reflect urothelial bladder-tumor pathologies (e.g., grade, stage, metastatic capacity, mutational load, and genetic heterogeneity), different multivariate approaches were employed, including the PLS-DA (SIMCA-P), KODAMA (R package), and Breiman's Random-Forest (BR-F) (StatTarget) tools. The results obtained from multivariate analyses were evaluated based on their multi-ROC (Receiver Operating Characteristic) values (calculated for every MS feature) and are summarized in Table 2, wherein the features with an Area Under Curve (AUC) > 0.9 and their respective ranking after employing the different methodologies are shown. Loadings and Kruskal–Wallis ranking are the different platforms used by the Knowledge Discovery by Accuracy Maximization Analysis (KODAMA) algorithm for variable selection. The results described in Table 2 strongly suggest that KODAMA loadings and BF-R classification exhibit better performance for the four-group UBC-member comparisons than the classical PLS-DA model. Figure 5 presents the scores plot constructed using the three models. It is observed that the obtained results are in accordance with the ones derived from NMR analysis, with the grade III (T24) UBC cell group showing the highest separation on the first principal component in all three methods used. Detailed results for testing each variable's importance using the different methodologies KODAMA, PLS-DA, and multi-ROC AUC are shown in Supplementary Table S2, while the first 50 ranked variables using BF-R are summarized in Supplementary Table S3.

Table 2. MS features with multi-ROC AUC > 0.9 and their ranking, based on different multivariate approaches. Knowledge Discovery by Accuracy Maximization Analysis (KODAMA) loadings and Breiman's Random-Forest (BF-R) classification exhibit better performance for the four-group UBC-member comparisons than the classical PLS-DA model.

Feature	Multi-ROC AUC	Variable Importance in Projection (VIP) (PLS-DA)	Loadings Ranking	Kruskal Ranking	Random Forest (RF) (p-Value)
993.7033_3.7	0.995	56	11	54	2
828.2532_3.71	0.982	77	6	58	5
129.1015_3.71	0.98	79	4	61	2
993.3025_3.7	0.973	66	5	53	6
348.7831_0.69	0.972	22	3	1	7
993.5029_3.7	0.972	58	13	66	11
828.0866_3.71	0.96	69	9	57	20
136.0611_3.3	0.955	1	66	11	8
827.9193_3.71	0.952	71	14	65	12
828.4207_3.71	0.95	74	7	33	9
696.5591_0.69	0.942	49	52	17	41
823.9269_3.79	0.938	55	12	24	16
824.0938_3.8	0.938	52	32	70	13
120.08_2.03	0.935	99	57	4	15
823.4258_3.79	0.932	51	2	3	16
823.5929_3.8	0.932	41	15	31	5
823.7596_3.8	0.928	53	23	25	18
380.7729_0.69	0.925	86	49	28	38
118.0643_2.01	0.922	39	37	16	28
988.1106_3.8	0.917	54	20	12	1
828.7551_3.7	0.913	67	10	69	18
622.646_0.68	0.912	65	16	8	34
350.7812_0.69	0.91	47	26	20	31
212.8509_0.69	0.908	19	38	36	30
828.5893_3.79	0.908	112	30	55	14
988.7121_3.78	0.907	62	17	47	26
330.7728_0.66	0.902	36	33	13	45
486.713_0.66	0.902	34	28	6	>50
827.7527_3.7	0.9	84	21	79	22

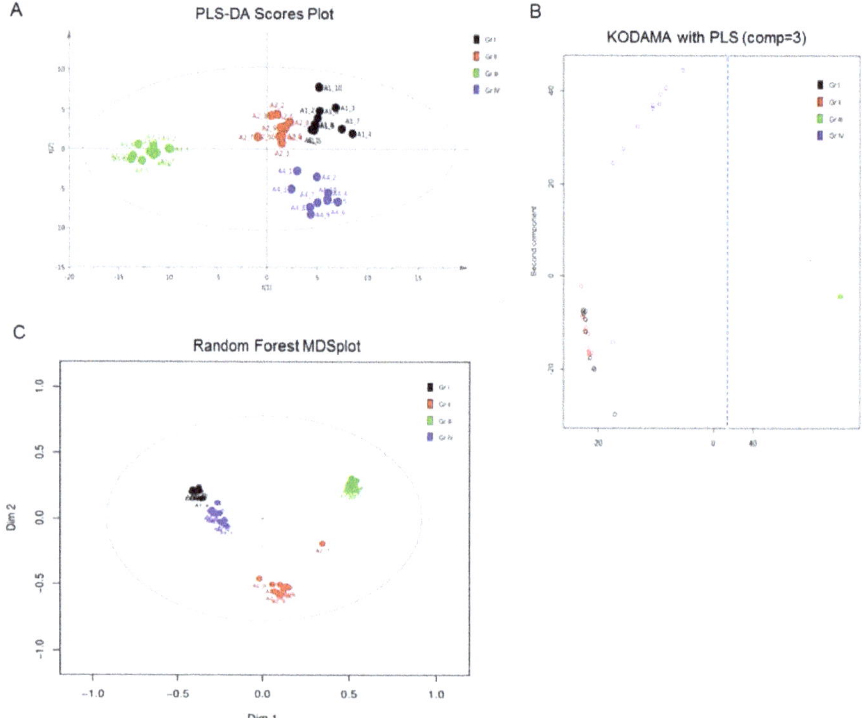

Figure 5. Comparison of the PLS-DA modeling of MS analysis, with KODAMA and Random Forest methods for the four UBC cell lines herein examined. All methods presented the greatest separation for the grade III (T24) group, highlighting T24 as the most suitable cell line to study the metabolic signature of highly malignant and strongly metastatic UBC disease. Black: grade I (RT4), Red: grade II (RT112), Green: grade III (T24), and Blue: grade IV (TCCSUP). (**A**) Principal Component (PC) scores plot from PLS-DA model. (**B**) PC scores plot from the KODAMA-PLS model. Figure is cut on the x-axis (dashed line), as grade III (T24) is far removed from the initial conditions. (**C**) Multidimensional Scaling (MDS) plot from the Random Forest model. Gr: (malignancy) grade.

Among the top ranked variables, peaks corresponding to two peptides have been herein identified, after deconvolution of multiple charged peaks and isotope clusters. Accordingly, for the first peptide, penta- (*m/z* 993.5027), exa- (*m/z* 828.0855), and epta- (*m/z* 709.9307) charged ions of *N*-Acetyl Thymosin $\beta4$ (T$\beta4$) were recognized, while the monoisotopic mass M + H = 4961.4792 was also obtained after deconvolution of the Electro-Spray Ionization (ESI) spectra. For the second peptide, Thymosin $\beta10$ (T$\beta10$), penta- (*m/z* 988.2166), exa- (*m/z* 823.5936), and epta- (*m/z* 705.7941) charged ions were identified, with the deconvoluted mass of 4934.5153 corresponding again to the *N*-Acetyl form of T$\beta10$ peptide. The previous identification of thymosin-type peptides [29] has revealed that the fragmentation of T$\beta4$ generates mainly fragments of the b series, while that of T$\beta10$ generates mainly fragments of the y series. The respective ions were searched in the MS/MS spectra of the penta- and exa-charged ions, using the peptide-fragmentation tool of mMass after noise filtering. The matched ions for T$\beta4$ and T$\beta10$ are described in Table 3.

Table 3. Matched ions of b series, with the MS/MS fragmentation profile of the penta- (*m/z* 993.5027) and exa- (*m/z* 828.0855) charged (acetylated) thymosin $\beta4$ (T$\beta4$), and matched ions of the y series, with the MS/MS fragmentation profile of the penta- (*m/z* 988.2166) and exa- (*m/z* 823.5936) charged (acetylated) thymosin $\beta10$ (T$\beta10$).

			Ions of b Series, (Acetylated) Thymosin $\beta4$ (T$\beta4$)		
m/z	Ion	z	Sequence	Error (Da)	Deconvoluted Mass
774.9006	b13	2	.SDKPDMAEIEKFD.k [1xAcetyl]	0.053	1547.696
946.616	b16	2	.SDKPDMAEIEKFDKSK.l [1xAcetyl]	0.157	1890.9178
1067.2304	b18	2	.SDKPDMAEIEKFDKSKLK.k [1xAcetyl]	0.182	2132.097
831.2934	b21	3	.SDKPDMAEIEKFDKSKLKKTE.t [1xAcetyl]	0.197	2490.2895
355.2822	b27	9	.SDKPDMAEIEKFDKSKLKKTETQEKNP.l [1xAcetyl]	0.096	3187.6722
850.3742	b29	4	.SDKPDMAEIEKFDKSKLKKTETQEKNPLP.s [1xAcetyl]	−0.069	3397.7732
936.3339	b32	4	.SDKPDMAEIEKFDKSKLKKTETQEKNPLPSKE.t [1xAcetyl]	−0.152	3741.9428
869.5772	b37	5	.SDKPDMAEIEKFDKSKLKKTETQEKNPLPSKETIEQE.k [1xAcetyl]	0.132	4342.2255
1086.6825	b37	4	.SDKPDMAEIEKFDKSKLKKTETQEKNPLPSKETIEQE.k [1xAcetyl]	0.128	4342.218
1164.2402	b40-NH$_3$	4	.SDKPDMAEIEKFDKSKLKKTETQEKNPLPSKETIEQEKQA.g [1xAcetyl]	0.145	4669.4134
788.6117	b41	6	.SDKPDMAEIEKFDKSKLKKTETQEKNPLPSKETIEQEKQAG.e [1xAcetyl]	−0.129	4726.4448
1182.801	b41	4	.SDKPDMAEIEKFDKSKLKKTETQEKNPLPSKETIEQEKQAG.e [1xAcetyl]	0.194	4726.4304
971.9887	b42	5	.SDKPDMAEIEKFDKSKLKKTETQEKNPLPSKETIEQEKQAGE.s [1xAcetyl]	−0.107	4855.48
			Ions of y Series, (Acetylated) Thymosin $\beta10$ (T$\beta10$)		
m/z	Ion	z	Sequence	Error (Da)	Deconvoluted Mass
839.5505	y14	2	p.TKETIEQEKRSEIS.	0.1142	1676.8726
592.5017	y15	3	l.PTKETIEwebQEKRSEIS.	0.1909	1773.9327
1775.0578	y15	1	l.PTKETIEQEKRSEIS.	0.1397	1790.9491
944.3809	y16	2	t.LPTKETIEQEKRSEIS.	−0.1239	1887.0094
663.8185	y17	3	n.TLPTKETIEQEKRSEIS.	0.1304	1988.0643
994.9422	y17	2	n.TLPTKETIEQEKRSEIS.	−0.0864	1988.0572
1052.2492	y18	2	k.NTLPTKETIEQEKRSEIS.	0.1992	2119.131
1244.6476	y21	2	t.QEKNTLPTKETIEQEKRSEIS.	−0.0005	2504.3272
863.8784	y22	3	e.TQEKNTLPTKETIEQEKRSEIS.	0.0947	2605.3821
1295.2735	y22	2	e.TQEKNTLPTKETIEQEKRSEIS.	0.1016	2605.3748
983.2832	y25	3	k.KTETQEKNTLPTKETIEQEKRSEIS.	0.1044	2946.5364
1130.0686	y29	3	k.AKLKKTETQEKNTLPTKETIEQEKRSEIS.	0.1194	3403.8786
1172.5977	y30	3	d.KAKLKKTETQEKNTLPTKETIEQEKRSEIS.	−0.0498	3531.9735
630.6308	y32	6	s.FDKAKLKKTETQEKNTLPTKETIEQEKRSEIS.	0.1209	3777.0594
756.3638	y32	5	s.FDKAKLKKTETQEKNTLPTKETIEQEKRSEIS.	−0.0466	3777.0525
945.1581	y32	4	s.FDKAKLKKTETQEKNTLPTKETIEQEKRSEIS.	−0.1031	3777.0452
810.8174	y35	5	e.IASFDKAKLKKTETQEKNTLPTKETIEQEKRSEIS.	0.1763	4048.2055
807.212	y35-NH$_3$	5	e.IASFDKAKLKKTETQEKNTLPTKETIEQEKRSEIS.	−0.0238	4048.21
1059.3714	y37	4	m.GEIASFDKAKLKKTETQEKNTLPTKETIEQEKRSEIS.	−0.1943	4251.2934
744.6523	y39-H$_2$O	6	p.DMGEIASFDKAKLKKTETQEKNTLPTKETIEQEKRSEIS.	−0.07	4480.3443
1116.7269	y39-H$_2$O	4	p.DMGEIASFDKAKLKKTETQEKNTLPTKETIEQEKRSEIS.	0.1471	4479.3502
916.6534	y40	5	k.PDMGEIASFDKAKLKKTETQEKNTLPTKETIEQEKRSEIS.	0.1754	4594.421
965.1255	y42	5	a.DKPDMGEIASFDKAKLKKTETQEKNTLPTKETIEQEKRSEIS.	0.0231	4837.5425
1206.0731	y42	4	a.DKPDMGEIASFDKAKLKKTETQEKNTLPTKETIEQEKRSEIS.	−0.053	4837.5354
801.7036	y42-NH3	6	a.DKPDMGEIASFDKAKLKKTETQEKNTLPTKETIEQEKRSEIS.	0.1215	4820.5236

Pairwise comparisons, using OPLS-DA models and univariate analysis, have also been performed. Hence, T24 (grade III) were compared to RT4 (grade I) that serve as reference cells. Figure 6 presents the pairwise comparison between the lower (I) and higher (III) UBC grade, using both multivariate and univariate approaches.

OPLS-DA analysis of these two UBC cell lines (RT4 and T24) was carried out to unveil important variables for their grade-specific and metabolic signature-dependent discrimination. In the OPLS-DA derived S-plot, features with the highest variation and reliability were selected. T$\beta4$ and T$\beta10$ were found to be strikingly elevated in the grade III (T24) UBC cell group. In the univariate analysis of the grade I (RT4) versus grade III (T24) UBC group, comparably similar results were obtained. T$\beta10$ peaks exhibit a $\log_2$ (FC) < -5, indicating a ca. 40-fold (x) increase in the grade III (T24) UBC cell group, while T$\beta4$ shows a $\log_2$ (FC) $= -3$, corresponding to a ca. 10-fold (x) increase for T24 cells, again.

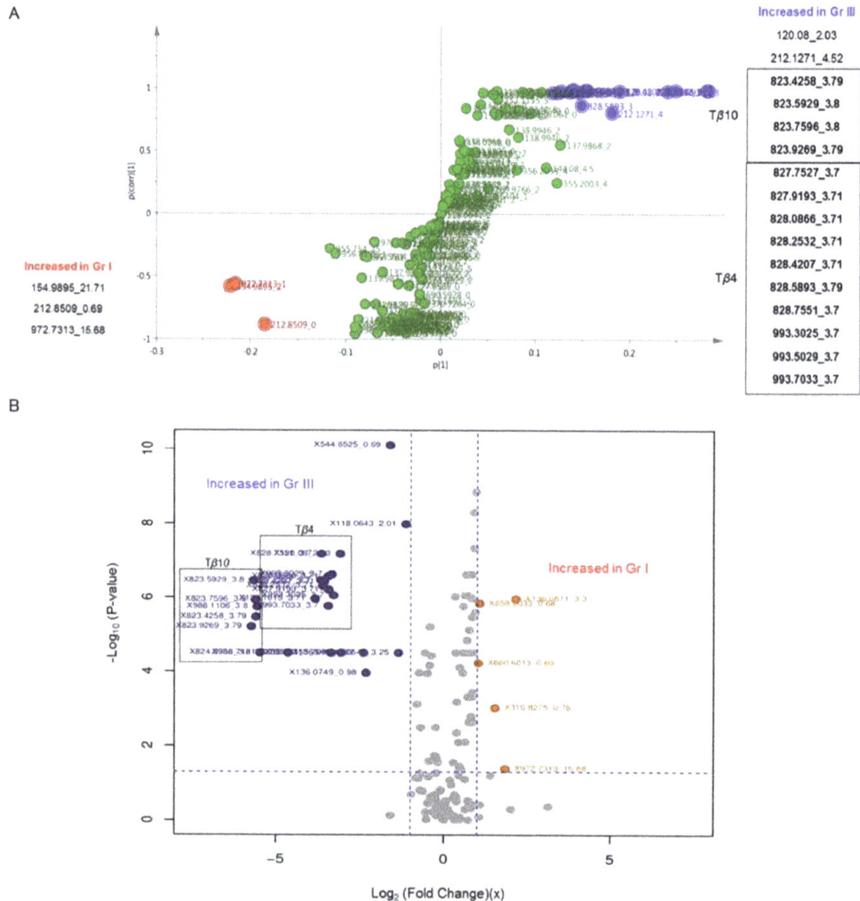

Figure 6. Comparison of the grade I (RT4) versus grade III (T24) cell groups and the significant MS analysis features. Tβ4 and Tβ10 charged peaks, and their respective isotopes, were found to be elevated in the grade III (T24) UBC cell group, using both univariate and multivariate approaches. Blue: increased in grade III (T24), Red: increased in grade I (RT4). (**A**) S-plot from OPLS-DA modeling multivariate approach. (**B**) Volcano plot of $\log_2$ [fold change (FC) (x)] versus *p*-values, and the selected variables with $p < 0.05$ and FC > 2, or < 0.5 (univariate approach). Gr: (malignancy) grade.

3. Discussion

Cancer research has considerably benefited from cultured-cell metabolomics, which offers a number of advantages, such as minor ethical issues, cost-efficiency merit, and low biological variation, as compared to human biofluids [30,31]. In vitro metabolomics approaches facilitate the more integrated, systemic, and reliable experimental design, and, most importantly, the successful investigation of metabolic alterations that are directly and/or mechanistically linked to the tumorigenic process, and these may not be captured by blood and/or urine classical biochemical examination. However, there are still some challenges to cope with, such as the fast quenching of metabolism and data normalization [32,33]. To successfully encounter these challenges, we have chosen a grade-specific unique collection of UBC human cell lines that are able to largely maintain and thus mimic the pathology of the disease, including both its clinical features and molecular subtypes. Immediate freezing of UBC cultured cells ensured metabolism's fast quenching equally for all the four cell lines examined, with RT4 (grade I) serving as the line of reference (control), due to its lowest malignancy grade among all. Data statistical processing, via the engagement of advanced algorithmic platforms, unearthed the major biological importance of our results to UBC progression toward tissue metastasis and refractory responses to chemotherapies.

To our knowledge, this is the first time all major UBC malignancy-grade cell types, I, II, III, and IV, with different mutational loads and metastatic proficiencies, are being metabolically fingerprinted, combining both NMR and LC-MS state-of-the-art technologies. Powerful and multifaceted statistical processing of the metabolic data ensures their biological validity and highlights the role of metabolomics pathways in UBC progression toward metastasis in vivo. Remarkably, each grade-specific UBC cell line has proved to carry its own unique metabolic signature that diagnostically, mechanistically, and therapeutically typifies each distinct tumorigenic phenotype examined. The question is whether the grade-dependent metabolome governs UBC pathology and aggressiveness, or, vice versa, the advancement to metastatic state(s) compels the acquisition of metabolic aberrations and the generation of derailed UBC metabolomes. It must be the grade-specific molecular signature of each UBC cell type that defines its unique metabolic landscape. However, the four cell lines herein examined carry different mutational profiles, with some mutations being likely unrelated (due to their generation stochasticity) to UBC aggressiveness. Hence, the possibility that these (non-causative for tumor features) mutations could be linked to some of the observed metabolic alterations cannot be excluded. Nevertheless, the major mutation contents of the cell lines used are indeed grade dependent, and they can be classified according to the UBC grade, metastatic capacity, and general disease pathology. In any case, the high grade-specific oncometabolomes (e.g., of T24) seem to contain a number of critical metabolites that can serve as novel and powerful biomarkers for both the diagnosis and drug-mediated clinical management of UBC disease.

In this study, a four-cell-line group of a human UBC model has been in vitro engaged to thoroughly investigate the metabolic alterations that tumor cells likely undergo during UBC advancement, thus highlighting the importance of a malignancy grade, mutational signature, de-differentiation state and metastatic activity to "diagnostic biomarkering" and "targeted therapeutic drugging" of the disease. The four human UBC cell lines that have been analyzed critically reflect the distinct de-differentiation state and malignancy grade (I–IV) of UBC in vivo. Our results clearly indicate that T24 (grade III) can serve as a powerful, informative, and versatile cell-line system that can be successfully exploited to illuminate the role of metabolic reprogramming in UBC progression toward metastasis. It seems that the elevated contents of most metabolites specifically identified in T24 are tightly associated with the highly oncogenic character of the cells. Notably, PCA analysis showed that the grade III-specific T24-cell group exhibits the clearest separation on the first principal component, both in NMR and MS analysis, thus explaining the maximal amount of variation for its discrimination among the four cell groups. These results are strongly supported by biological data interpretations, since T24 cells bear a heavy mutational load and strong tumorigenic capacity. They are characterized by the mutant, oncogenic, form H-RAS^{G12V} and the disruption of stress-induced activation of mutant p53 ($\Delta\Upsilon^{126}$) protein [34]. Hence, the aberrant signaling activity of H-RAS^{G12V}, in a cellular environment that lacks the genome-protecting properties of p53, may render T24 cells susceptible to severe metabolic reprogramming, with grade III-specific metabolites fostering and promoting highly tumorigenic features and pathologies, including genetic instability, clonal heterogeneity, chemoresistance, immune escape, and organ metastasis (tissue invasion). Interestingly, a role of *H-RAS*^{G12V} oncogene (*RAS*) in metabolic reprogramming during early mammary carcinogenesis has been previously reported, with the MCF10A-*RAS* transfected human breast epithelial cells exhibiting enhanced glycolytic activity and lactate production [35], consistently with the cancer hallmark of the classic "Warburg effect" [36,37]. Comparative genomics evidence that indicates that the T24 cell line (https://depmap.org/portal/cell_line/ACH-000018?tab=mutation) reliably reflects the mutational profile of muscle-invasive bladder cancer patients (https://www.cbioportal.org; Bladder Cancer, TCGA Cell 2017, 413 Total Samples) supports and increases the utilization of T24 as a valid, pre-clinical, cell-model system for advanced bladder cancer research in diagnosis and therapy. Remarkably, besides the *H-RAS* and *TP53* (encodes p53) mutated oncogenes, T24 cells share with muscle-invasive UBC patients multiple genes carrying molecular alterations, including (among others) the *KDM6A*, *MAGEF1*, *DIDO1*, and *EP300* ones, with 37%, 31%, 30% and 30% of detection frequency, respectively, in the UBC patient cohort studied (Supplementary Table S4).

Among all UBC–cell pairs, embracing different grades being compared [e.g., II versus I, III versus I, and IV versus I; I (RT4) herein serves as the cell line of reference], only the grade III (T24) versus grade I (RT4) proved to significantly differ in the majority of metabolite contents examined, thus indicating the major role of the T24-specific mutational signature (including H-RAS^{G12V} and p53$^{\Delta Y126}$) in metabolome composition and its oncogenic proficiency. The surprising resemblance between grade I (RT4) and grade IV (TCCSUP) metabolic profiles strongly suggests the engagement of a "metabolic inversion" process that likely favors late-metastasis cells to successfully encounter energetic challenges, nutritional demands, and oxygen deprivations. It is possible that a pre-metastatic UBC cell, after it becomes metastatic and invades other (proximal or/and distal) tissues/organs, will undergo a dramatic metabolic reprogramming to suppress its ability for a second metastasis event. If so, it may always be the primary tumor mass that feeds metastasis, with a metastatic-cell clonal population likely colonizing tissues outside the urinary bladder only once. In accordance, cell dissemination seems to occur during the early stages of tumor evolution, with cells from early and low-density lesions displaying more "stemness" features, migrating more and founding more metastases than cells derived from dense and advanced tumors [38–40].

The majority of previous UBC metabolomics reports have underlined the importance of amino acids to urothelium oncometabolome, with most amino acid levels being upregulated compared to controls; similar differential patterns were described for advanced UBC stage(s) compared to early stage(s). Interestingly, increased contents of glutathione were found in UBC cell lines, while glycine was elevated in the tumorigenic cells as well [21,22]. Alanine was also increased in the TCCSUP (high-grade) cell line compared to the RT4 (low grade) one [28]. An abundance of amino acids is important for the proliferative cancer cells, not only as substrates of protein synthesis, but also for energy generation, cellular redox homeostasis, and nucleotide biosynthesis [41]. Pyruvate consumption and alterations in glycolytic profile have also been related to UBC aggressiveness, as anaerobic conditions in high(er) grade UBC favor the conversion of pyruvate to lactate, or alanine [28]. In our study, and in accordance with previous results, T24 (grade III) exhibited elevated contents of totally 17 amino acids and derivatives, with the highest increase being detected for N-acetylglutamine, glutathione, alanine, and glutamate, together with a 3x increase of lactate. Nucleotides are also involved in biomass build-up observed in cancer cells and in the changes of ATP concentrations that indicate the energetic status (usually crisis) of tumors [42]. In serum samples of UBC patients, the raised levels of hypoxanthine and reduced levels of uracil indicated a perturbed breakdown of purine nucleotides, favoring the purine synthesis pathway (reviewed in ref. [17]). Notably, herein, purine metabolism has emerged as one of the most important networks in our *in silico* analysis (Figure 4), thus highlighting its major contribution to UBC aggressiveness and progression toward metastasis. Increased contents of hypoxanthine and adenosine nucleotides (AMP/ADP/ATP), with up to a 34x striking increase for AMP, were observed in T24 (grade III), but they were surprisingly restored (again) to the initial (RT4-like) levels in TCCSUP (grade IV) cells. In a study of urine samples derived from UBC patients, it has been suggested that the high(er) levels of choline phosphate may reflect increased lipid membrane remodeling, which has also been reported for other cancers [24,42]. Choline phosphate and, to lower extent, choline contents were also increased in our T24 (grade III) cell-line group, with a 6x and 2x rise, respectively. As expected, the elevated contents of these metabolites were reduced in TCCSUP (grade IV) cells, indicating the activation of a "metabolic inversion" effect. Regarding the two major metabolites involved in osmoregulation and volume regulation, taurine and myo-inositol, contradictory results were previously reported, with either upregulated or downregulated levels detected (reviewed in ref. [17,42]), likely implicating the role of cellular micro-environments in metabolome compositions. Interestingly, herein, significantly elevated contents of myo-inositol (12x) and taurine (5x) were observed in T24 (grade III), indicating the high grade-dependent ability of UBC to regulate osmosis and volume, in favor of promoting cell motility and tumor metastasis.

Taking into account that the majority of the identified metabolites (40 out of 42) were increased in the grade III (T24) group, multivariate analysis and the use of pairwise ratios were employed in order to highlight metabolites with major alterations. Notably, multivariate analysis of the obtained NMR data indicated the importance of, among others, glutamate and myo-inositol level deregulations to UBC pathology, while AXPs (AMP, ADP and ATP), GTP, oxypurinol, and creatine phosphate content increases were presented with the strongest statistical significance in the grade III/I cell pair (III/I). The use of pairwise ratios allowed us to account for dilution and signal instability effects and to unveil alterations that are masked by the "metabolic inversion" phenomenon. Increased ratios were found in III/I for metabolites that were also profiled with a "metabolic inversion" effect in IV/I (e.g., AMP, oxypurinol, myo-inositol, and creatine phosphate); thus, they might critically contribute to UBC advancement. On the other hand, decreased ratios were observed in III/I for several metabolites that were also presented with downregulated proportions in IV/I (e.g., uracil and propylene glycol) and, as such, they could presumably function as UBC-specific "oncosuppressing" modulators/inducers. Further discussion will focus on those metabolites that were herein identified as the most important by both (NMR and LC-MS) applied technologies, and especially the ones with the highest fold change (x) in metabolite levels and the highest alterations in all pairwise metabolic ratios.

Regarding the top two metabolites with the highest elevation contents in grade III (T24) versus grade I (RT4) UBC cells, creatine phosphate and AMP, they were remarkably presented with 23x and 34x positive change (upregulation), respectively (Table 1). Strikingly, by taking uracil as the metabolite of reference (since it was downregulated both in III/I and IV/I cell pairs), their respective fold changes (x) were further increased up to 32x and 50x values (Supplementary Table S5). Since colon cancer-derived liver metastases carry higher creatine kinase brain type (CKB) levels compared to primary tumors [43,44], UBC metastatic populations, in order to overcome hypoxia and other metabolic stresses, may also upregulate CKB expression or/and activity. This allows (after CKB secretion) energy to be likely captured from the extracellular ATP-mediated generation of creatine phosphate and its subsequent SLC6A8-dependent import into metastatic cells to regenerate ATP. Similarly to colon cancer cells [45], hypoxic UBC cells, in the absence of functional Hypoxia-Inducible Factor 1-alpha (HIF1α) (a key regulator of hypoxia response) pathway, could adapt their energy metabolism via the upregulation of creatine metabolism (and synthesis), thus opening a new chemotherapeutic window for metastatic UBC targeting and management in the clinic. Most importantly, T24 (grade III) cells contain a mutant version of the EP300 (KAT3B/p300) transcriptional co-activator (Supplementary Table S4) (https://depmap.org/portal/cell_line/ACH-000018?tab=mutation), which, in its wild-type form, is required for the transcriptional activation of HIF1α-target genes [46]. This indicates their competence to survive and grow in adverse hypoxic environments through the engagement of HIF1α-independent, but likely creatine-dependent, metabolic pathways. Given that the calculated fold change (x) in the III/I pair for ADP is 20.76x, which is a value close to the 22.99x of creatine phosphate (Table 1) (an approximately 1:1 molecular stoichiometry), T24 (grade III) cells may utilize intracellular creatine phosphate as a phosphate donor to the available ADP to finally produce ATP.

The remarkably elevated content of AMP in T24 (grade III) versus RT4 (grade I) cells indicates its major value for UBC progression toward chemoresistance and metastasis. High levels of ADP and AMP in a cell undergoing energetic stress/crisis cause significant increase in the AMPK kinase activity [47]. Activated AMPK phosphorylates a number of target substrates to regulate cell growth, metabolism, and autophagy [48]. Interestingly, activated H-RAS (G12V) requires autophagy for the maintenance of tumorigenesis [49]. Therefore, it seems that the major AMP/ADP/ATP (AXPs) metabolic reprogramming specifically observed in grade III (T24) cells may be tightly related to the aberrant signaling of the H-RAS^{G12V} mutant oncoprotein. If so, H-RAS^{G12V}–AMP/ADP–AMPK–autophagy must operate as an indispensable axis for UBC cell survival and growth in unfavorable and adverse (e.g., hypoxic or nutritionally deprived) environments. Since we have previously shown that T24 cells are characterized by constitutively activated basal autophagy [34], the H-RAS^{G12V}-induced intracellular energetic stress, in the form of AMP (and ADP) highly upregulated levels (this study), serves as a valuable and powerful metabolic biomarker, with its implicated enzymes/regulators likely opening a new therapeutic window for UBC metastasis and drug tolerance.

Intriguingly, propylene glycol and uracil herein emerged as metabolites that were downregulated in both III/I and IV/I grade cell pairs. Especially for propylene glycol, a prominent reduction in its intracellular contents was observed for both T24 (grade III) and TCCSUP (grade IV) compared to RT4 (grade I) cells of reference. Propylene glycol is produced by the conversion of pyruvaldehyde to lactaldehyde, which is then converted to propylene glycol via the aldehyde reductase mediation. Aldo-keto reductases family 1 members A1 and B1 (AKR1A1 and AKR1B1) are part of the Aldo-keto reductase superfamily and catalyze the reduction of several aldehydes. Data derived from the TCGA (The Cancer Genome Atlas) platform (https://www.cbioportal.org) strengthen our interpretation for perturbed (compromised) aldehyde reductase activities in advanced metastatic UBC disease, with 16% and 7% of the examined muscle-invasive UBC patients (Bladder Cancer, Cell 2017, z: 1.5) exhibiting deregulated expression/activity of the AKR1A1 and AKR1B1 enzymes, respectively, and 2.67% of them bearing low mRNA levels of the *AKR1A1* gene (https://www.cbioportal.org). Thereby, it seems that T24 may have originated from a patient with a molecular signature of downregulated *AKR1A1* gene expression in the tumor cells.

A major advantage (and novelty) of the present study is the employment of two complementary, state-of-the-art, analytical platforms: Nuclear Magnetic Resonance (NMR) and Mass Spectrometry (MS). Their successful combination offers a comprehensive metabolic characterization that covers a variety of chemical structures and concentrations of profiled metabolites. Strikingly, application of the MS-based metabolomics technology led to the detection and identification of novel molecules that could significantly contribute to UBC progression toward metastasis. Two peptides, Tβ4 and Tβ10, were identified with a high confidence level, and proved to be statistically significant both in the discrimination of the four (I, II, III, and IV) groups and of the low(er) or high(er) malignancy grade pairwise comparisons. Members of the β thymosin family form a (1:1) complex with the monomeric G-Actin protein, acting as its sequestration peptides, thus critically controlling actin cytoskeleton dynamics [50]. Furthermore, in contrast to Tβ4, Tβ10 can also directly bind to RAS, inhibiting its signaling activity, in an endothelial cell environment [51]. Nevertheless, in a T24-specific cellular setting, Tβ10 could no longer interact with the mutant H-RAS^{G12V} form, thus presumably releasing its aberrant signaling function(s) to drive the oncogenic and metastatic phenotypes of grade III UBC cells. Hence, the strikingly elevated contents of Tβ4 (10x) and Tβ10 (40x) in T24 (grade III) compared to RT4 (grade I; reference) cell line strongly suggest their actin cytoskeleton remodeling-dependent role in UBC advancement to metastasis, with oncogenic H-RAS^{G12V} (after its presumable release from Tβ10) also orchestrating UBC aggressiveness and drug/radiation resistance. Accordingly, Tβ10 overexpression correlates with the poor prognosis and progression of UBC disease [52], while Tβ4 expression is associated with clinical outcomes and clinicopathological parameters of UBC patients (it is significantly increased in UBC patients versus normal (control) volunteers) [53]. Most importantly, TCGA-derived data unveiled 6% of muscle-invasive UBC cases (bladder cancer, "amplification" and "mRNA high", Cell 2017, z: 1.5) to be carrying upregulated levels of *TMSB10* gene (encodes Tβ10) expression (https://www.cbioportal.org), thus indicating the in vivo importance of Tβ10 (and Tβ4) to UBC progression toward high-malignancy grades and aggressive metastatic stages that are characterized by resistance to (chemo/radio)therapy, shorter survival of patients, and, generally, poor prognosis.

4. Materials and Methods

4.1. Chemicals and Reagents

The detailed information for chemicals and reagents is listed in Supplementary Materials.

4.2. Cell Lines and Culture Conditions

The UBC human cell lines RT4, RT112, T24, and TCCSUP were used in the present study. RT4 was obtained from ECACC-Sigma-Aldrich (Munich, Germany). RT112 was kindly provided by Professor J.R. Masters (London, England, UK). T24 and TCCSUP were purchased from ATCC-LGC Standards GmbH (Wesel, Germany). All cell lines were derived from urothelial cell carcinomas of human urinary bladder, with RT4 being classified as malignancy grade I, RT112 as grade I–II (II), T24 as grade III, and TCCSUP as grade IV. All four UBC cell lines were authenticated mainly using in-house established technologies. Cell authentication was based on several combinational criteria, such as the cell-specific morphology, growth rate, nutritional requirement, mitotic index, immunofluorescence pattern (e.g., Epithelial–Mesenchymal Transition (EMT) phenotype), mutational load (e.g., *H-RAS* and *TP53*), signaling activity (e.g., Akt and p44/42 MAPK {ERK1/2}), protein content, gene-expression profiling, drug response, motility (e.g., wound-healing assay) and tumorigenicity (e.g., xenograft in Severe Combined ImmunoDeficient (SCID) mouse). All four UBC human cell lines were being tested periodically, but, most importantly, they were thoroughly examined just before the commencement of their large-scale growth for the herein implemented metabolomics analysis. The detailed culture conditions are described in the Supplementary Materials.

4.3. Cell Collection and Storage

The analytical protocols of cell collection and storage are described in the Supplementary Materials.

4.4. Metabolomics Experiments

The detailed protocols of metabolomics experiments (e.g., metabolite extraction, sample preparation, NMR, and MS analysis) are described in the Supplementary Materials.

4.5. Data Preprocessing

The binning of NMR spectra was conducted (0.001/0.02 ppm) using the AMIX software. Regions of water and contaminations being observed at the blank solutions were removed from the analysis. Pairwise ratios of the metabolites identified in NMR analysis were also calculated ($42 \times 42 = 1.764$ metabolic traits). In MS analysis, data preprocessing was performed using the XCMS online. Peak-based normalization was applied in order to correct data within the batch experiment. Specifically, a QC-based signal-correction method (QC-RLSC), engaging the non-linear local polynomial regression (LOESS), was performed using the MetaX R package [54]. KNN (*K*-Nearest Neighbor) imputation for missing values and filtering of features based on the % Relative Standard Deviation (RSD) in QCs were applied.

4.6. Metabolite/Pathway Identification

The Chenomx NMR suite (Chenomx Inc., Alberta, Canada) was utilized for the NMR-mediated metabolite identification. For the recognition of peptides, the mMass peptide tool v. 5.5.0 was suitably employed [55]. The Cytoscape platform was engaged for visualizing molecular networks of significant metabolites derived from the NMR analysis [56,57].

4.7. Statistical Analysis

Principal Component Analysis (PCA), Partial Least Square-Discriminant Analysis (PLS-DA), and Orthogonal Partial Least Square-Discriminant Analysis (OPLS-DA), using SIMCA-P 14.0 (Umetrics, Umea, Sweden), were suitably applied. The quality of obtained models was assessed via R2X (variance explained by X Matrix) and Q2 (Goodness of prediction) obtained by 7x cross-validation, parameters, and permutation test results (100 random permutations for the PLS-DA and OPLS-DA models). The Knowledge Discovery by Accuracy Maximization Analysis (KODAMA) R package [58] was performed for the unsupervised extraction of variables in the MS analysis. The selected classifier was PLS-DA, and the procedure was repeated 100 times. Two methods implemented in the same package were used for the ranking of variables' importance; Kruskal–Wallis test and the model's loadings. Breiman's Random-Forest (BR-F) algorithm was also evaluated using the StatTarget tool [59]. A number of 500 grown trees and 20 permutations were imported as model parameters. Multi-ROC AUC was used for the evaluation of methods performance using the multi-ROC R package [60].

5. Conclusions

In the present study, the metabolic landscapes of grade I, II, III, and IV UBC human cell lines were extensively mapped. Obtained results indicated a prominently perturbed amino acid and purine/pyrimidine metabolism with a remarkable increase of most metabolites being identified in grade III (T24) UBC cells, using RT4 (grade I) as the line of reference. Surprisingly, insignificant changes were observed for grade IV (TCCSUP) cells, thus implying the activation of a "metabolic inversion" process. T24 (grade III) has proved the most powerful and versatile cell line, which is able to accurately and reliably unveil the metabolic signature of highly malignant and strongly metastatic UBC pathology. "Metabolic inversion" has to be mechanistically investigated, in order to open new chemotherapeutic windows for UBC advancement to drug-resistant metastasis. Analysis of NMR-derived metabolite contents and ratios showed significant perturbations in purine and pyrimidine metabolism, while MS analysis demonstrated the importance of Tβ4 and Tβ10 peptides to UBC progression toward metastasis. AMP (and ADP) highly upregulated levels indicate the H-RAS^{G12V}-induced intracellular energetic stress/crisis, and they can serve as valuable metabolic biomarkers, while the remarkably elevated contents of Tβ4 and Tβ10 in the T24 (grade III) compared to RT4 (grade I) cell line strongly suggest their actin cytoskeleton remodeling-dependent role in UBC advancement to metastasis and drug tolerance. Furthermore, decreased levels of propylene glycol are indicative of dysregulated *AKR1A1* gene expression in the tumor cells of urinary bladder, thus rendering it (propylene glycol) as a potentially significant biomarker.

Our work also made use of novel statistical approaches for metabolomics data analysis. Metabolic ratios are strongly suggested to account for the size effect present in the data and to highlight novel metabolic pathways. Hence, their combined employment and biological interpretation are crucial in order to avoid erroneous results. A common bottleneck in the untargeted MS analysis is the selection of important variables. We herein compared the typical PLS-DA method used in metabolomics analyses with other statistical tools carrying different merits and drawbacks (e.g., KODAMA and BF-R). Our results underline the importance of either pairwise comparisons or the implementation of more sophisticated multivariate approaches, such as the Random Forest models, which may exhibit better performances.

Most importantly, the integration of high-resolution metabolic maps with high-scale proteomic profiles containing enzymes/regulators that are able to control the homeostasis of grade-dependent UBC intracellular metabolites will shed light on mechanisms of urothelial bladder tumorigenesis, and they will benefit our tools in terms of the safe, efficient, and generally successful (including reduced medical costs) diagnostic and therapeutic management of the advanced UBC disease in the clinic.

Supplementary Materials: Supplementary materials can be found at http://www.mdpi.com/1422-0067/21/5/1892/s1. References [61,62] are cited in the Supplementary Materials.

Author Contributions: Conceptualization, D.J.S.; methodology, A.I., A.P., A.F.G., D.B., E.G., E.M. and D.J.S.; software, A.I., A.P., D.B., M.K., E.G. and E.M.; validation, A.I., A.P., A.F.G., D.B., M.K., A.D.V., O.E.T., I.S.P., G.E.V., E.G.K., E.G., E.M. and D.J.S.; resources, E.M. and D.J.S.; writing—original draft preparation, A.I., E.G., E.M. and D.J.S.; writing—review and editing, E.M. and D.J.S.; supervision, D.B., E.M. and D.J.S.; project administration, D.B., E.G., E.M. and D.J.S.; funding acquisition, A.I., E.M. and D.J.S. All authors have read and agreed to the published version of the manuscript.

Funding: Financial support was kindly provided by the: (a) "European Social Fund UoA-MIS 375784" (European Union and Greek National Funds 2012–2015/"THALIS" Program) and (b) "Bodossaki Foundation Donation Program" 2013–2014, Athens, Greece (GR), to Dimitrios J. Stravopodis (DJS). The work herein presented was carried out within the framework of a Stavros Niarchos Foundation (SNF) grant to Aikaterini Iliou (AI) at the National and Kapodistrian University of Athens (NKUA), Athens, Greece (GR).

Acknowledgments: Dimitrios J. Stravopodis (DJS) at NKUA devotes the present article to the memory of his beloved mother who suddenly passed away in October 2015.

Conflicts of Interest: The authors declare no conflict of interest.

Abbreviations

AKR1A1/AKR1B1	Aldo-keto Reductases Family 1 Member(s) A1/B1
AUC-ROC	Area Under the Receiver Operating Characteristic Curve
BR-F	Breiman's Random-Forest
KEGG	Kyoto Encyclopedia of Genes and Genomes
KODAMA	Knowledge Discovery by Accuracy Maximization Analysis
OPLS-DA	Orthogonal Partial Least Squares-Discriminant Analysis
PCA	Principal Component Analysis
PLS-DA	Partial Least Squares-Discriminant Analysis
QC-RLSC	QC-based Signal-correction Method
QCs	Quality Control Samples
UBC	Urothelial Bladder Cancer
VIP	Variable Importance in Projection

References

1. Burger, M.; Catto, J.W.; Dalbagni, G.; Grossman, H.B.; Herr, H.; Karakiewicz, P.; Kassouf, W.; Kiemeney, L.A.; La Vecchia, C.; Shariat, S.; et al. Epidemiology and risk factors of urothelial bladder cancer. *Eur. Urol.* **2013**, *63*, 234–241. [CrossRef]

2. Huang, Z.; Lin, L.; Gao, Y.; Chen, Y.; Yan, X.; Xing, J.; Hang, W. Bladder cancer determination via two urinary metabolites: A biomarker pattern approach. *Mol. Cell. Proteom.* **2011**, *10*. [CrossRef] [PubMed]

3. Montironi, R.; Cheng, L.; Scarpelli, M.; Lopez-Beltran, A. Pathology and genetics: Tumours of the urinary system and male genital system: Clinical implications of the 4th edition of the who classification and beyond. *Eur. Urol.* **2016**, *70*, 120–123. [CrossRef] [PubMed]

4. Hurle, R.; Losa, A.; Manzetti, A.; Lembo, A. Upper urinary tract tumors developing after treatment of superficial bladder cancer: 7-year follow-up of 591 consecutive patients. *Urology* **1999**, *53*, 1144–1148. [CrossRef]

5. Hansen, R.P.; Vedsted, P.; Sokolowski, I.; Søndergaard, J.; Olesen, F. Time intervals from first symptom to treatment of cancer: A cohort study of 2,212 newly diagnosed cancer patients. *BMC Health Serv. Res.* **2011**, *11*, 284. [CrossRef] [PubMed]

6. James, A.C.; Gore, J.L. The costs of non-muscle invasive bladder cancer. *Urol. Clin. N. Am.* **2013**, *40*, 261–269. [CrossRef]

7. Vlachostergios, P.J.; Faltas, B.M. Treatment resistance in urothelial carcinoma: An evolutionary perspective. *Nat. Rev. Clin. Oncol.* **2018**, *15*, 495–509. [CrossRef] [PubMed]

8. Giannopoulou, A.F.; Velentzas, A.D.; Konstantakou, E.G.; Avgeris, M.; Katarachia, S.A.; Papandreou, N.; Kalavros, N.; Mpakou, V.E.; Iconomidou, V.A.; Anastasiadou, E.; et al. Revisiting histone deacetylases in human tumorigenesis: The paradigm of urothelial bladder cancer. *Int. J. Mol. Sci.* **2019**, *20*, 1291. [CrossRef]

9. Nicholson, J.K.; Lindon, J.C.; Holmes, E. Metabonomics: Understanding the metabolic responses of living systems to pathophysiological stimuli via multivariate statistical analysis of biological nmr spectroscopic data. *Xenobiotica* **1999**, *29*, 1181–1189. [CrossRef]

10. Locasale, J.W.; Cantley, L.C.; Heiden, M.G.V. Cancer's insatiable appetite. *Nat. Biotechnol.* **2009**, *27*, 916–917. [CrossRef]

11. Hanahan, D.; Weinberg, R.A. Hallmarks of cancer: The next generation. *Cell* **2011**, *144*, 646–674. [CrossRef] [PubMed]

12. Aboud, O.A.; Weiss, R.H. New opportunities from the cancer metabolome. *Clin. Chem.* **2013**, *59*, 138–146. [CrossRef] [PubMed]

13. DeBerardinis, R.J.; Chandel, N.S. Fundamentals of cancer metabolism. *Sci. Adv.* **2016**, *2*, e1600200. [CrossRef] [PubMed]

14. Boroughs, L.K.; DeBerardinis, R.J. Metabolic pathways promoting cancer cell survival and growth. *Nat. Cell Biol.* **2015**, *17*, 351–359. [CrossRef] [PubMed]

15. Sahu, D.; Lotan, Y.; Wittmann, B.; Neri, B.; Hansel, D.E. Metabolomics analysis reveals distinct profiles of nonmuscle-invasive and muscle-invasive bladder cancer. *Cancer Med.* **2017**, *6*, 2106–2120. [CrossRef] [PubMed]

16. Denkert, C.; Budczies, J.; Kind, T.; Weichert, W.; Tablack, P.; Sehouli, J.; Darb-Esfahani, S.; Könsgen, D.; Dietel, M.; Fiehn, O. Mass spectrometry-based metabolic profiling reveals different metabolite patterns in invasive ovarian carcinomas and ovarian borderline tumors. *Cancer Res.* **2006**, *66*, 10795–10804. [CrossRef]

17. Rodrigues, D.; Jerónimo, C.; Henrique, R.; Belo, L.; Bastos, M.D.L.; De Pinho, P.G.; Carvalho, M. Biomarkers in bladder cancer: A metabolomic approach using in vitro and ex vivo model systems. *Int. J. Cancer* **2016**, *139*, 256–268. [CrossRef]

18. Catchpole, G.; Platzer, A.; Weikert, C.; Kempkensteffen, C.; Johannsen, M.; Krause, H.; Jung, K.; Miller, K.; Willmitzer, L.; Selbig, J.; et al. Metabolic profiling reveals key metabolic features of renal cell carcinoma. *J. Cell. Mol. Med.* **2011**, *15*, 109–118. [CrossRef]

19. Cheng, Y.; Xie, G.; Chen, T.; Qiu, Y.; Zou, X.; Zheng, M.; Tan, B.; Feng, B.; Dong, T.; He, P.; et al. Distinct urinary metabolic profile of human colorectal cancer. *J. Proteom. Res.* **2012**, *11*, 1354–1363. [CrossRef]

20. Huang, Q.; Tan, Y.; Yin, P.; Ye, G.; Gao, P.; Lu, X.; Wang, H.; Xu, G. Metabolic characterization of hepatocellular carcinoma using nontargeted tissue metabolomics. *Cancer Res.* **2013**, *73*, 4992–5002. [CrossRef]

21. Pendyala, L.; Velagapudi, S.; Toth, K.; Zdanowicz, J.; Glaves, D.; Slocum, H.; Perez, R.; Huben, R.; Creaven, P.J.; Raghavan, D. Translational studies of glutathione in bladder cancer cell lines and human specimens. *Clin. Cancer Res.* **1997**, *3*, 793–798.

22. Pasikanti, K.K.; Norasmara, J.; Cai, S.; Mahendran, R.; Esuvaranathan, K.; Ho, P.C.; Chan, E.C.Y. Metabolic footprinting of tumorigenic and nontumorigenic uroepithelial cells using two-dimensional gas chromatography time-of-flight mass spectrometry. *Anal. Bioanal. Chem.* **2010**, *398*, 1285–1293. [CrossRef] [PubMed]

23. Bansal, N.; Gupta, A.; Mitash, N.; Shakya, P.S.; Mandhani, A.; Mahdi, A.A.; Sankhwar, S.N.; Mandal, S.K. Low- and high-grade bladder cancer determination via human serum-based metabolomics approach. *J. Proteom. Res.* **2013**, *12*, 5839–5850. [CrossRef] [PubMed]

24. Wittmann, B.M.; Stirdivant, S.M.; Mitchell, M.; Wulff, J.E.; McDunn, J.E.; Li, Z.; Dennis-Barrie, A.; Neri, B.P.; Milburn, M.V.; Lotan, Y.; et al. Bladder cancer biomarker discovery using global metabolomic profiling of urine. *PLoS ONE* **2014**, *9*, e115870. [CrossRef] [PubMed]

25. Tan, G.; Wang, H.; Yuan, J.; Qin, W.; Dong, X.; Wu, H.; Meng, P. Three serum metabolite signatures for diagnosing low-grade and high-grade bladder cancer. *Sci. Rep.* **2017**, *7*, 46176. [CrossRef]

26. Kouznetsova, V.L.; Kim, E.; Romm, E.L.; Zhu, A.; Tsigelny, I. Recognition of early and late stages of bladder cancer using metabolites and machine learning. *Metabolomics* **2019**, *15*, 94. [CrossRef]

27. Rodrigues, D.; Pinto, J.; Araujo, A.M.; Jerónimo, C.; Henrique, R.; Bastos, M.D.L.; De Pinho, P.G.; Carvalho, M. Gc-ms metabolomics reveals distinct profiles of low- and high-grade bladder cancer cultured cells. *Metabolites* **2019**, *9*, 18. [CrossRef]

28. Conde, V.R.; Oliveira, P.F.; Nunes, A.R.; Rocha, C.S.; Ramalhosa, E.; Pereira, J.A.; Alves, M.G.; Silva, B.M. The progression from a lower to a higher invasive stage of bladder cancer is associated with severe alterations in glucose and pyruvate metabolism. *Exp. Cell Res.* **2015**, *335*, 91–98. [CrossRef]

29. Inzitari, R.; Cabras, T.; Pisano, E.; Fanali, C.; Manconi, B.; Scarano, E.; Faa, G. Hplc-esi-ms analysis of oral human fluids reveals that gingival crevicular fluid is the main source of oral thymosins β4 and β10. *J. Sep. Sci.* **2009**, *32*, 57–63. [CrossRef]

30. León, Z.; García-Cañaveras, J.C.; Donato, M.T.; Lahoz, A. Mammalian cell metabolomics: Experimental design and sample preparation. *Electrophoresis* **2013**, *34*, 2762–2775. [CrossRef]

31. Kalluri, U.; Naiker, M.; Myers, M.A. Cell culture metabolomics in the diagnosis of lung cancer-the influence of cell culture conditions. *J. Breath Res.* **2014**, *8*, 027109. [CrossRef] [PubMed]

32. Čuperlović-Culf, M.; Barnett, D.; Culf, A.S.; Chute, I. Cell culture metabolomics: Applications and future directions. *Drug Discov. Today* **2010**, *15*, 610–621. [CrossRef] [PubMed]

33. Bi, H.; Krausz, K.W.; Manna, S.K.; Li, F.; Johnson, C.H.; Gonzalez, F.J. Optimization of harvesting, extraction, and analytical protocols for uplc-esi-ms-based metabolomic analysis of adherent mammalian cancer cells. *Anal. Bioanal. Chem.* **2013**, *405*, 5279–5289. [CrossRef] [PubMed]

34. Konstantakou, E.G.; Voutsinas, G.E.; Velentzas, A.D.; Basogianni, A.-S.; Paronis, E.; Balafas, E.; Kostomitsopoulos, N.; Syrigos, K.; Anastasiadou, E.; Stravopodis, D.J. 3-brpa eliminates human bladder cancer cells with highly oncogenic signatures via engagement of specific death programs and perturbation of multiple signaling and metabolic determinants. *Mol. Cancer* **2015**, *14*, 135. [CrossRef] [PubMed]

35. Zheng, W.; Tayyari, F.; Gowda, G.N.; Raftery, D.; McLamore, E.S.; Porterfield, D.M.; Donkin, S.; Bequette, B.; Teegarden, R. Altered glucose metabolism in harvey-ras transformed mcf10a cells. *Mol. Carcinog.* **2015**, *54*, 111–120. [CrossRef] [PubMed]

36. Gatenby, R.A.; Gillies, R.J. Why do cancers have high aerobic glycolysis? *Nat. Rev. Cancer* **2004**, *4*, 891–899. [CrossRef] [PubMed]

37. Koppenol, W.H.; Bounds, P.L.; Dang, C.V. Otto warburg's contributions to current concepts of cancer metabolism. *Nat. Rev. Cancer* **2011**, *11*, 325–337. [CrossRef]

38. Harper, K.L.; Sosa, M.S.; Entenberg, D.; Hosseini, H.; Cheung, J.F.; Nobre, R.; Farias, E.F. Mechanism of early dissemination and metastasis in her2 mammary cancer. *Nature* **2016**, *540*, 588–592. [CrossRef]

39. Hosseini, H.; Obradović, M.M.S.; Hoffmann, M.; Harper, K.L.; Sosa, M.S.; Werner-Klein, M.; Nanduri, S.L.K.; Werno, C.; Ehrl, C.; Maneck, M.; et al. Early dissemination seeds metastasis in breast cancer. *Nature* **2016**, *540*, 552–558. [CrossRef]

40. Yachida, S.; Jones, S.; Bozic, I.; Antal, T.; Leary, R.; Fu, B.; Kamiyama, M.; Hruban, R.H.; Eshleman, J.R.; Nowak, M.A.; et al. Distant metastasis occurs late during the genetic evolution of pancreatic cancer. *Nature* **2010**, *467*, 1114–1117. [CrossRef]

41. Vettore, L.; Westbrook, R.L.; Tennant, D.A. New aspects of amino acid metabolism in cancer. *Br. J. Cancer* **2020**, *122*, 150–156. [CrossRef] [PubMed]

42. Griffin, J.L.; Shockcor, J.P. Metabolic profiles of cancer cells. *Nat. Rev. Cancer* **2004**, *4*, 551–561. [CrossRef] [PubMed]

43. Loo, J.M.; Scherl, A.; Nguyen, A.; Man, F.Y.; Weinberg, E.; Zeng, Z.; Saltz, L.B.; Paty, P.B.; Tavazoie, S.F. Extracellular metabolic energetics can promote cancer progression. *Cell* **2015**, *160*, 393–406. [CrossRef] [PubMed]

44. Sullivan, W.J.; Christofk, H.R. The metabolic milieu of metastases. *Cell* **2015**, *160*, 363–364. [CrossRef]

45. Valli, A.; Morotti, M.; Zois, C.E.; Albers, P.K.; Soga, T.; Feldinger, K.; Fischer, R.; Frejno, M.; McIntyre, A.; Bridges, E.; et al. Adaptation to hif1α deletion in hypoxic cancer cells by upregulation of glut14 and creatine metabolism. *Mol. Cancer Res.* **2019**, *17*, 1531–1544. [CrossRef]

46. Kung, A.; Zabludoff, S.D.; France, D.S.; Freedman, S.J.; Tanner, E.A.; Vieira, A.; Cornell-Kennon, S.; Lee, J.; Wang, B.; Wang, J.; et al. Small molecule blockade of transcriptional coactivation of the hypoxia-inducible factor pathway. *Cancer Cell* **2004**, *6*, 33–43. [CrossRef]

47. Hardie, D.G.; Ross, F.A.; Hawley, S.A. Ampk: A nutrient and energy sensor that maintains energy homeostasis. *Nat. Rev. Mol. Cell Biol.* **2012**, *13*, 251–262. [CrossRef]

48. Mihaylova, M.M.; Shaw, R.J. The ampk signalling pathway coordinates cell growth, autophagy and metabolism. *Nat. Cell Biol.* **2011**, *13*, 1016–1023. [CrossRef]

49. Guo, J.Y.; Chen, H.-Y.; Mathew, R.; Fan, J.; Strohecker, A.M.; Karsli-Uzunbas, G.; Kamphorst, J.J.; Chen, G.; Lemons, J.M.; Karantza, V.; et al. Activated ras requires autophagy to maintain oxidative metabolism and tumorigenesis. *Genes Dev.* **2011**, *25*, 460–470. [CrossRef]

50. Sribenja, S.; Wongkham, S.; Wongkham, C.; Yao, Q.C.; Chen, C. Roles and mechanisms of β-thymosins in cell migration and cancer metastasis: An update. *Cancer Investig.* **2013**, *31*, 103–110. [CrossRef]

51. Lee, S.H.; Son, M.J.; Oh, S.H.; Rho, S.B.; Park, K.; Kim, Y.J.; Lee, J.H. Thymosin β10 inhibits angiogenesis and tumor growth by interfering with ras function. *Cancer Res.* **2005**, *65*, 137–148. [PubMed]

52. Wang, B.; Wang, Z.; Zhang, T.; Yang, G. Overexpression of thymosin β10 correlates with disease progression and poor prognosis in bladder cancer. *Exp. Ther. Med.* **2019**, *18*, 3759–3766. [CrossRef]

53. Wang, Z.Y.; Zhang, W.; Yang, J.; Song, D.K.; Wei, J.X.; Gao, S. Association of thymosin β4 expression with clinicopathological parameters and clinical outcomes of bladder cancer patients. *Neoplasma* **2016**, *63*, 991–998. [CrossRef]

54. Wen, B.; Mei, Z.; Zeng, C.; Liu, S. Metax: A flexible and comprehensive software for processing metabolomics data. *BMC Bioinform.* **2017**, *18*, 183. [CrossRef] [PubMed]

55. Strohalm, M.; Kavan, D.; Novák, P.; Volny, M.; Havlicek, V. Mmass 3: A cross-platform software environment for precise analysis of mass spectrometric data. *Anal. Chem.* **2010**, *82*, 4648–4651. [CrossRef] [PubMed]

56. Gao, J.; Tarcea, V.G.; Karnovsky, A.; Mirel, B.R.; Weymouth, T.E.; Beecher, C.W.; Cavalcoli, J.D.; Athey, B.; Omenn, G.S.; Burant, C.; et al. Metscape: A cytoscape plug-in for visualizing and interpreting metabolomic data in the context of human metabolic networks. *Bioinformatics* **2010**, *26*, 971–973. [CrossRef] [PubMed]

57. Shannon, P.; Markiel, A.; Ozier, O.; Baliga, N.S.; Wang, J.T.; Ramage, D.; Amin, N.; Schwikowski, B.; Ideker, T. Cytoscape: A software environment for integrated models of biomolecular interaction networks. *Genome Res.* **2003**, *13*, 2498–2504. [CrossRef]

58. Cacciatore, S.; Tenori, L.; Luchinat, C.; Bennett, P.R.; MacIntyre, D.A. Kodama: An r package for knowledge discovery and data mining. *Bioinformatics* **2017**, *33*, 621–623. [CrossRef]

59. Luan, H.; Ji, F.; Chen, Y.; Cai, Z. Stattarget: A streamlined tool for signal drift correction and interpretations of quantitative mass spectrometry-based omics data. *Anal. Chim. Acta* **2018**, *1036*, 66–72. [CrossRef]

60. Robin, X.; Turck, N.; Hainard, A.; Tiberti, N.; Lisacek, F.; Sanchez, J.-C.; Müller, M. Proc: An open-source package for r and s+ to analyze and compare roc curves. *Bmc Bioinform.* **2011**, *12*, 77. [CrossRef]

61. Wu, H.; Southam, A.D.; Hines, A.; Viant, M.R. High-throughput tissue extraction protocol for NMR- and MS-based metabolomics. *Anal. Biochem.* **2008**, *372*, 204–212. [CrossRef] [PubMed]

62. Dunn, W.B.; Broadhurst, D.; Begley, P.; Zelena, E.; Francis-McIntyre, S.; Anderson, N.; Brown, M.; Knowles, J.D.; Halsall, A.; Haselden, J.N.; et al. Procedures for large-scale metabolic profiling of serum and plasma using gas chromatography and liquid chromatography coupled to mass spectrometry. *Nat. Protoc.* **2011**, *6*, 1060–1083. [CrossRef] [PubMed]

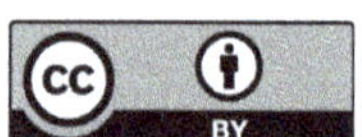

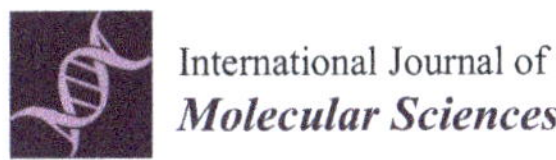

International Journal of
Molecular Sciences

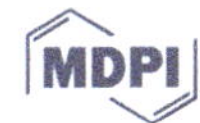

Article

ITIH5 and *ECRG4* DNA Methylation Biomarker Test (EI-BLA) for Urine-Based Non-Invasive Detection of Bladder Cancer

Michael Rose [1,2,*], Sarah Bringezu [1], Laura Godfrey [1], David Fiedler [1], Nadine T. Gaisa [1], Maximilian Koch [1], Christian Bach [3], Susanne Füssel [4], Alexander Herr [5], Doreen Hübner [4], Jörg Ellinger [6], David Pfister [3,7], Ruth Knüchel [1], Manfred P. Wirth [4], Manja Böhme [5] and Edgar Dahl [1,2,*]

[1]   Institute of Pathology, RWTH Aachen University, 52074 Aachen, Germany; bringezu.sarah@gmail.com (S.B.); laura.dierichs@rwth-aachen.de (L.G.); david@fiedler.online (D.F.); ngaisa@ukaachen.de (N.T.G.); maximilian.koch@uk-koeln.de (M.K.); rknuechel-clarke@ukaachen.de (R.K.)

[2]   RWTH Centralized Biomaterial Bank (RWTH cBMB), Medical Faculty, RWTH Aachen University, 52074 Aachen, Germany

[3]   Department of Urology, RWTH Aachen University, 52074 Aachen, Germany; chbach@ukaachen.de (C.B.); david.pfister@uk-koeln.de (D.P.)

[4]   Department of Urology, University Hospital Carl Gustav Carus, Technische Universität Dresden, 01307 Dresden, Germany; Susanne.Fuessel@uniklinikum-dresden.de (S.F.); Huebner-Doreen@gmx.de (D.H.); Manfred.Wirth@uniklinikum-dresden.de (M.P.W.)

[5]   Biotype GmbH, 01109 Dresden, Germany; alx.herr@gmail.com (A.H.); m.boehme@biotype.de (M.B.)

[6]   Department of Urology, University Hospital Bonn, 53105 Bonn, Germany; joerg.ellinger@ukb.uni-bonn.de

[7]   Department of Urology, Uro-Oncology, Robot Assisted and Reconstructive Urologic Surgery, University Hospital Cologne, 50937 Cologne, Germany

*   Correspondence: mrose@ukaachen.de (M.R.); edahl@ukaachen.de (E.D.); Tel.: +49-241-808-9715 (M.R.); +49-241-808-8431 (E.D.); Fax: +49-241-808-2439 (M.R.); +49-241-808-2439 (E.D.)

Received: 16 December 2019; Accepted: 5 February 2020; Published: 7 February 2020

Abstract: Bladder cancer is one of the more common malignancies in humans and the most expensive tumor for treating in the Unites States (US) and Europe due to the need for lifelong surveillance. Non-invasive tests approved by the FDA have not been widely adopted in routine diagnosis so far. Therefore, we aimed to characterize the two putative tumor suppressor genes *ECRG4* and *ITIH5* as novel urinary DNA methylation biomarkers that are suitable for non-invasive detection of bladder cancer. While assessing the analytical performance, a spiking experiment was performed by determining the limit of RT112 tumor cell detection (range: 100–10,000 cells) in the urine of healthy donors in dependency of the processing protocols of the RWTH cBMB. Clinically, urine sediments of 474 patients were analyzed by using quantitative methylation-specific PCR (qMSP) and Methylation Sensitive Restriction Enzyme (MSRE) qPCR techniques. Overall, *ECRG4-ITIH5* showed a sensitivity of 64% to 70% with a specificity ranging between 80% and 92%, i.e., discriminating healthy, benign lesions, and/or inflammatory diseases from bladder tumors. When comparing single biomarkers, *ECRG4* achieved a sensitivity of 73%, which was increased by combination with the known biomarker candidate *NID2* up to 76% at a specificity of 97%. Hence, *ITIH5* and, in particular, *ECRG4* might be promising candidates for further optimizing current bladder cancer biomarker panels and platforms.

Keywords: bladder cancer detection; urinary biomarkers; DNA methylation; ECRG4; ITIH5

---

1. Introduction

Bladder cancer is the most frequent urogenital malignant tumor concerning both sexes worldwide, with an estimated ~549,400 new cases and 200,000 deaths in 2018 [1], which causes the highest costs of all cancers per patient [2]. In the European Union (EU) alone, the costs were €4.9 billion, with health care accounting for €2.9 billion in 2012 [3] due to long-term survival with the need for lifelong surveillance by cost-intensive diagnostically tools [2]. Cystoscopy, the "gold standard" for the detection of bladder cancer, is an invasive and time-consuming procedure, achieving an operator-dependent sensitivity and specificity of approximately 90% [4]. In particular, repeating cystoscopy for patients with non-muscle invasive bladder cancer (NMIBC) to determine whether their disease has recurred or progressed to muscle invasive bladder cancer (MIBC) represents a major cost associated with treating bladder cancer patients [5]. Nevertheless, only 10% of haematuria patients are faced with a diagnosis of bladder cancer [6], a fact that did not increase the compliance of undergoing cystoscopy. Complementary to these procedures, the current guidelines recommend completion by non-invasive urine cytology, which, however, is characterized by poor sensitivity varying between 20 to 53% [7]. Additional non-invasive urinary assays have been developed, which could help to minimize the invasive procedure of cystoscopy and reduce its economic burden (for an overview see: [8]). Although such assays have been shown to increase the sensitivity of urine cytology, they have not been widely adopted in routine practice: either they are characterized by cost-intensive performances, like UroVysion [9], or failed as point of-care tests due to limited sensitivity or specificity, such as the NMP22-based "BladderCheck^{TM} Test" [10,11]. Given that, none of the currently available urinary biomarkers that have been approved by the FDA can absolutely be recommended as a stand-alone test to replace cystoscopy in the clinic. Recently, several commercially available tests have been developed with improved sensitivity and specificity by using mRNA (e.g., "Xpert BC" [12]) or protein-based ELISA assay technology (e.g., "UBC" [13]), but these data must be independently be confirmed in further studies. Therefore, it is still of great interest to identify novel tumor biomarkers for urine-based early detection of bladder cancer, which might optimize existing panels and platforms to improve both the initial detection of bladder cancer and detection of its recurrence.

For several decades now, epigenetic alterations are an excellent source of biomarker candidates for cancer detection, diagnosis, and prognosis [14]. In particular, aberrant DNA hypermethylation of putative tumor suppressor genes emerged as a potential biomarker source for assessing early cancer detection, which has recently moved towards clinical practice, for instance, in colorectal cancer [15]. For non-invasive detection of bladder cancer, promising DNA methylation biomarkers have been described in various studies [16], but the FDA has approved none of the presented methylation biomarkers (panels) for routinely diagnostic procedures so far. In the presented study, we focused on two putative tumor suppressor genes in bladder cancer that may also hold a prognostic impact, namely inter-α-trypsin inhibitor heavy chain 5 (*ITIH5*) and esophageal cancer-related gene 4 (*ECRG4* or *C2orf40*). *ITIH5* has previously been shown to be epigenetically silenced in various cancer entities [17–19], including bladder cancer [20], where its expression was associated with tumor recurrence of the clinical important group of high-grade pT1 patients. In addition, *ITIH5* was characterized as a putative metastasis suppressor gene in breast [21,22] and pancreatic cancers [23]. *ECRG4* has also been described to be a candidate tumor suppressor gene that is inactivated by DNA methylation in cancers, like esophageal squamous cell carcinoma [24,25], breast cancer [26], renal cell cancer [27], and colorectal cancer [28,29], but not in bladder cancer so far.

We now provide evidence that *ECRG4* and *ITIH5* DNA methylation could be useful as urinary biomarkers for non-invasive bladder cancer detection. Biomarkers were assessed by comparing different techniques, i.e., bisulfite-pyrosequencing, qMSP, and MSRE qPCR in comprehensive cohorts of patients with bladder diseases and controls, overall composing 474 urine samples, including a significant number of benign and inflammatory diseases. In particular, we demonstrate strong biomarker performance for *ECRG4*, which might be a suitable candidate to complete and improve current non-invasive biomarker panels and platforms.

2. Results

2.1. Analytical Performance of ITIH5 and ECRG4 qMSP and Pyrosequencing Biomarker Assays

ITIH5 and *ECRG4* have been previously identified as putative class II tumor suppressor genes, which are epigenetically silenced in various tumor entities. In the presented study, we aimed to assess the biomarker quality of both candidates to detect bladder tumors *via* urine samples. The analytical performance of quantitative methylation-specific PCR (qMSP) and pyrosequencing assays was assessed involving standard biobank processing procedure of the RWTH cBMB biobank prior to assessing the biomarker performance of ECRG4 and ITIH5 by patient materials.

For *ECRG4*, Figure 1A shows the genomic location of the qMSP and pyrosequencing assays. Both of the assays spanned CpG sites, which were characterized by strong median hypermethylation in bladder tumors within the TCGA data set [30] as compared to normal controls. CpG sites of the *ECRG4* target region showed a significant inverse correlation between DNA methylation and *ECRG4* mRNA expression (Figure 1A). Subsequently, a spiking experiment was performed to assess both sensitivity and reproducibility in dependence on a distinct number of RT112 tumor cells (range: 100–10,000 cells), i.e., RT112 bladder cancer cells harboring methylated *ECRG4* (see Supplementary Figure S1) and *ITIH5* [20] genes were spiked into 20 mL pooled urine of healthy donors ($n = 4$), respectively. Urine samples that were spiked with RT112 cells were processed according to the standard operating protocol of the RWTH cBMB. Urine pellets were either directly used for DNA extraction (probe set A) or urine sediments were stored according to the RWTH cBMB conditions ($-80\,°C$) for two weeks (probe set B) (Figure 1B). We found that DNA yield was significantly higher in freshly processed samples when compared to those processed after two weeks of storage at $-80\,°C$ (probe set B, Figure 1C). However, this was not associated with significant changes in the detection sensitivity of *ECRG4* methylation by both assays, qMSP and pyrosequencing). Overall, the *ECRG4* qMSP assay showed the highest sensitivity with a detection limit of 25 tumor cells/ml (equivalent to 89.75 pg tumor DNA), whereas pyrosequencing-based detection of *ECRG4* methylation required 45 tumor cells/ml (161.55 pg tumor DNA) urine (Figure 1D). Furthermore, the *ECRG4* qMSP assay exhibited a robust reproducibility when comparing methylation detection rates of the two storage time points, i.e., the qMSP assay convinced with high sensitivity and strong reliability (Spearman r: 0.955, $p < 0.001$) (Figure 1E). In contrast, pyrosequencing missed a significant correlation of *ECRG4* methylation levels of spiking samples, which were directly used for DNA extraction and those processed after two weeks (Supplementary Figure S2).

qMSP and pyrosequencing assays for the detection of the *ITIH5* promoter methylation were established similar to *ECRG4*. In Figure 2A, the relative location of qMSP and pyrosequencing primers are indicated. TCGA BLCA data analyses confirmed differences in median DNA methylation level for the targeted region of the *ITIH5* qMSP and pyrosequencing assay, which spanned the CpG site (#10119075), showing an inverse correlation between *ITIH5* DNA methylation and corresponding gene expression (Figure 2A). Of clinical significance, *ITIH5* hypermethylation of the CG site #10119075 was associated with shorter overall survival in advanced (pT > 2) bladder tumors (Figure 2B). In concordance with the results that were observed for *ECRG4*, pyrosequencing-based detection of *ITIH5* methylation failed to perform with a suitable reproducibility when using samples of both storage time points (directly processed vs. two weeks biobank storage). The *ITIH5* qMSP assay achieved strong reliability (Spearman correlation: 0.902, $p < 0.001$, Figure 2C,D) and high sensitivity being characterized by a detection limit that ranged between 25 and 30 tumor cells/mL (89.75 pg/107.70 pg tumor DNA), whereas a robust detection of *ITIH5* methylation by pyrosequencing required at least 125 tumor cells/mL (448.75 pg tumor DNA) urine (Supplementary Figure S2). Hence, qMSP assays of both genes were selected for assessment in a clinical cohort setting.

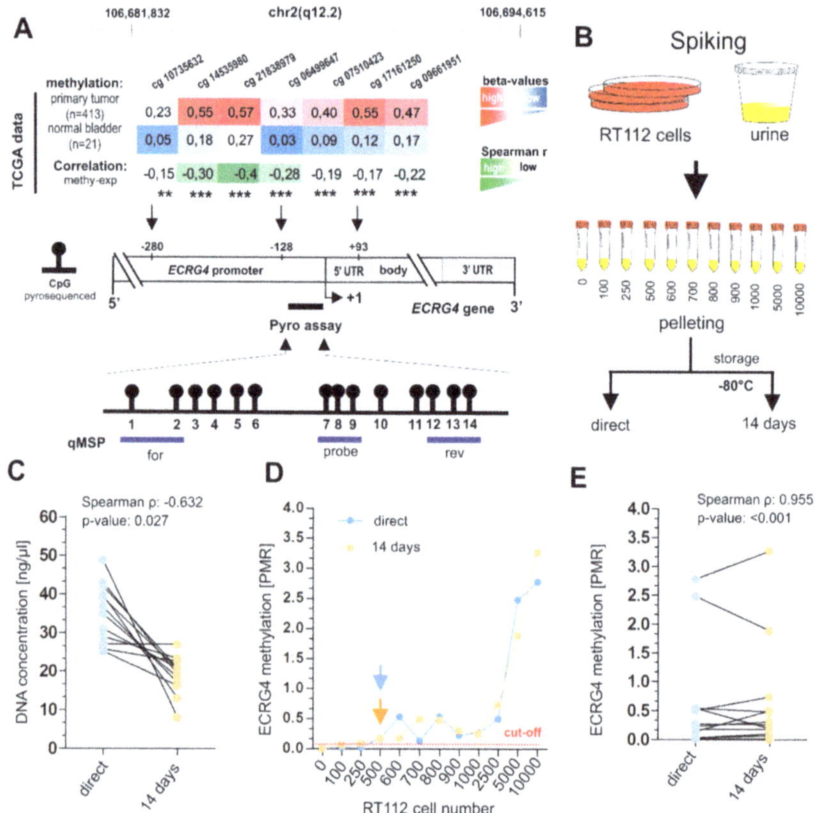

Figure 1. Analytical performance of the Quantitative Methylation-Specific PCR (qMSP) *ECRG4* DNA methylation biomarker assay. (**A**) Schematic map of the human *ECRG4* gene, including the relative positions and median β-values (of normal and tumor samples) of seven CpG sites based on 450K methylation arrays of the bladder cancer (BLCA) TCGA data set and corresponding Spearman correlation between *ECRG4* methylation (colored scale bar red to white; red: high methylation, white: low methylation) and *ECRG4* mRNA expression (colored scale bar green to white; green: strong correlation, white: no correlation) for each CpG site; ** $p \leq 0.01$, *** $p \leq 0.001$. +1: *ECRG4* transcription start site (TSS). Relative position of the promoter area analyzed by bisulfite-pyrosequencing that comprises 14 single CpG sites (black dots) is shown as a black line. CpG sites analyzed by qMSP (blue lines) were indicated covering the pyrosequenced promoter region close to the TSS. (**B**) Cartoon illustrating the spiking experiment using cultured RT112 tumor cells and urine pooled from four healthy donors. Distinct cell numbers of RT112 tumor cells (100-10,000) were spiked into 20 mL urine, respectively. Afterwards, urine samples were processed according to the standard operating protocol of the RWTH cBMB biobank. Pellets of probe set A were directly used for DNA extraction while urine sediments of probe set B were stored according to the RWTH cBMB conditions ($-80\ °C$) for two weeks before further processing. (**C**) Comparison of DNA concentrations (=yield) achieved of samples from probe set A (direct processing) and B (after 14 days). DNA yield was significantly higher in freshly processed urine samples. (**D**) *ECRG4* promoter methylation determined by using qMSP of spiked urines samples. Red dotted line: threshold value for positive detection; orange and blue arrow: stably exceeding the threshold (detection limit) (**E**) Correlation of *ECRG4* DNA methylation for spiked urine samples of probe set A and B.

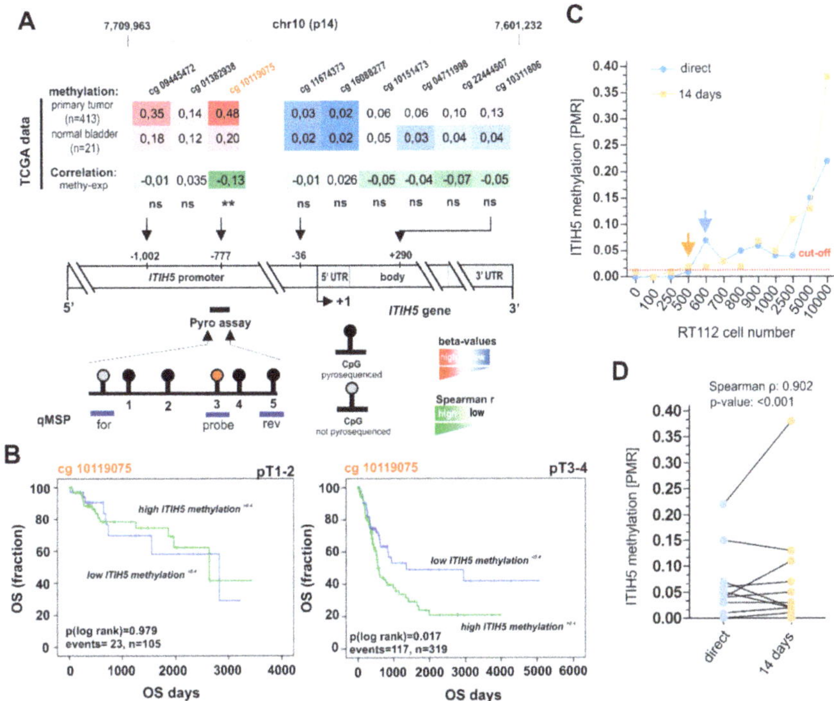

Figure 2. Analytical performance of the qMSP *ITIH5* DNA methylation biomarker assay. (**A**) Schematic map of the human *ITIH5 gene* including the relative positions and median median *β*-values (of normal and tumor samples) of nine CpG sites based on 450K methylation arrays of the BLCA TCGA data set and corresponding Spearman correlation between *ITIH5* methylation (colored scale bar red to white; red: high methylation, white: low methylation) and *ITIH5* mRNA expression (colored scale bar green to white; green: strong correlation, white: no correlation) for each CpG site; ** $p \leq 0.01$. +1: *ITIH5* transcription start site (TSS). Relative position of the upstream promoter area analyzed by bisulfite-pyrosequencing that comprises five single CpG sites (black dots) is shown as a black line. CpG sites analyzed by qMSP (blue lines) were indicated largely covering the pyrosequenced promoter region. (**B**) Kaplan–Meier survival curves display overall survival (OS) of patients with high ITIH5 methylation (*β*-value of CG #10119075 > 0.4, green curve) compared to low ITIH5 methylation (*β*-value of CG #10119075 ≤ 0.4, blue curve) based on TCGA data. (**C**) *ITIH5* promoter methylation determined by using qMSP of spiked urine samples. Red dotted line: threshold value for positive detection; orange and blue arrow: stably exceeding the threshold (detection limit) (**D**) Correlation of *ITIH5* DNA methylation for spiked urine samples of probe set A and B.

2.2. Clinical Biomarker Performance of the ECRG4-ITIH5 qMSP Test for Accurate Non-Invasive Detection of Bladder Cancer

ECRG4 and *ITIH5* performance was initially assessed in a clinical cohort of urine samples (total *n* = 263) comprising 116 urine samples that were derived from bladder cancer patients. Patients with urological malignancies of other origin (testis, prostate, kidney) as well as benign and inflammatory urological-diseases (prostate hyperplasia, renal stones, chronic cystitis) and healthy (without pathological finding) donors that were included as controls (cohort 1a: benign - inflammatory, cohort 1b: all controls including urological cancers). *ECRG4* and *ITIH5* methylation for each urine sample is shown as the mean percentage of methylated reference (PMR) in the scatter plots of Figure 3A,B. *ECRG4* and *ITIH5* methylation were both significantly increased in the urine samples from patients with cancers of the bladder (*ECRG4* mean PMR: 5.011, 95% CI: 2.118–7.905; *ITIH5* mean PMR: 2.634, 95% CI: 0.730–4.539), the prostate (*ECRG4* mean PMR: 1.306, 95% CI: 0.178–2.434; *ITIH5* mean PMR: 1.018, 95% CI: 0.441–1.720), and the kidney (*ECRG4* mean PMR: 0.985, 95% CI: 0.188–1.781, *ITIH5* mean PMR: 1.311, 95% CI: 0.147–2.475) when compared to healthy controls (*ECRG4* mean PMR: 0.017, 95% CI: <0.001–0.033, *ITIH5* mean PMR: 0.031, 95% CI: 0.009–0.070). In benign and inflammatory diseases, a single statistical outlier was detected, respectively, however, diagnosis had been done in a clinical setting and, thus, a true malignancy in this few cases cannot be completely excluded. No associations were found between both *ECRG4* and *ITIH5* promoter methylation and clinical-pathological characteristics, including tumor size, histological grade, age at diagnosis, and gender (Supplementary Table S1 and S2). Calculating the optimal cut-off value for a combined *ECRG4-ITIH5* (EI-BLA) qMSP application with robust specificity by using ROC statistics (Table 1), we demonstrated significant discrimination of bladder cancer patients from non-malignant controls (control cohort 1a) with a sensitivity of 64.3% and a specificity of 81.5% (AUC: 0.783, 95% CI: 0.716–0.850, *p* < 0.0001) (Figure 3C).

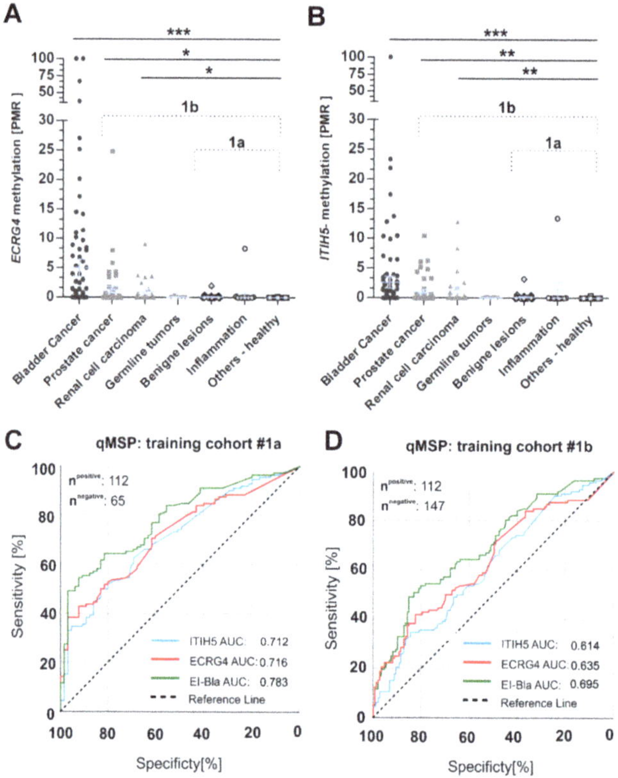

Figure 3. Performance of the *ECRG4* and *ITIH5* biomarker panel using qMSP technique and training cohort #1. (**A,B**) Scatterplots show the PMR methylation values for *ECRG4* (**A**) and *ITIH5* (**B**) in urine sediments of urological tumors, benign lesions, inflammatory diseases and healthy samples; *** *p* < 0.001, ** *p* < 0.01, * *p* < 0.05. 1a: training cohort excluding other urological malignancies 1b: training cohort including other urological malignancies. (**C,D**) ROC-curve analysis illustrating *ECRG4* (red curve), *ITIH5* (blue curve) and *ECRG4-ITIH5* (green curve) biomarker performance based on qMSP in cohort 1a (being and inflammatory controls (**C**)) and cohort 1b (further urological cancer entities as controls (**D**)), *AUC*: Area under the curve.

Table 1. EI-BLA biomarker performance based on training cohort #1 as compared to different control groups.

EI-BLA qMSP					
Cut-Off	Specificity	Sensitivity	AUC	*p*-Value	Control Group
0.54	81.5%	64.3%	0.783	<0.001	1a
0.38	81.6%	50.9%	0.695	<0.001	1b

Additionally, *ECRG4-ITIH5* in combination were able to distinguish bladder cancer patients from patients with neoplasms of other urological origin (control cohort 1b) with similar specificity (81.6%, AUC: 0.695, 95% CI: 0.631–0.760, $p < 0.0001$) but reduced sensitivity (50.9%) (Figure 3D). The application of both biomarker candidates in combination achieved the most reliable results as compared with single biomarker performances.

Next, the biomarker quality of *ECRG4* and *ITIH5* promoter methylation was tested and then compared to a known putative bladder cancer methylation biomarker (*NID2*) by Methylation Sensitive Restriction Enzyme (MSRE) qPCR at the independent laboratories of Biotype GmbH (Dresden, Germany). The independent urine cohort (overall $n = 211$) included 130 urines of patients that were diagnosed with primary bladder cancer as well as 81 control urines (benign lesions, inflammatory diseases, and healthy controls). *ECRG4-ITIH5* methylation was found to be significantly increased in the urines of bladder cancer patients (mean methylation: 10.31, 95% CI: 6.132–14.50) as compared to all control groups, i.e., benign lesions (mean methylation: 0.143), inflammatory diseases (mean methylation: 2.900), and healthy donors (mean methylation: 0.203) (Figure 4A). In this independent cohort, a close association of both *ECRG4* and *ITIH5* with increased tumor size (pTa vs. pT1-4) and age at diagnosis was determined by Fisher's exact test (Tables 2 and 3).

Table 2. Clinico-pathological parameters in relation to ITIH5 methylation in training cohort #2.

		ITIH5 Methylation [b]		
	n [a]	Low	High	*p*-Value [c]
Age at diagnosis				
≤70 years	111	65	46	0.001
>70 years	106	39	67	
Gender				
male	143	57	56	0.150
female	42	22	20	
Histological tumor grade [d]				
low grade	19	4	15	0.174
high grade	113	42	71	
Tumor stage [d]				
pTa	76	33	43	0.024
pT1-pT4	54	13	41	

[a] Urines of cohort #2; [b] cut-off level MSRE = 0.22 representing >90% specificity in ROC curve statistic; [c] Fisher's exact test; [d] According to WHO 2004 classification; Significant *p*-values are marked in bold face.

Table 3. Clinico-pathological parameters in relation to ECRG4 methylation in training cohort #2.

		ECRG4 Methylation [b]		
	n [a]	Low	High	*p*-Value [c]
Age at diagnosis				
<70 years	111	84	27	**<0.001**
≥70 years	106	55	51	
Gender				
male	143	82	61	0.802
female	42	25	17	
Histological tumor grade [d]				
low grade	19	10	9	0.645
high grade	113	53	60	
Tumor stage[d]				
pTa	76	45	31	**0.007**
pT1-pT4	54	19	35	

[a] Urines of cohort #2; [b] cut-off level MSRE = 0.52 representing >90% specificity in ROC curve statistic; [c] Fisher's exact test; [d] According to WHO 2004 classification; Significant *p*-values are marked in bold face.

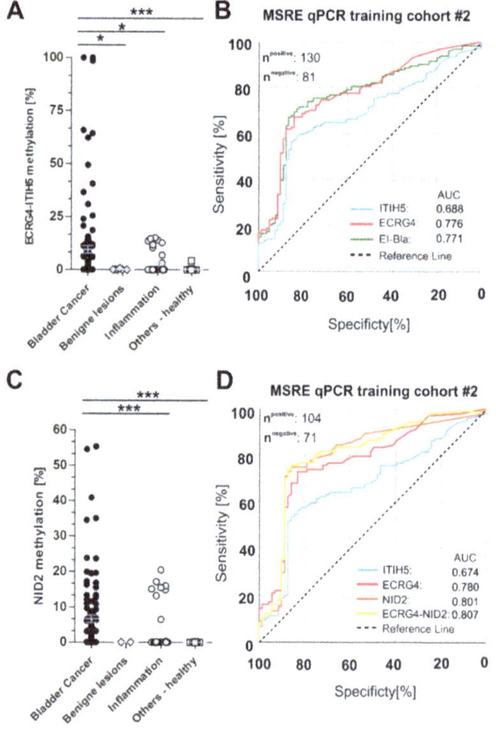

Figure 4. Biomarker performance of *ECRG4*, *ITIH5*, and the *ECRG4-ITIH5* panel assessed by an independent urine cohort (training cohort #2) and compared to *NID2* using MSRE qPCR. (**A**) Scatter plot illustrates significant increased methylation levels for *ECRG4* and *ITIH5* in urine sediments of bladder cancer compared to benign lesions, inflammatory and healthy samples; *** $p < 0.001$, * $p < 0.05$. (**B**) ROC-curve analysis illustrating *ECRG4* (red curve), *ITIH5* (blue curve) and *ECRG4-ITIH5* (green curve) biomarker performance based on MSRE qPCR in cohort #2. (**C**) Scatter plot showed significant increased methylation values for *NID2* in urine sediments of bladder cancer compared to benign lesions, inflammatory and healthy samples; *** $p < 0.001$. (**D**) ROC-curve analysis compares *ECRG4* (red curve), ITIH5 (blue curve), and *NID2* (orange curve) and combined ECRG4-NID2 biomarker performance based on MSRE qPCR in cohort #2. *AUC*: Area under the curve.

The ROC analyses showed that *ECRG4-ITIH5* combination achieved a sensitivity of 71.6% at a specificity of 80.2% (AUC: 0.771, 95% CI: 0.706–0.836) in a cohort that included benign lesions and inflammatory diseases of the urinary tract (Figure 4B), whereas specificity was increased up to 92% with minimally decreased sensitivity (69%) focusing on healthy controls. When comparing our single biomarkers, i.e., *ITIH5* and *ECRG4*, with the recently proposed biomarker candidate *NID2* [31], we revealed a similar biomarker performances of *ECRG4* and *NID2*, achieving a sensitivity of 73.1% (AUC: 0.780, 95% CI: 0.709–0.851) and 75% (AUC: 0.801, 95% CI: 0.729–0.873) at a specificity of 83.1%, respectively (Table 4).

Table 4. Biomarker performances based on training cohort #2.

EI-BLA MRSE qPCR					
Cut-Off	Specificity	Sensitivity	AUC	*p*-Value	Control Group
0.52	80.2%	71.6%	0.771	<0.001	all
0.53	91.9%	69.2%	0.850	<0.001	healthy
Single markers MSRE qPCR (control group "all")					
Cut-Off	Specificity	Sensitivity	AUC	*p*-Value	Marker
0.94	83.1%	73.1%	0.780	<0.001	*ECRG4*
0.77	83.1%	56.7%	0.674	<0.001	*ITIH5*
0.11	83.1%	75.0%	0.801	<0.001	*NID2*
Combined ECRG4-NID2 MSRE qPCR					
Cut-Off	Specificity	Sensitivity	AUC	*p*-Value	Control Group
0.49	85.9%	75.0%	0.807	<0.001	all
0.49	97.3%	76.0%	0.884	<0.001	healthy

According to that, *ITIH5* was characterized by reduced sensitivity (56.7%, AUC: 0.674, 95% CI: 0.592–0.755), which did not lead to improved biomarker performance when combining with ECRG4. While considering that, we were able to increase sensitivity for bladder cancer detection up to 75% with improved specificity (85.9%; AUC: 0.807, 95% CI: 0.737–0.877) in a cohort comprising benign lesions and inflammatory diseases of the urinary tract when combining *ECRG4* with the known biomarker *NID2* (Figure 4C,D). In comparison to healthy controls, the panel set of *ECRG-NID2* achieved 76% sensitivity with 97.3% specificity (AUC: 0.884, 95% CI: 0.831–0.937) (Table 4).

3. Discussion

The field of liquid biopsy-based cancer detection systems is rapidly evolving, as novel (epi)genetic biomarkers have been characterized, which can be detected in biological fluids, like blood or urine, offering an easy and non-invasive application for cancer detection, prognosis, and therapy prediction. In colorectal cancer (CRC), for instance, a blood-based screening was realized by targeting Septin 9 (*SEPT9*) hypermethylation, whose Epi proColon®test has been approved by the FDA in 2016 [32]. In bladder cancer, liquid biopsy still needs improvement [33], as various molecular (epi)genetic biomarker candidates and signatures have been described, but none of those assays are FDA-approved for routine diagnostic so far.

In the current study, we present two novel biomarker candidates, *ITIH5* and *ECRG4*, which show strong potential for improving or even completing existing non-invasive biomarker panels and platforms. Already in the year 2010, Renard and colleagues identified *TWIST1* and *NID2* as putative biomarker candidates while using qMSP [31]. In the same year, Costa et. al. showed three novel gene loci, i.e., *GDF15*, *TMEFF2*, and *VIM*, whose DNA methylation could be suitable for detecting bladder cancers in urine samples [34]. Meanwhile, many more putative candidates have been presented [16], but most of the studies were characterized by small sample cohorts without taking into account crucial cohorts of non-malignant diseases like chronic inflammation. Hence, only a handful of biomarkers such as *TMEFF2*, *NID2* and *TWIST1* meet to some degree the needed requirements and, thus, were independently studied and validated [35]. Therefore, we took great care to implement suitable steps and criteria for biomarker validation from the beginning of the study. In the first step, established biomarker assays were assessed by comparing the reliability of different detection methods (qMSP and pyrosequencing) in dependency on the urine sample processing *in vitro*. Of importance, we demonstrated that the regular procedure of urine processing analogue to SOPs of the centralized biomaterial bank (cBMB) of the RWTH Aachen University (i.e., storage at −80 °C) did not impair biomarker detection. However, the DNA yield was considerably higher when fresh urine samples were processed. Beyond that, the qMSP technique showed both the highest sensitivity and reproducibility, which is in line with previous studies demonstrating high levels of accuracy and lower rates of false negatives as compared with other techniques [36]. In a second step, we validated the clinical performance of both biomarkers by independent cohorts and laboratories. In this setting, we included high numbers of urological benign and inflammatory diseases as controls that can be endemically and frequently found in larger population groups, thereby reflecting a much more real-world scenario. We achieved a sensitivity ranging between 64 to 72% at a specificity of over 80% by combined performance of the *ECRG4-ITIH5* DNA methylation biomarker panel. Importantly, we still detect approximately 50% of bladder tumors with a robust true-negative rate (>80% specificity) by including urological malignancies of other origins supporting a liquid biopsy application in the field of bladder cancer. However, a putative benefit of both biomarker candidates being further useful for future assays dealing with the non-invasive detection of other urothelial malignancies, like prostate or renal cell carcinomas, should not be excluded at this stage. Interestingly, in our independent training cohort from Dresden, *ECRG4* reached a sensitivity of over 73% as single biomarker. Hence, a suitable impact was suggested, in particular for *ECRG4*, for discriminating BPH or urocystitis from bladder tumors, which is comparable with proposed biomarker candidates, like *NID2* or *TWIST1* [33]. *CFTR*, *SAL3*, and *TWIST1* have been recently shown to be useful for monitoring bladder cancer in a real clinical scenario, as a sensitivity of 96% was achieved by pyrosequencing in combination with urine cytology—however with low specificity (40%) [35]. In our cohort, the ECRG4-ITIH5 biomarker performance also reached over 90% sensitivity at a specificity of 40%, however, we finally focused on the best panel according to their specificity: combining *ECRG4* and *NID2* led to an increased sensitivity (76%) at a specificity of 97% when compared to healthy controls, encouraging validation studies of this biomarker setting in the future.

In view of novel diagnostic platforms, *ECRG4* and *ITIH5* could also be part of NGS-based gene signatures, which are currently considered to be at the cutting edge of the technical development of future diagnostic applications. In 2017, the multiplex bisulfite NGS-based sequencing concept "UroMark" was described achieving 98% sensitivity and 97% specificity [37]. However, this NGS assay should be confirmed in comprehensive cohorts and the usability of a 150 CpG loci comprising biomarker assay for routinely and cost-effective diagnosis, in particular as a population-based screening tool, in a real-world scenario must be further considered. So far, real-world application of available urinary markers has not reduced any bladder cancer treatment costs, as predicted by decision-analytic economic models [2]. Still, biomarkers are missing, which serve as the basis for decision-making of risk stratification. According to that, DNA methylation of our markers, in particular *ITIH5*, might hold a prognostic impact, as both candidates have been characterized as putative tumor suppressor genes whose silencing could be triggered by DNA promoter hypermethylation [20]. In 2008, *ITIH5* was described to be epigenetically silenced in breast cancer [17] and five years later *ITIH5* DNA methylation has been identified as a putative blood-based biomarker for the early detection of breast cancer [38]. Since then functionally studies revealed, for instance, ITIH5 mediated suppression of breast [21,22] and pancreatic cancer metastases [23] *in vitro* and *in vivo*. Interestingly, in aggressive mammary cancer cells, ITIH5 triggered an epigenetic reprogramming which was associated with a demethylation of various promoter regions, including that of *DAPK1*, a tumor suppressor gene and putative blood-based biomarker in several tumor entities [21]. In bladder carcinogenesis, the downregulation of ITIH5 was also associated with worse prognosis while functionally high-grade bladder cancer cells showed reduced growth *in vitro* after ITIH5 overexpression [20]. Of clinical interest, ITIH5 protein expression was shown to predict tumor relapse of the clinical important subgroup of pT1 high-grade patients [20], of which 30% never displayed recurrence after transurethral resection of the bladder, while a further 30% died due to metastatic disease [39]. In the present study, we now confirmed a putative prognostic impact as *ITIH5* promoter hypermethylation was associated with poor patients' outcome in the subgroup of advanced tumors (pT > 2) of the TCGA bladder cancer data set, while increased *ITIH5* methylation was further shown to correlate with a higher pT status in our second urine cohort. These findings may support our hypothesis that *ITIH5* could be a useful biomarker for risk stratification, helping to monitor patients for the recurrence and/or progression of bladder tumors.

In conclusion, we provide two novel DNA methylation biomarkers for non-invasive detection of bladder carcinomas. As *ITIH5* might keep prognostic information for bladder cancer risk stratification, while *ECRG4* showed a convincing diagnostic performance, in particular in combination with the known biomarker candidate *NID2*, both biomarkers, *ECRG4* and *ITIH5*, may be promising candidates to complete and improve current biomarker panels and platforms. For instance, the "Bladder EpiCheck™" urine assay that combines 15 DNA methylation biomarkers leading to an overall sensitivity of 68.2% and a specificity of 80.0% [40] may benefit from our biomarker candidates to reduce the number of biomarkers while also improving the overall performance. Future studies should be conducted to clarify which of our biomarkers, is suitable for which clinical application, e.g. as a guidance tool for early detection, risk stratification, surveillance, and/or therapeutic management.

4. Materials and Methods

4.1. Cell Line

The bladder cancer cell line J82 was originally obtained from the American Type Culture Collection (ATCC, Manassas, VA, USA). The urothelial bladder cancer cell line RT112 was used for studies of the analytical performance, a gift from Dr. Alexander Buchner (LMU München, München, Germany). All of the cell lines successfully underwent an identity check (Multiplexion GmbH, Immenstadt, Germany) prior to the experiments.

4.2. Urine Samples

In total, 474 urine samples were assessed in this study. The Departments of Urology of the University Hospitals of Aachen, Bonn, and Dresden provided the voided urine samples. The samples that were collected in Aachen were obtained from the RWTH centralized biomaterial bank (RWTH cBMB). The collection of tissue samples was performed within the framework of the Biobank of the Center for Integrated Oncology Köln Bonn. All of the patients gave written consent for asservation and analysis of their samples according to local Institutional Review Board (IRB)-approved protocols of the Medical Faculty of RWTH Aachen University (EK 206/09, 05 Jan 2010), the University of Bonn (EK 205/13, 16 Mar 2013), and the University of Dresden (EK 96032012, 15 Jul 2014). The urine samples derived from patients diagnosed with a primary bladder tumor (*n* = 246) were used to assess biomarker performance, while samples with a known second malignancy, such as prostate cancer, were excluded from this study. Urines from healthy donors (*n* = 49) and samples derived from patients with inflammatory (chronic cystitis), benign (benign prostate hyperplasia), and urological malignant diseases of other tissue origin (testicular tumors, prostate cancer, renal cell carcinoma) served as the controls (overall *n* = 179). For the characteristics of training cohort I (Aachen–Bonn) and training cohort II (Dresden) see Table 5. Unless otherwise stated, 10–20 mL of urines were centrifuged for 10 min. at 2000 × g, washed with PBS and sediments were stored at −80 °C.

Table 5. The clinico-pathological parameters of 474 patients whose urine samples were analyzed in this study.

	Categorization	*n*	% Analyzable
Controls		228	100%
Age (median 61.0; range: 23–82 years)			
	<61.0 years	72	31.6%
	≥61.0 years	80	35.1%
	na	76	33.3%
Gender			
	male	96	42.1%
	female	24	10.5%
	na	108	47.4%
Diagnosis			
	Healthy	49	21.5%
	Uro-stones	13	5.7%
	Inflammatory—Uro-cystitis	38	16.7%
	Inflammatory—other	8	3.5%
	Benign—BPH	23	10.1%
	Benign—other	17	7.5%
	PCa	48	21.1%
	GTR	5	2.2%
	RCC	27	11.8%
BCa-Asscociated [a]		246	100%
Age (median 70; range: 27–89 years)			
	<70 years	119	48.4%
	≥70 years	127	51.6%
Gender			
	male	195	79.3%
	female	51	20.7%
Histological tumor grade [b]			
	low grade	42	17.1%
	high grade	172	69.9%
	na	32	13.0%
Tumor stage [b]			
	pTa	106	43.1%
	pTis	8	3.3%
	pT1	54	22.0%
	pT2	37	15.0%
	pT3	19	7.7%
	pT4	8	3.3%
	pTx	8	3.3%
	na	6	2.4%

[a] Only urine samples of patients preoperatively diagnosed with primary, bladder cancer (BCa, without any other malignancy) were included; [b] According to WHO 2004 classification; BPH: prostate hyperplasia; PCa: prostate cancer; GRT: germline tumor; RCC: renal cell carcinoma; na: not available

4.3. DNA Extraction from Urines

The urine sediments of training cohort I (Aachen–Bonn) stored at −80 °C were subjected to DNA extraction by using the ZR Urine DNA Isolation Kit (ZR, Zymo Research, Freiburg, Germany), following the manufacturer's instructions. DNA extraction from the urine sediments of training cohort II (Dresden) stored at −80 °C in RLT buffer was performed by using the QIAamp DNA Mini Kit (Qiagen, Hilden, Germany), according to the manufacturer's instructions. The DNA yield (ng/mL urine) and purity (A_{260}/A_{280}) were determined by using the NanoDrop (Thermo Fisher Scientific, Waltham, MA, USA). Only extractions from urines with a minimal total amount of 100 ng genomic DNA and a ratio of ≥1.5 were finally used for qMSP, pyrosequencing, and MSRE qPCR analyses.

4.4. DNA Bisulfite Conversion

100 to 250 ng of the genomic DNA (training cohort I) were bisulfite-converted for 14 to 16 h by using the EZ DNA Methylation™ kit (Zymo Research) according to the manufacturer's instructions. Bisulfite-converted DNA was eluted in 20 μL of TRIS-EDTA buffer.

4.5. Bisulfite-Pyrosequencing

The pyrosequencing of bisulfite-converted DNA was performed by using the PyroMark PCR Kit, the PyroMark96 ID device, and the PyroGoldSQA reagent Kit (Qiagen), as reported previously [20]. *ECRG4* and *ITIH5* pyrosequencing assays were designed by using the Pyromark Assay Design Software (Qiagen), and Supplementary Table S3 lists all of the primers. Primers and sequence of interest meet the following criteria: Based on TCGA data analyses, sequences of interest should cover promoter regions that a) are characterized by strong differences in mean DNA methylation between urothelial normal and bladder cancer samples and b) are located in important gene regulatory sequences, i.e., a statistically significant inverse correlation between *ECRG4/ITIH5* gene expression and the corresponding DNA methylation had to be observed. The EpiTect®PCR Control DNA Set (Qiagen) was used as the positive controls for unmethylated and methylated DNA in each run.

4.6. Quantitative Methylation-Specific PCR (qMSP)

Bisulfite-modified DNA was used as a template for fluorescence-based real-time PCR amplified in an iCycler iQ5 (Biorad, Munich, Germany), as previously described [37] with slight modifications: The designed primers and probes were specific for amplifying bisulfite-converted DNA for the genes of interest (*ECRG4* and *ITIH5*) (for cycle conditions, primer sequences, and annealing temperatures, see Supplementary Table S4). The reference gene *GAPDH* was used for internal normalization. Eight calibration dilutions of *in vitro* methylated human leukocyte DNA (0.1%, 1%, 5%, 10%, 20%, 30%, 50%, 100%) and unmethylated sequence (human leukocyte DNA from a healthy donor), as well as multiple water blanks were included in each run. The gene of interest was called methylated if the cycle threshold (Ct) of at least two of three qPCR replicates for each specimen had a value of less than 45 cycles. The amount of methylated DNA (percentage of methylated reference, PMR) at a specific locus was calculated by dividing the GENE/*GAPDH* ratio of a sample by the GENE/*GAPDH* ratio of SssI-treated human leukocyte DNA and multiplying by 100, as specified [37]. The primer binding sites of the qMSP assays were located in the same genomic promoter region as covered by pyrosequencing. The efficiencies of real time MSP were calculated according to the equation: $E = 10^{[-1/\text{slope of calibration dilutions}]}$ [41] and the mean efficacy of ECRG4 and ITIH5 qMSP was 76.57% and 77.76%, respectively.

4.7. Methylation Sensitive Restriction Enzyme qPCR (MSRE) qPCR

Isolated genomic DNA (125 ng) was used for double restriction digest. Methylation-sensitive restriction enzymes AciI and HpaII (New England Biolabs, NEB, MA, USA) were selected based on their capacity to distinguish methylated from unmethylated DNA sequences. Two independent digestion reactions (test reaction and control) were prepared for each patient DNA. Restriction digest was performed within a total volume of 25 μL in CutSmart Buffer (NEB) for 1 h at 37 °C and followed by heat inactivation for 20 min. at 80 °C. The control samples were treated in the same way but without the addition of the enzymes, 50% glycerol was added instead. Finally, DNA digest was diluted with 1x TE buffer before MSRE qPCR. The designed primers and probes for MSRE qPCR are specific for amplifying unrestricted DNA for the genes of interest (ECRG4, ITIH5, and NID2).

MSRE qPCRs were carried out while using the Roche LightCycler 480 II Real-Time PCR detection system. Mono color hydrolysis probe detection (FAM) was used. All of the samples were done in duplicate in 25 μL reactions containing 5 μL Reaction Mix B (Biotype GmbH, Dresden), 3 U Multi Taq 2 (Biotype), 1.5 μL primers and probes (5 μM each), nuclease-free water (Biotype), and 2 μL of digested DNA (2.5 ng/μL, test or control template). For *ECRG4* and *NID2*, the addition of Combinatorial Enhancer Solution (1× CES, [42]) was necessary due to the very high GC content of the amplified region.

For cycle conditions, primer sequences and annealing temperatures, see Supplementary Table S5. Ct values were analyzed while using LightCycler 480 Software (Hoffmann-La Roche AG, Basel, Switzerland).

Undetected Ct values were normalized to 47 for calculations. The methylation level of the amplified region was calculated by using the following equation: percent methylation = $100 \times 2^{-\Delta Ct}$, where ΔCt is the average Ct value from the test reaction minus the average Ct values from the control reaction. Methylation values exceeding 100% were set to 100%.

4.8. Analytical Assay Performances

RT112 wildtype bladder cancer cells harboring a methylated *ECRG4* and *ITIH5* promoter were cultured for two weeks. After cell counting RT112 cells were spiked into pooled urine of healthy donors ($n = 4$). Serial dilutions (10 to 10.000) of RT112 cells were added to 20 mL pooled urine, respectively, which was subsequently processed at the RWTH cBMB laboratories according to its standard operating protocol. Afterwards, urine pellets were either directly used for DNA extraction (probe set A) or urine sediments were stored according to the RWTH cBMB conditions by using two-dimensional (2D) barcoded LVL tubes (LVL technologies, Crailsheim, Germany) at −80 °C for two weeks (probe set B). Pooled urines without any spiked RT112 cells served as the control for normalization and threshold calculation by defining methylation cut-offs. Next, DNA was bisulfite-treated, as mentioned earlier, and the *ECRG4* and *ITIH5* qMSP as well as pyrosequencing assays were performed for *ECRG4* and *ITIH5*, respectively. The gene of interest was called methylated if the PMR (qMSP) or mean percent of CpG methylation (pyrosequencing) stably exceed the background noise and certainly maintained this threshold (=cut-off).

4.9. TCGA BLCA Data Set

Infinium HumanMethylation450 BeadChip data (level 2) and RNASeqV2 data (level 3) of the tumor and normal tissue samples were obtained from the TCGA data portal [30] and analyzed, as previously described [43].

4.10. Statistical Data Acquisition

Two-sided p-values that were less than 0.05 were considered to be significant. The non-parametric Mann–Whitney U-test was applied in order to compare two groups, whereas, in the case of more than two groups, the Dunn's multiple comparison test was used. Correlation analysis was performed by calculating a non-parametric *Spearman's rank* correlation coefficient. Statistical associations between clinico-pathological parameters and DNA methylation of *ITIH5* and *ECRG4* were determined by Fisher's exact test by using SPSS software version 25.0 (SPSS Inc., Chicago, IL, USA). Survival curves for overall survival (OS) were calculated using the Kaplan–Meier method with log-rank statistics. OS was measured from surgery until death and it was censored for patients alive without evidence of death at the last follow-up date. The receiver operating characteristics (ROC) curves and AUC values were calculated to assess the biomarker performance of *ECRG4* and *ITIH5* methylation similar to our previous report [43]. The ROC curves of combined biomarkers were based on the binary logistic regression model using the probability as test variable.

Supplementary Materials: Supplementary materials can be found at http://www.mdpi.com/1422-0067/21/3/1117/s1.

Author Contributions: Conceptualization, M.R., N.T.G., M.B. and E.D.; Methodology, M.R., S.B., L.G., D.F., M.K., A.H., M.B.; Software and Statistics, M.R.; Resources, C.B., S.F., D.H., J.E., D.P.; Writing—Original Draft Preparation, M.R.; Writing–Editing, S.F. and M.B.; Writing—Review, all authors; Visualization, M.R.; Supervision, M.R., R.K., M.B., M.P.W. and E.D. All authors have read and agreed to the published version of the manuscript.

Acknowledgments: The authors appreciate the excellent technical support of Sonja von Sérenyi. Genomic 450K methylation and RNA seq. data used in this study were provided by the TCGA Research Network BLCA datasets (http://cancergenome.nih.gov). This work was supported by a grant from the Medical Faculty of the RWTH Aachen University (START program project 149/08).

Conflicts of Interest: M.R. and E.D. have been inventors of a patent application (Biomarker for Bladder Cancer. US Patent App. 14/389,393, 2016) that was later dropped by RWTH Aachen University for reasons of costs. All other authors declare that they have no conflict of interest.

References

1. Ferlay, J.; Colombet, M.; Soerjomataram, I.; Mathers, C.; Parkin, D.M.; Piñeros, M.; Znaor, A.; Bray, F. Estimating the global cancer incidence and mortality in 2018: GLOBOCAN sources and methods. *Int. J. Cancer* **2019**, *144*, 1941–1953. [CrossRef]

2. Yeung, C.; Dinh, T.; Lee, J. The health economics of bladder cancer: An updated review of the published literature. *Pharmacoeconomics* **2014**, *32*, 1093–1104. [CrossRef]

3. Leal, J.; Luengo-Fernandez, R.; Sullivan, R.; Witjes, J.A. Economic Burden of Bladder Cancer Across the European Union. *Eur. Urol.* **2016**, *69*, 438–447. [CrossRef]

4. Schlake, A.; Crispen, P.L.; Cap, A.P.; Atkinson, T.; Davenport, D.; Preston, D.M. NMP-22, urinary cytology, and cystoscopy: A 1 year comparison study. *Can. J. Urol.* **2012**, *19*, 6345–6350.

5. National Collaborating Centre for Cancer (UK). *Bladder Cancer: Diagnosis and Management*; National Institute for Health and Care Excellence: London, UK, 2015. Available online: https://www.ncbi.nlm.nih.gov/books/NBK305022/ (accessed on 5 February 2020).

6. Sarosdy, M.F.; Kahn, P.R.; Ziffer, M.D.; Love, W.R.; Barkin, J.; Abara, E.O.; Jansz, K.; Bridge, J.A.; Johansson, S.L.; Persons, D.L.; et al. Use of a multitarget fluorescence in situ hybridization assay to diagnose bladder cancer in patients with hematuria. *J. Urol.* **2006**, *176*, 44–47. [CrossRef]

7. Lotan, Y.; Roehrborn, C.G. Sensitivity and specificity of commonly available bladder tumor markers versus cytology: Results of a comprehensive literature review and meta-analyses. *Urology* **2003**, *61*, 109–118. [CrossRef]

8. Bhat, A.; Ritch, C.R. Urinary biomarkers in bladder cancer: Where do we stand? *Curr. Opin. Urol.* **2019**, *29*, 203–209. [CrossRef] [PubMed]

9. Bubendorf, L. Multiprobe fluorescence in situ hybridization (UroVysion) for the detection of urothelial carcinoma - FISHing for the right catch. *Acta Cytol.* **2011**, *55*, 113–119. [CrossRef] [PubMed]

10. Behrens, T.; Stenzl, A.; Brüning, T. Factors influencing false-positive results for nuclear matrix protein 22. *Eur. Urol.* **2014**, *66*, 970–972. [CrossRef]

11. Wang, Z.; Que, H.; Suo, C.; Han, Z.; Tao, J.; Huang, Z.; Ju, X.; Tan, R.; Gu, M. Evaluation of the NMP22 BladderChek test for detecting bladder cancer: A systematic review and meta-analysis. *Oncotarget* **2017**, *8*, 100648–100656. [CrossRef]

12. Pichler, R.; Fritz, J.; Tulchiner, G.; Klinglmair, G.; Soleiman, A.; Horninger, W.; Klocker, H.; Heidegger, I. Increased accuracy of a novel mRNA-based urine test for bladder cancer surveillance. *BJU Int.* **2018**, *121*, 29–37. [CrossRef] [PubMed]

13. Ecke, T.H.; Weiß, S.; Stephan, C.; Hallmann, S.; Arndt, C.; Barski, D.; Otto, T.; Gerullis, H. UBC®Rapid Test-A Urinary Point-of-Care (POC) Assay for Diagnosis of Bladder Cancer with a focus on Non-Muscle Invasive High-Grade Tumors: Results of a Multicenter-Study. *Int. J. Mol. Sci.* **2018**, *19*, 3841. [CrossRef] [PubMed]

14. Baylin, S.B.; Jones, P.A. A decade of exploring the cancer epigenome-biological and translational implications. *Nat. Rev. Cancer.* **2011**, *11*, 726–734. [CrossRef] [PubMed]

15. Molnár, B.; Tóth, K.; Barták, B.K.; Tulassay, Z. Plasma methylated septin 9: A colorectal cancer screening marker. *Expert Rev. Mol. Diagn.* **2015**, *15*, 171–184. [CrossRef]

16. Larsen, L.K.; Lind, G.E.; Guldberg, P.; Dahl, C. DNA-Methylation-Based Detection of Urological Cancer in Urine: Overview of Biomarkers and Considerations on Biomarker Design, Source of DNA, and Detection Technologies. *Int. J. Mol. Sci.* **2019**, *20*, 2657. [CrossRef]

17. Veeck, J.; Chorovicer, M.; Naami, A.; Breuer, E.; Zafrakas, M.; Bektas, N.; Dürst, M.; Kristiansen, G.; Wild, P.J.; Hartmann, A.; et al. The extracellular matrix protein ITIH5 is a novel prognostic marker in invasive node-negative breast cancer and its aberrant expression is caused by promoter hypermethylation. *Oncogene* **2008**, *27*, 865–876. [CrossRef]

18. Kloten, V.; Rose, M.; Kaspar, S.; von Stillfried, S.; Knüchel, R.; Dahl, E. Epigenetic inactivation of the novel candidate tumor suppressor gene ITIH5 in colon cancer predicts unfavorable overall survival in the CpG island methylator phenotype. *Epigenetics* **2014**, *9*, 1290–1301. [CrossRef]

19. Dötsch, M.M.; Kloten, V.; Schlensog, M.; Heide, T.; Braunschweig, T.; Veeck, J.; Petersen, I.; Knüchel, R.; Dahl, E. Low expression of ITIH5 in adenocarcinoma of the lung is associated with unfavorable patients' outcome. *Epigenetics* **2015**, *10*, 903–912. [CrossRef]

20. Rose, M.; Gaisa, N.T.; Antony, P.; Fiedler, D.; Heidenreich, A.; Otto, W.; Denzinger, S.; Bertz, S.; Hartmann, A.; Karl, A.; et al. Epigenetic inactivation of ITIH5 promotes bladder cancer progression and predicts early relapse of pT1 high-grade urothelial tumours. *Carcinogenesis* **2014**, *35*, 727–736. [CrossRef]

21. Rose, M.; Kloten, V.; Noetzel, E.; Gola, L.; Ehling, J.; Heide, T.; Meurer, S.K.; Gaiko-Shcherbak, A.; Sechi, A.S.; Huth, S.; et al. ITIH5 mediates epigenetic reprogramming of breast cancer cells. *Mol. Cancer* **2017**, *16*, 44. [CrossRef]

22. Rose, M.; Meurer, S.K.; Kloten, V.; Weiskirchen, R.; Denecke, B.; Antonopoulos, W.; Deckert, M.; Knüchel, R.; Dahl, E. ITIH5 induces a shift in TGF-β superfamily signaling involving Endoglin and reduces risk for breast cancer metastasis and tumor death. *Mol. Carcinog.* **2018**, *57*, 167–181. [CrossRef] [PubMed]

23. Sasaki, K.; Kurahara, H.; Young, E.D.; Natsugoe, S.; Ijichi, A.; Iwakuma, T.; Welch, D.R. Genome-wide in vivo RNAi screen identifies ITIH5 as a metastasis suppressor in pancreatic cancer. *Clin. Exp. Metastasis* **2017**, *34*, 229–239. [CrossRef] [PubMed]

24. Yue, C.M.; Deng, D.J.; Bi, M.X.; Guo, L.P.; Lu, S.H. Expression of ECRG4, a novel esophageal cancer-related gene, downregulated by CpG island hypermethylation in human esophageal squamous cell carcinoma. *World J. Gastroenterol.* **2003**, *9*, 1174–1178. [CrossRef] [PubMed]

25. Li, L.W.; Yu, X.Y.; Yang, Y.; Zhang, C.P.; Guo, L.P.; Lu, S.H. Expression of esophageal cancer related gene 4 (ECRG4), a novel tumor suppressor gene, in esophageal cancer and its inhibitory effect on the tumor growth in vitro and in vivo. *Int. J. Cancer* **2009**, *125*, 1505–1513. [CrossRef]

26. Tang, G.Y.; Tang, G.J.; Yin, L.; Chao, C.; Zhou, R.; Ren, G.P.; Chen, J.Y.; Zhang, W. ECRG4 acts as a tumor suppressor gene frequently hypermethylated in human breast cancer. *Biosci. Rep.* **2019**, *39*, BSR20190087. [CrossRef]

27. Luo, L.; Wu, J.; Xie, J.; Xia, L.; Qian, X.; Cai, Z.; Li, Z. Downregulated ECRG4 is associated with poor prognosis in renal cell cancer and is regulated by promoter DNA methylation. *Tumour Biol.* **2016**, *37*, 1121–1129. [CrossRef]

28. Götze, S.; Feldhaus, V.; Traska, T.; Wolter, M.; Reifenberger, G.; Tannapfel, A.; Kuhnen, C.; Martin, D.; Müller, O.; Sievers, S. ECRG4 is a candidate tumor suppressor gene frequently hypermethylated in colorectal carcinoma and glioma. *BMC Cancer* **2009**, *9*, 447. [CrossRef]

29. Cai, Z.; Liang, P.; Xuan, J.; Wan, J.; Guo, H. ECRG4 as a novel tumor suppressor gene inhibits colorectal cancer cell growth in vitro and in vivo. *Tumour Biol.* **2016**, *37*, 9111–9120. [CrossRef]

30. Cancer Genome Atlas Research Network. Comprehensive molecular characterization of urothelial bladder carcinoma. *Nature* **2014**, *507*, 315–322. [CrossRef]

31. Renard, I.; Joniau, S.; van Cleynenbreugel, B.; Collette, C.; Naômé, C.; Vlassenbroeck, I.; Nicolas, H.; de Leval, J.; Straub, J.; Van Criekinge, W.; et al. Identification and validation of the methylated TWIST1 and NID2 genes through real-time methylation-specific polymerase chain reaction assays for the noninvasive detection of primary bladder cancer in urine samples. *Eur. Urol.* **2010**, *58*, 96–104. [CrossRef]

32. Song, L.; Jia, J.; Peng, X.; Xiao, W.; Li, Y. The performance of the SEPT9 gene methylation assay and a comparison with other CRC screening tests: A meta-analysis. *Sci. Rep.* **2017**, *7*, 3032. [CrossRef] [PubMed]

33. Lodewijk, I.; Dueñas, M.; Rubio, C.; Munera-Maravilla, E.; Segovia, C.; Bernardini, A.; Teijeira, A.; Paramio, J.M.; Suárez-Cabrera, C. Liquid Biopsy Biomarkers in Bladder Cancer: A Current Need for Patient Diagnosis and Monitoring. *Int. J. Mol. Sci.* **2018**, *19*, 2514. [CrossRef]

34. Costa, V.L.; Henrique, R.; Danielsen, S.A.; Duarte-Pereira, S.; Eknaes, M.; Skotheim, R.I.; Rodrigues, A.; Magalhães, J.S.; Oliveira, J.; Lothe, R.A.; et al. Three epigenetic biomarkers, GDF15, TMEFF2, and VIM, accurately predict bladder cancer from DNA-based analyses of urine samples. *Clin. Cancer Res.* **2010**, *16*, 5842–5851. [CrossRef] [PubMed]

35. Van der Heijden, A.G.; Mengual, L.; Ingelmo-Torres, M.; Lozano, J.J.; van Rijt-van de Westerlo, C.C.M.; Baixauli, M.; Geavlete, B.; Moldoveanud, C.; Ene, C.; Dinney, C.P.; et al. Urine cell-based DNA methylation classifier for monitoring bladder cancer. *Clin. Epigenetics* **2018**, *10*, 71. [CrossRef] [PubMed]

36. Hernández, H.G.; Tse, M.Y.; Pang, S.C.; Arboleda, H.; Forero, D.A. Optimizing methodologies for PCR-based DNA methylation analysis. *Biotechniques* **2013**, *55*, 181–197. [CrossRef] [PubMed]

37. Feber, A.; Dhami, P.; Dong, L.; de Winter, P.; Tan, W.S.; Martínez-Fernández, M.; Paul, D.S.; Hynes-Allen, A.; Rezaee, S.; Gurung, P.; et al. UroMark-a urinary biomarker assay for the detection of bladder cancer. *Clin. Epigenetics* **2017**, *9*, 8. [CrossRef] [PubMed]

38. Kloten, V.; Becker, B.; Winner, K.; Schrauder, M.G.; Fasching, P.A.; Anzeneder, T.; Veeck, J.; Hartmann, A.; Knüchel, R.; Dahl, E. Promoter hypermethylation of the tumor-suppressor genes ITIH5, DKK3, and RASSF1A as novel biomarkers for blood-based breast cancer screening. *Breast Cancer Res.* **2013**, *15*, R4. [CrossRef]

39. Shahin, O.; Thalmann, G.N.; Rentsch, C.; Mazzucchelli, L.; Studer, U.E. A retrospective analysis of 153 patients treated with or without intravesical bacillus Calmette-Guerin for primary stage T1 grade 3 bladder cancer: Recurrence, progression and survival. *J. Urol.* **2003**, *169*, 96–100. [CrossRef]

40. Witjes, J.A.; Morote, J.; Cornel, E.B.; Gakis, G.; van Valenberg, F.J.P.; Lozano, F.; Sternberg, I.A.; Willemsen, E.; Hegemann, M.L.; Paitan, Y.; et al. Performance of the Bladder EpiCheck™ Methylation Test for Patients Under Surveillance for Non-muscle-invasive Bladder Cancer: Results of a Multicenter, Prospective, Blinded Clinical Trial. *Eur. Urol. Oncol.* **2018**, *1*, 307–313. [CrossRef]

41. Pfaffl, M.W. A new mathematical model for relative quantification in real-time RT-PCR. *Nucleic Acids Res.* **2001**, *29*, e45. [CrossRef]

42. Ralser, M.; Querfurth, R.; Warnatz, H.J.; Lehrach, H.; Yaspo, M.L.; Krobitsch, S. An efficient and economic enhancer mix for PCR. *Biochem. Biophys. Res. Commun.* **2006**, *347*, 747–751. [CrossRef] [PubMed]

43. Mijnes, J.; Veeck, J.; Gaisa, N.T.; Burghardt, E.; de Ruijter, T.C.; Gostek, S.; Dahl, E.; Pfister, D.; Schmid, S.C.; Knüchel, R.; et al. Promoter methylation of DNA damage repair (DDR) genes in human tumor entities: RBBP8/CtIP is almost exclusively methylated in bladder cancer. *Clin. Epigenetics* **2018**, *10*, 15. [CrossRef] [PubMed]

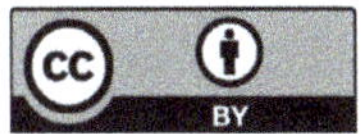

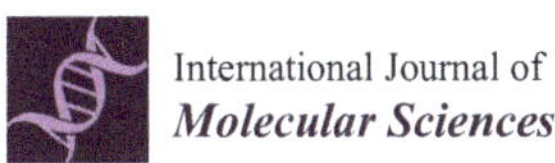
International Journal of
Molecular Sciences

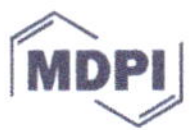

Article

STAT3/5 Inhibitors Suppress Proliferation in Bladder Cancer and Enhance Oncolytic Adenovirus Therapy

Sruthi V. Hindupur [1,†], Sebastian C. Schmid [1,†], Jana Annika Koch [1], Ahmed Youssef [1,2], Eva-Maria Baur [1], Dongbiao Wang [1], Thomas Horn [1], Julia Slotta-Huspenina [3], Juergen E. Gschwend [1], Per Sonne Holm [1] and Roman Nawroth [1,*]

[1] Department of Urology, Klinikum rechts der Isar, Technical University of Munich, 81675 Munich, Germany; sruthi.hindupur@tum.de (S.V.H.); sebastian.schmid@tum.de (S.C.S.); jana.koch@tum.de (J.A.K.); ahmed0122@med.bsu.edu.eg (A.Y.); e-m.baur@gmx.de (E.-M.B.); dongbiao.wang@tum.de (D.W.); t.horn@tum.de (T.H.); juergen.gschwend@tum.de (J.E.G.); per.holm@tum.de (P.S.H.)
[2] Department of Urology, Beni-suef University, Beni Suef 62511, Egypt
[3] Department of Pathology, Klinikum rechts der Isar, Technical University of Munich, 81675 Munich, Germany; julia.slotta-huspenina@tum.de
* Correspondence: roman.nawroth@tum.de; Tel.: +49-089-4140-2553
† These authors contributed equally to this work.

Received: 17 January 2020; Accepted: 5 February 2020; Published: 7 February 2020

Abstract: The JAK-STAT signalling pathway regulates cellular processes like cell division, cell death and immune regulation. Dysregulation has been identified in solid tumours and STAT3 activation is a marker for poor outcome. The aim of this study was to explore potential therapeutic strategies by targeting this pathway in bladder cancer (BC). High STAT3 expression was detected in 51.3% from 149 patient specimens with invasive bladder cancer by immunohistochemistry. Protein expression of JAK, STAT and downstream targets were confirmed in 10 cell lines. Effects of the JAK inhibitors Ruxolitinib and BSK-805, and STAT3/5 inhibitors Stattic, Nifuroxazide and SH-4-54 were analysed by cell viability assays, immunoblotting, apoptosis and cell cycle progression. Treatment with STAT3/5 but not JAK1/2 inhibitors reduced survival, levels of phosphorylated STAT3 and Cyclin-D1 and increased apoptosis. Tumour xenografts, using the chicken chorioallantoic membrane (CAM) model responded to Stattic monotherapy. Combination of Stattic with Cisplatin, Docetaxel, Gemcitabine, Paclitaxel and CDK4/6 inhibitors showed additive effects. The combination of Stattic with the oncolytic adenovirus XVir-N-31 increased viral replication and cell lysis. Our results provide evidence that inhibitors against STAT3/5 are promising as novel mono- and combination therapy in bladder cancer.

Keywords: bladder cancer; JAK-STAT pathway; combination therapy; oncolytic adenovirus; virotherapy; STAT3/5 inhibitor; JAK inhibitor; XVir-N-31

---

1. Introduction

Bladder cancer (BC) is the 10th most common cancer in the world, as of 2018 [1]. Approximately 25% of patients present as muscle invasive bladder cancer (MIBC) at time of diagnosis. Metastasized BC patients face a poor outcome with median survival time of approximately 14 months and the survival rates have remained largely unchanged for the past 30 years until the emergence of immune checkpoint inhibitors (ICB). Checkpoint inhibitors targeting programmed cell death protein 1 (PD-1) or programmed cell death 1 ligand 1 (PD-L1) have demonstrated durable responses in patients with cisplatin-refractory metastasized BC [2]. However, only 13–21% of patients with metastatic BC respond to immune checkpoint inhibition [3–5].

To find new therapeutic approaches, a plethora of compounds are being tested in clinical trials targeting various signalling pathways in MIBC, including inhibitors of EGFR, HER2, VEGF and the

PI3K/AKT/mTOR pathway [6]. Clinical trials so far have demonstrated that only sub-cohorts of patients benefit from those treatment strategies, probably due to required molecular alterations for therapy response [6]. In 2019, the FGFR inhibitor Balversa (Erdafitinib) was approved by the FDA (Food and Drug Administration) for treatment of patients with metastatic bladder cancer harbouring molecular alterations in FGFR2/3, marking it to be the first targeted therapy to be approved in bladder cancer [7]. Most targeted therapies have shown inconsistent results in early phase clinical trials, which could be attributed to suboptimal selection criteria and biomarker selection, and molecular heterogeneity of the disease [6,8]. Thus, it is not only necessary to identify suitable molecular targets but also predictive markers and combination therapies that broaden the spectrum of responders to treatment.

The JAK-STAT pathway is one of the most studied pathways in cellular signal transduction with diverse roles in physiological processes including cell growth and differentiation and immune response via cytokine signalling [9]. Dysregulations in this pathway are implicated in carcinogenesis and are also associated with poor prognosis in various cancers including kidney cancer [10], lung cancer [11], cervical cancer [12] and bladder cancer [13,14]. The JAK (Janus Kinase) protein family consists of JAK1-3 and Tyk2 in mammals. These proteins are non-receptor tyrosine kinases that are associated with transmembrane cytokine receptors. Signalling is initiated upon binding of a wide range of cytokines (interleukins, interferons, growth factors) to their appropriate receptor. This leads to the dimerization of receptors, bringing the JAKs into close proximity and facilitating transphosphorylation. These activated JAK proteins mediate phosphorylation of STAT proteins. The STAT (signal transducer and activator of transcription) protein family comprises of 7 family members (STAT-1, 2, 3, 4, 5a, 5b and 6). The phosphorylated state results in dimerization and eventual translocation to the nucleus where STATs can activate transcription of target genes. STAT3, in particular, plays a role in cell cycle regulation, cytokine signalling and apoptosis. Increased protein level and constitutive activation of STAT3 have also been reported in bladder cancer [13–17]. Elevated and increased nuclear level of STAT3 and p-STAT3 have been reported to be associated with invasiveness of the disease and advanced stages of the cancer [13,17–21]. Using a STAT3 transgenic mouse model, chemical induction of bladder cancer by N-butyl-N-(4-Hydroxybutyl) nitrosamine (BBN) directly resulted in the development of invasive carcinoma from carcinoma in situ, asserting the role of STAT3 in bladder cancer progression [18].

Considering these findings, we explored targeting of the JAK1/2 and STAT3/5 proteins using specific small molecule inhibitors and combined these inhibitors with standard chemotherapy, inhibitors of cell cycle progression and oncolytic adenovirus in preclinical models of bladder cancer. Several inhibitors for JAK and STAT proteins have been developed and JAK inhibitors were approved by the FDA for treatment of auto-immune disorders and myelofibrosis [22,23]. STAT3 inhibitors have shown anti-tumour activity in pre-clinical stages and have been successfully tested in phase-I clinical trials for safety and efficacy in solid tumours [24,25].

Application of targeted therapies as monotherapy has been shown to be largely influenced by a specific genetic background of patients or acquired resistance mechanisms in the clinical setting. These limitations can be improved by the use of combination therapies. STAT3 is implicated in the development of chemotherapy resistance in various cancers. Targeting STAT3 in combination with chemotherapeutics sensitises cells to chemotherapy in oral squamous cell carcinoma [26]. The interference with STAT3 activity has also been linked to cell cycle arrest either in G0/1 or in G2 phase [27,28]. Thus, we addressed the question if the combination of STAT3/5 inhibitors and inhibitors of cell cycle progression might be beneficial for therapy response. Targeted therapies against CDK4/6 pathway in bladder cancer showed promising data in various preclinical studies [29]. CDK4/6 inhibitors were approved by the FDA for the treatment of Hormone Receptor (HR)-positive and Human Epidermal Growth Factor Receptor 2 (HER2)-negative breast cancer. However, most patients inevitably develop resistance for multifactorial reasons [30,31]. Recently, our group demonstrated that the JAK-STAT pathway plays a role in acquired resistance of CDK4/6 inhibitors in bladder cancer [32]. In this study, we extended these data to show the efficiency of CDK4/6 inhibition by combining it with STAT3/5 inhibitors.

In recent years, there has been a surge in oncolytic virotherapy with several oncolytic viruses showing anti-cancer activity in patients [33]. The use of oncolytic viruses is a very promising new strategy in which native or modified viruses selectively target cancer cells and cause tumour elimination not only by viral spread but also by elicitation of an anti-tumour immune response [34]. As one example, Talimogene laherparepvec (T-Vec), a modified type I Herpes simplex virus for the treatment of advanced melanoma, was approved by the FDA [35]. A multitude of viruses from vesicular stomatitis virus, vaccinia virus or adenovirus are at various stages in clinical trials and most of them have a remarkable safety profile. Most side effects are infection-related or nausea and are easily manageable [36]. At preclinical level, it has been shown that oncolytic adenoviruses are successful in treating MIBC [37]. Several other oncolytic viruses have shown efficacy in urothelial carcinomas and some are currently tested in clinical trials [38]. Combination of oncolytic viruses with immune checkpoint inhibitors and targeted therapies has been proven to be a successful strategy to enhance the efficiency of therapy response to oncolytic virus [39,40]. There are studies showing that targeting the JAK-STAT pathway in combination with the oncolytic herpes simplex virus and vesicular stomatitis viruses could enhance their efficiency possibly by modulating IFN signalling [41,42]. Hence, in this study we investigated also the effects upon combining oncolytic adenovirus with STAT3/5 inhibitors in bladder cancer.

2. Results

2.1. JAK-STAT Pathway is Dysregulated in Bladder Cancer

Activation of JAK-STAT signalling, mostly by phosphorylation and protein level of STAT3/5 has been described in bladder cancer by several groups [14,15,20,43,44]. We wanted to specifically focus on involvement of JAK-STAT proteins as prognostic marker and also as potential targets for therapy. Thus, we included the 4 JAK family proteins and 7 STAT family proteins and analysed the data in the TCGA cohort consisting of 412 bladder cancer patients to identify molecular alterations in the JAK-STAT signalling pathway related genes (Table S1) [45]. In 54% of the patients, we found alterations in the selected genes (Figure 1A). The alterations in the JAK-STAT pathway did not have a significant effect on overall survival in patients with bladder cancer (Figure 1B). The TCGA cohort analysis showed that alterations in STAT3 were observed in 7%, STAT5A in 8% and STAT5B in 7% of patients. Alterations in JAK1 were observed in 8% and in JAK2 in 15% of patients indicating, that these genes are frequently altered in bladder cancer (Figure 1C). STAT3 and STAT5 are shown to interact majorly with JAK1 and 2. Statistically significant co-occurrence was found in between JAK2-STAT5A, STAT3-STAT5A and STAT3-STAT5B among others (Table S2). As for mutual exclusivity, none of the genes showed any significance.

Subsequently, considering the TCGA analysis results, we also performed immunohistochemistry to determine STAT3 expression. Here, we wanted to confirm that increased expression level of STAT3 protein might serve as a prognostic marker. We used a previously described tissue microarray including tissue specimen from urothelial carcinoma patients with metastatic disease limited to lymph nodes from 149 patients from January 2003 until December 2012. The clinical characteristics of the patients are described in a prior publication [46]. We analysed STAT3 staining in sections from tumour centre. In total, 14/149 showed no staining, 18/149 showed low intensity staining, 34/149 had moderate staining and 74/149 had high intensity staining (Figure 1D). It was established that 9/149 sections were not evaluable due to a technical reason. When correlating the expression with cancer specific survival, we could not observe any significant difference in survival among no/low staining vs. moderate/high staining (Figure 1E). This also correlates with the survival data from the TCGA cohort. However, the high number of patients positively expressing STAT3 qualifies this protein as a potential molecular target.

Inhibitors against JAK1/2 and STAT3/5 are most advanced in clinical use and molecular alterations in STAT3 and STAT5 genes have previously been shown to be altered in various solid cancers [10,12,47,48]. Based on the TCGA results, we decided to analyse expression and activation level of JAK1/2 and STAT3 in a panel of 10 different bladder cancer derived cell lines. Constitutive expression of JAK1/2 protein was detected in all cell lines (Figure 1G). However, phosphorylation of JAK1/2 could not be detected. In all cell lines, expression of STAT3 protein and also its constitutive phosphorylation was detected although at different level in between cell lines.

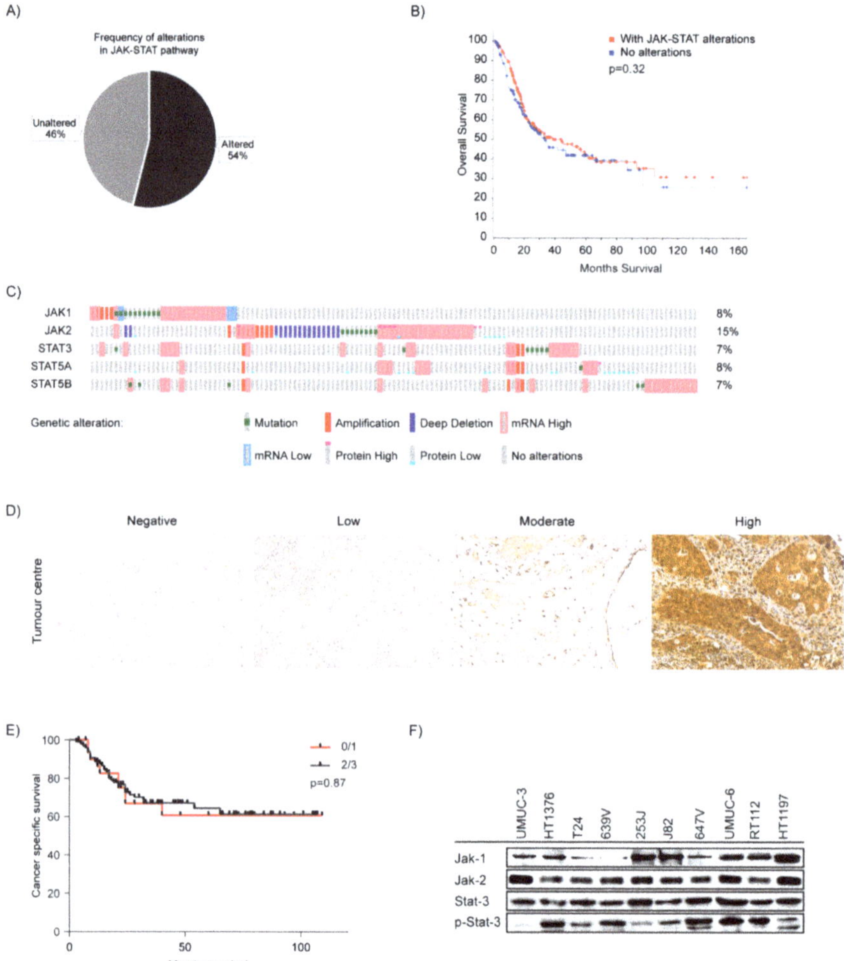

Figure 1. JAK-STAT pathway in bladder cancer: (**A**) TCGA cohort of 412 patients (413 samples) was analysed using cBioPortal. JAK-STAT pathway was altered in 54% of bladder cancer specimens. (**B**) Kalpan-Meier plot depicting overall survival analysis among patients with and without alterations in JAK-STAT pathway in the TCGA cohort. (**C**) Alterations in JAK1, JAK2, STAT3, STAT5A and STAT5B genes—OncoPrint indicates tumours altered with mutations (green bars), amplification (red bars), homozygous deletion (blue bars), high mRNA (red—outlined bars), mRNA low (blue-outlined bars), protein high (bars with red cap), protein low (blue-bottomed bars) and no alterations (grey bars). (**D**) Immunohistochemistry of patient tissues stained for STAT3- images showing staining intensities- Negative (Score-0), Low (Score-1), Moderate (Score-2), High (Score-3). Tissue sections were imaged at 200× magnification. (**E**) Kaplan-Meier plots for cancer specific survival analysis among patients with no or low STAT3 staining vs. moderate/high STAT3 staining. (**F**) Cell lines were analysed for Jak1, Jak2, Stat3 expression and Stat3 phosphorylation by immunoblotting.

2.2. JAK1/2 Inhibitors Have No Effect on Proliferation in Bladder Cancer Cell Lines

We wanted to explore whether upstream inhibition of the JAK-STAT pathway would affect cell viability and used the inhibitors Ruxolitinib targeting JAK1/2 and BSK805 which is a specific JAK2 inhibitor. The effect of these drugs on cell viability was tested in a bladder cancer cell panel of 10 different cell lines. Cells were treated with serial concentrations of Ruxolitinib (0.015–10 μM) and BSK805 (0.0125 to 1 μM). Ruxolitinib did not have any effect on cell viability (Figure 2A and Figure S1). The JAK2 inhibitor, BSK-805 diminished cell growth only on the cell lines T24, J82 and RT112, whereas the other cell lines did not respond (Figure 2B and Figure S2). Overall, the inhibition of JAK1/2 proteins did not substantially interfere with cell growth which might be due to the observation that JAK1/2 protein was also not phosphorylated and thus not activated.

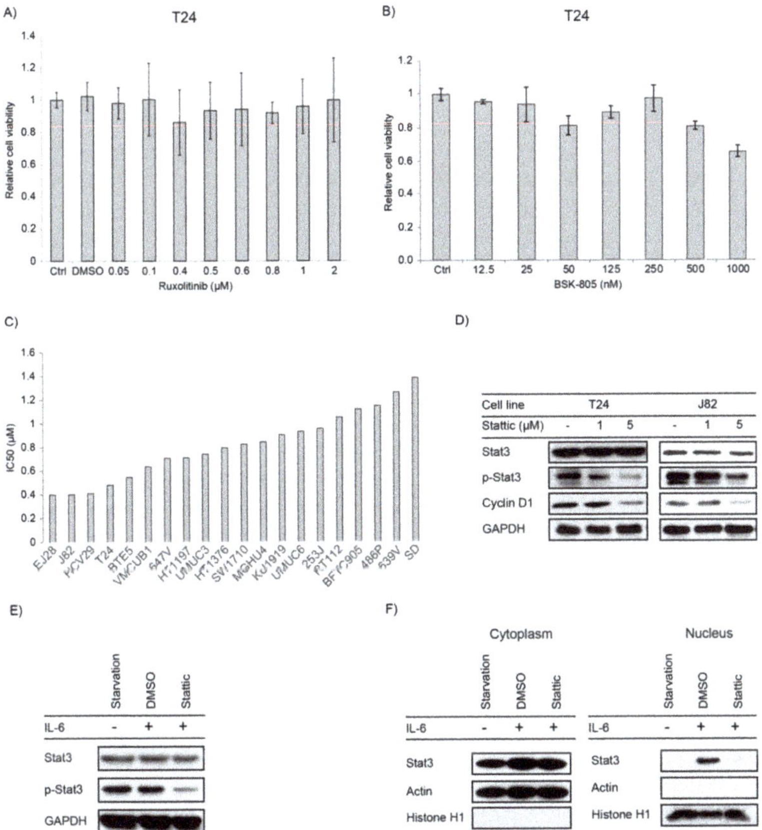

Figure 2. A) JAK inhibition by specific inhibitors: T24 cells were treated with increasing concentrations of (**A**) Ruxolitinib and (**B**) BSK-805 and cell viability was assessed by CellTiter-Blue® Cell Viability Assay 72 h after treatment. Error bars S.E. STAT3 inhibition by Stattic: (**C**) Cell viability was assessed by CellTiter-Blue® Cell Viability Assay 72 h after treatment with Stattic and IC50 was determined. Cell lines arranged according to IC50 values. (**D**) T24 and J82 cells were starved for 4 h then activated with 25% FBS and simultaneously treated with serial concentrations of Stattic and DMSO as a control followed by immunoblotting. (**E**) T24 cells were serum starved overnight, treated with 5 μM Stattic (or DMSO) for 3 hours then activated with IL-6 (25 ng/mL) for 30 min before being harvested; protein expression and phosphorylation were analysed by Immunoblotting. (**F**) Cells were treated the same as in (**E**). Compartmental protein extraction was performed, and the lysates were analysed by Immunoblotting.

2.3. STAT3/5 Inhibitors Reduced Proliferation and Downstream Signaling in Bladder Cancer Cell Lines

We also examined effects of STAT3/5 inhibitors on bladder cancer cell growth. Therefore, we applied the specific STAT3/5 inhibitors Stattic and SH-4-54 to 10 different bladder cancer cell lines, and Nifuroxazide in T24 and RT112 cell lines. All inhibitors resulted in dose dependent reduction in cell proliferation in the cell lines tested (Figures S3 and S4). As for Stattic, we extended the number of cell lines to 20 and all cell lines showed a dose-dependent response to Stattic treatment (Figure 2C and Figure S5).

We investigated also the molecular response to Stattic treatment by examining protein levels of total and phosphorylated STAT3. Therefore, we first examined the effect of STAT3 on the constitutive phosphorylation level on T24 and J82 cells which could be suppressed upon treatment in a dose dependent manner (Figure 2D). This effect of Stattic was also confirmed by analysis of the STAT3 downstream effector molecule Cyclin D1, which was downregulated upon treatment.

We also confirmed activity of Stattic on phosphorylation level of STAT3 and its subcellular localization upon an extracellular stimulus, using IL-6. Cells were serum starved, followed by interleukin-6 (IL-6) stimulation. IL-6 stimulation did not result in a further increase in the constitutive STAT3 phosphorylation, but STAT3 phosphorylation could still be suppressed by Stattic (Figure 2E). We then tested the nuclear translocation of STAT3 upon Stattic treatment to evaluate the molecular mechanism of Stattic inhibition. Nuclear and cytoplasmic protein fractions were isolated and the level of total STAT3 and activated STAT3 were analysed. As for control of the purity of the protein compartments, presence of Histone H1 and actin was examined. Interestingly, only after IL-6 treatment we detected a nuclear translocation of STAT3 that was suppressed by Stattic (Figure 2F).

2.4. Stattic Induced G2/M Arrest and Apoptosis in Bladder Cancer Cell Lines

STAT3 and 5 have diverse roles in cells including cell cycle regulation and apoptosis [49]. To investigate whether Stattic influences cell cycle in bladder cancer cells, we treated T24 with Stattic in increasing doses and performed cell cycle analysis measuring BrdU incorporation by flow cytometry, 24 h after treatment. We observed that Stattic induced a G2/M cell cycle arrest in cells (Figure 3A). We also investigated whether Stattic induces apoptosis in a concentration kinetic using T24 cells. Thus, 24 h after treatment, a dose dependent 9-fold increase in Caspase3/7 activity was determined (Figure 3B). From the above results, it is implied that Stattic is acting as a cytostatic and a cytotoxic agent in bladder cancer.

2.5. Stattic Reduced Tumour Growth in 3-Dimensional Xenografts

To further test the effect of Stattic on tumour xenografts, we used the chicken chorioallantoic membrane (CAM) model. As for the purpose of this study, this model reflects characteristics of an immunocompromised mouse model, including the development of a host derived vasculature and extracellular matrix [50]. Hence, we tested the effect of Stattic in vivo by using the CAM model to grow three-dimensional in vivo xenografts of RT112 cells. T24 cells could not be used in the CAM assay as they do not grow well and form very small tumours on the CAM. A significant weight reduction in tumour xenografts, reflecting tumour growth reduction of up to 50% was observed upon treatment with Stattic (Figure 3C). We also performed Ki-67 staining on the CAM tumour tissue sections to estimate the Stattic effect on tumour proliferation in the xenografts. A significant decrease in Ki-67 positive cells was observed in the Stattic treated tumours as compared to untreated tumours (Figure 3D). This correlates with the observed decrease in tumour cell proliferation in vitro.

2.6. Combination of Stattic and Chemotherapeutic Agents Showed Additivity

STAT3 has been shown to be activated in response to chemotherapeutic agents and mediating drug-resistance in several cancers. Hence, we wanted to explore potential options for combination therapy with Stattic and standard chemotherapeutic drugs. We chose 5 bladder cancer cell lines

(HT1376, J82, RT112, SD and T24) with different sensitivities to Stattic monotherapy: J82 as one of the best responder cell lines to Stattic, T24, HT1376 and RT112 as intermediate responder cell lines and SD as lowest responding cell line.

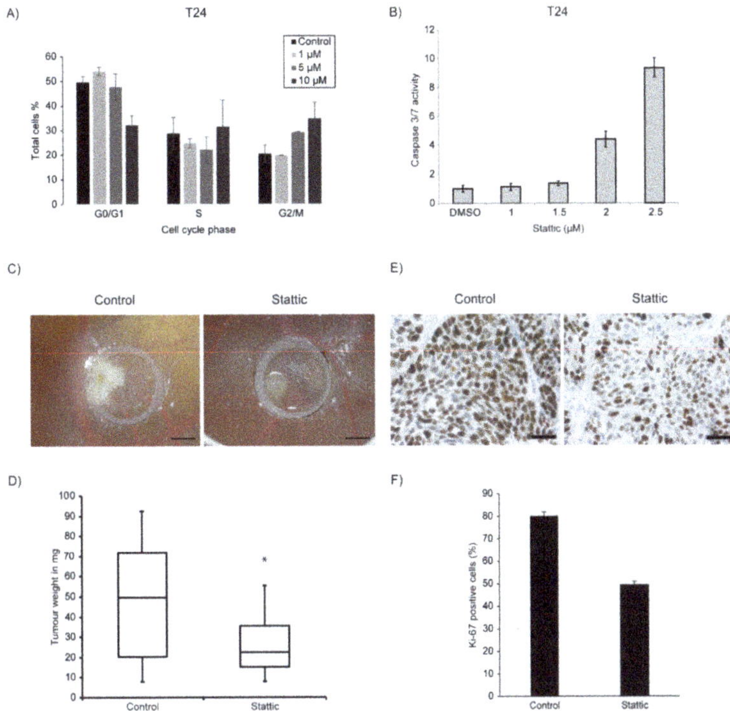

Figure 3. (**A**) Analysis of cell cycle progression in T24 treated with the indicated concentrations of Stattic for 24 h. An increase in G2 population was found with increasing concentration. (**B**) Caspase 3/7 assay for the apoptosis in T24 cells incubated for 24 h with the indicated concentrations of Stattic. The percentage of apoptotic cells was increased in a dose-dependent manner. (**C**) Stattic reduces the bladder cancer cell growth in vivo. Representative images of RT112 cells show tumour formation of Stattic versus control group on the CAM inside a silicone ring, 6 days after seeding of cells. Scale bar equals 2 mm. (**D**) Tumours from indicated cell line were harvested and weighed after Stattic ($n = 21$) or control (DMSO) ($n = 19$) treatment ('*' indicates $p = 0.0069$). (**E**) Tissue sections from the tumours were stained for Ki-67. (**F**) Number of Ki-67 positive cells were counted and compared between Control (DMSO) and Stattic-treated groups. Scale bar equals 4 μm. Error bars S.E.

The cell viability of bladder cancer cell lines in response to the increasing doses of single drugs and combination treatment of Stattic and Cisplatin, Docetaxel, Gemcitabine or Paclitaxel was investigated using the CellTiter-Blue® Cell Viability Assay. Dose response curves for the mono- and combination therapy were generated (Figure S6). Data were analysed using the Chou-Talalay theorem to generate a combination index (CI). According to the theorem, CI values less than 1 indicate a synergistic interaction, while values equal to or greater than 1 indicate additive or antagonistic effects respectively [51]. The combination index was calculated for the combination causing 50% inhibition of cell viability (Fa50). In HT1376 cells, the combination index for all the combinations of Stattic and chemotherapeutic agents were in the range of 1 indicating additivity. In SD cells, the combination index for most of the combinations of Stattic and chemotherapeutic agents were more than 1 indicating antagonism. In T24, J82 and RT112 cells, the combination index varies from additivity to antagonism depending on the combinations (Figure 4).

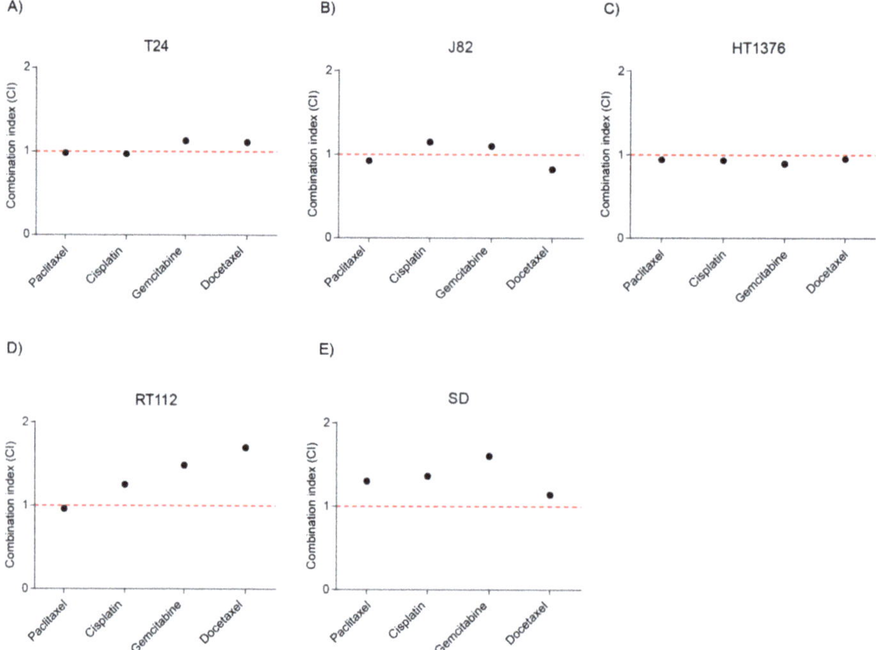

Figure 4. Combination therapy with Stattic and chemotherapeutics. Treatment of the respective cell lines was done for 72 h with Stattic alone and in a fixed ratio combination with Paclitaxel, Cisplatin, Gemcitabine or Docetaxel in (**A**) T24, (**B**) J82, (**C**) HT1376, (**D**) RT112, and (**E**) SD cell lines (See Materials and methods). Combination index (CI) for combining Stattic with Paclitaxel, Cisplatin, Gemcitabine or Docetaxel were plotted. Values were calculated using the Chou-Talalay theorem. CI < 1: synergy, CI = 1; additivity, CI > 1: antagonism.

2.7. Combination of Stattic and CDK4/6 inhibitor Palbociclib Showed Additivity

Our group has previously shown that STAT3 is one of the proteins contributing to therapy resistance to the CDK4/6 inhibitor Palbociclib. Palbociclib induces a G1 arrest in cells. The rational to combine both inhibitors was to induce both G1 and G2 arrest and using Stattic in a supportive role for enhancing Palbociclib activity. We tested this combination before in RT112 and T24 bladder cancer cell lines with slightly controversial results and included here additionally UMUC-3 cells [32]. UMUC-3 cells were treated with increasing doses of Stattic and a fixed concentration of Palbociclib and cell viability was assessed by sulphorhodamine-B assay and the CI was calculated. The combination index was around 1 indicating additive effect of the combination therapy (Figure 5A). In conclusion, the combination of both compounds results in additive activity but requires obviously also specific genetic predisposition as for substantial response limiting it to a subset of patients.

2.8. Stattic Enhanced Oncolytic Virotherapy of the Oncolytic Adenovirus XVir-N-31

Oncolytic virotherapy only recently entered clinical application and received FDA approval with a very favourable response rate and low adverse events [37]. It has been shown that the JAK-STAT pathway is activated upon adenoviral infection. As for viruses, such as vesicular stomatitis virus (VSV), inhibition of JAK by Ruxolitinib has been shown to support viral replication [41]. We combined Stattic with oncolytic adenovirus XVir-N-31 to suppress activation of STAT3/5 and analysed the effect on cell viability [37]. Cells were infected with XVir-N-31 24 h after treatment with Stattic. The combination treatment resulted in enhanced virus-induced cell death in both T24 and UMUC-3 cell lines (Figure 5B). We also observed increased viral replication in combination with Stattic which corresponded with an increase in viral particle formation (Figure 5C,D). Thus, inhibition of STAT3/5 substantially supports replication and viral particle production in cancer cells.

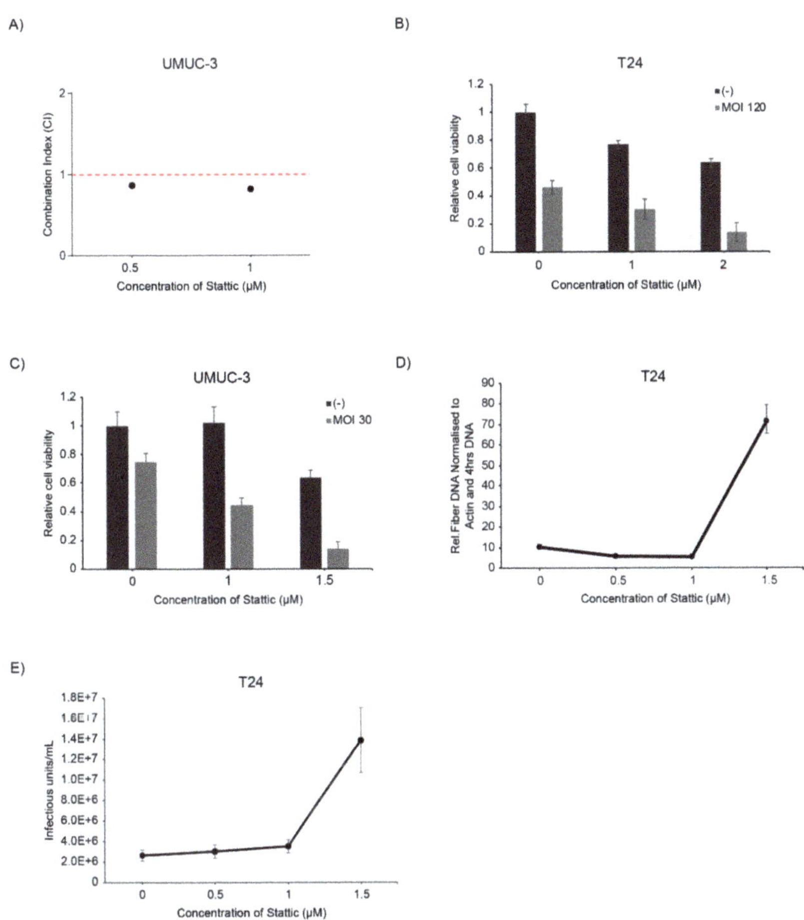

Figure 5. Combination therapy with Stattic and Palbociclib, and oncolytic virotherapy. (**A**) Treatment of the UMUC-3 cells was done for 72 h with Stattic alone at 0.5 μM and 1 μM and in a fixed concentration combination with 0.5 μM Palbociclib. Combination index (CI) for combining Stattic with Palbociclib were plotted. Values were calculated using the Chou-Talalay theorem. (**C**). Cells were treated with Stattic and infected with XVir-N-31 with corresponding multiplicity of infections (MOI) in T24 (**B**) and in UMUC-3 cells (**C**). The MOIs are indicated in the graphs. Cell viability was analysed at 4dpi by sulphorhodamine B assay. Error bars S.E. (**D,E**) T24 cells were infected with XVir-N-31 (MOI 50) and treated with increasing concentrations of Stattic (**D**) Viral replication was analysed at 48 h by qPCR of fibre DNA, and (**E**) the increase in viral titre upon Stattic inhibition is measured by hexon titre test and represented as infectious units/mL (IFU/mL).

3. Discussion

In this study, we analysed the potential use of targeting the JAK-STAT pathway for therapy in bladder cancer. It has been observed that expression level of STAT3 correlates with invasion and poor prognosis in bladder cancer [17–19,44]. However, other groups could not confirm the prognostic value of STAT3 expression level [14]. We analysed molecular alterations in JAK/STAT proteins in the TCGA dataset including 412 patient specimens of muscle invasive bladder cancer. This analysis revealed that genetic alterations in the molecular members of the JAK-STAT pathway are frequently found in bladder cancer but they are not suitable markers for prognosis. Analysis of STAT3 protein expression level on a TMA confirmed that most primary tumours of muscle invasive disease express high level of STAT3 but in this cohort STAT3 failed to be a prognostic marker for survival. In conclusion, the data presented here question the prognostic value of STAT3 in bladder cancer.

Previously, the JAK2 tyrosine kinase inhibitor AG490 has been tested in bladder cancer with positive results [52]. We wanted to further analyse if these data could be confirmed using the JAK1/2 inhibitor Ruxolitinib and the specific JAK2 inhibitor BSK-805. Surprisingly, our data are in contradiction to the described observations as we do not observe anti-tumour effects of JAK1/2 inhibition on cell proliferation. An explanation for the observed difference is the specificity of the inhibitors used. AG490 is a tyrosine kinase inhibitor that targets molecules such as EGFR, HER2 or STAT5a/b besides JAK2 whereas Ruxolitinib and BSK-805 are highly selective for JAK proteins [53,54]. Thus, the effects observed upon AG490 treatment could possibly be attributed to the broader spectrum of target molecules of this compound. This observation is very important, since a lower substrate specificity often results in a different response to a drug and is therefore not representative for interfering with a specific molecule which also complicates the identification of predictive biomarker [55]. Also, all bladder cancer cell lines tested by immunoblotting did not show any constitutive phosphorylation of JAK1/2 which might explain the lack of response. In conclusion, our data imply that JAK proteins are not suitable targets for monotherapy in bladder cancer therapy.

Furthermore, we analysed the role of STAT3/5 in bladder cancer cell lines using 3 different STAT3/5 inhibitors Stattic, SH-4-54 and Nifuroxazide. Stattic is a specific STAT3 inhibitor with a lower affinity towards STAT5 [56] and SH-4-54 is a dual inhibitor of STAT3/5 [57]. Nifuroxazide, besides being an inhibitor for STAT3 also inhibits JAK2 and TYK2 [58]. We observed that with these inhibitors proliferation in bladder cancer was greatly reduced which is in line with previous studies on STAT3 inhibition [13,59,60]. Some of the downstream target molecules of STAT3 include anti-apoptotic proteins Bcl-xL. Previously, studies have demonstrated that disrupting STAT3 signalling led to a decrease in anti-apoptotic proteins. Consistent with these findings, we observed a dose-dependent increase in the percentage of apoptotic cells and also a significant increase in cells in G2 phase, which is consistent with prior reports [27].

Combination therapies are a useful approach to overcome limitations of monotherapy options or to enhance the efficiencies. Over the years, there is growing evidence of a connection between STAT3 and chemotherapy resistance [26]. Several studies have shown STAT3 involvement in the development of resistance for chemotherapy in various cancers. It has been demonstrated that STAT3 inhibition sensitized for example squamous cell carcinoma to chemotherapy [61]. In our study, we show that STAT3 inhibition has an additive effect when combined with the most frequently used chemotherapeutic drugs approved for bladder cancer suggesting that this combination might be applicable in patients with STAT3 mediated chemo resistance.

Previously, our group applied a genome wide CRISPR-dCas9 screen to identify acquired resistance mechanisms to the CDK4/6 inhibitor Palbocicib in bladder cancer cell lines [32]. One of the results was an implication of the JAK-STAT signalling pathway in conferring resistance to CDK4/6 inhibitors. The combination therapy with Stattic and Palbociclib showed additive effects in T24 and UMUC-3 but antagonism in RT112 cell lines. Thus, the combination of STAT inhibitors with CDK4/6 inhibitors might not be a general treatment option but should be beneficial for a subset of patients that need to be defined by a detailed analysis of the underlying molecular mechanisms that regulate therapy response in this combination. In conclusion, we show that targeting of STAT3 along with chemotherapy or CDK4/6 inhibitors provide potential combination therapy options in order to improve therapy efficacy in bladder cancer.

In recent years, the development of oncolytic viruses entering clinical trials has dramatically gained momentum [33]. One of the obstacles for inducing an effective therapy response is successful replication of the virus in tumour cells [62]. Thus, a further aim of this study was to combine oncolytic virotherapy with JAK/STAT inhibitors and analyse the effects on virus induced cell death and viral replication. It has been shown that Ruxolitinib enhances replication of VSV but since we could not detect phosphorylation of JAK proteins nor effects on cell viability, we focused on STAT3 inhibitors. Numerous cytokines are released upon virus infection including IFNs and IL-6, which then stimulate the expression of genes that are involved in anti-viral response via direct or indirect mechanisms. It is shown that interferon signalling inhibits adenoviral DNA replication by inhibiting viral early gene expression in normal cells, but not in cancer cells [63,64]. In a STAT2 knockout Syrian hamster model, human adenovirus 5 replicated a 100–1000-fold higher than in the wildtype. The infected cells in the knockout hamsters show interrupted Type I interferon pathway which is implied to be the reason for enhanced replication of virus [65]. Pre-treatment with Ruxolitinib enhanced the viral replication of oncolytic Herpes Simplex Virus (oHSV) in malignant peripheral nerve sheath tumours. Pre-treatment of mice with Ruxolitinib reduced Interferon stimulated genes expression making the tumours susceptible to oHSV infection [42]. Combination of Ruxolitinib and oncolytic vesicular stomatitis virus therapy resulted in enhanced oncolysis and viral replication in non-small cell lung cancer [41].

In this study, combination of STAT3/5 inhibitors with an oncolytic adenovirus resulted in enhancement in virus induced cell death, viral replication and viral particle formation. STAT3/5 inhibition leads to reduction in expression of downstream molecules which also include interleukins and interferons. STAT3/5 inhibition also results in G2 arrest as described. There is evidence for enhanced adenoviral replication upon G2/M arrest [66], which might also be the reason for observed enhancement in viral replication and particle formation upon STAT3/5 inhibition. Further research is required to elucidate the exact mechanisms by which the adenovirus interacts with JAK-STAT pathway and cell cycle. It would also be beneficial to study the viral gene expression analysis to explore the interactions between the viral and cellular genes at various phases of infection.

In conclusion, our study shows that STAT3/5 inhibition reduces cell proliferation both in vitro and in vivo but specific JAK inhibition has no effect on bladder cancer cell lines. We show potential combination therapy options with Stattic and chemotherapeutics, and Stattic and CDK4/6 inhibitor Palbociclib. We also demonstrate enhancement in oncolytic effect of adenoviruses upon combination with STAT3/5 inhibitors. These results indicate that STAT3/5 inhibition, but not JAK1/2 inhibition could be a potentially effective therapeutic strategy in bladder cancer.

4. Materials and Methods

4.1. Patient Material, Tissue Microarray and Immunohistochemistry

Patient characteristics and the details of tissue microarray and immunohistochemistry have been published before [46].

4.2. Cell Lines and Adenovirus

UMUC-3, SW17110, MGHU4, UMUC-6, 639V, SD, J82, VMCUB-1, 647V and BFTC-805 were obtained from Düsseldorf. HCV-29 and KU19-19 were obtained from Leeds, UK. HT1197 was obtained from SIGMA/ECACC, England. BTE-5 were obtained from Uniklinik, Essen. HT-1376, 253J, RT112 and 486P were a kind gift from Homburg. T24, EJ28 and Hek293 cells were from ATCC, VA, USA. Cells were cultured in either RPMI supplemented with 10% foetal bovine serum (FBS), 1% NEAA (Biochrom, Berlin, Germany), penicillin and streptomycin or Dulbecco's modified Eagle's medium supplemented with

10% foetal bovine serum and penicillin-streptomycin, at 5% or 10% CO2, respectively. The oncolytic adenovirus XVir-N-31 was kindly provided by Prof. Holm [37].

4.3. Small Molecule Inhibitors and Chemotherapeutics

Stock solutions of Ruxolitinib, BSK-805, Stattic, SH-4- 54 and Nifuroxazide (Selleckchem, Munich, Germany) were prepared in dimethyl sulfoxide (DMSO). Palbociclib (Selleckchem, Munich, Germany) stock solution was prepared in water. Chemotherapeutic drugs Paclitaxel, Docetaxel and Gemcitabine (Sigma Aldrich Chemie GmbH, Munich, Germany) stock solutions were prepared in DMSO. Working concentrations were freshly prepared in medium for immediate use. Cisplatin (Sigma Aldrich Chemie GmbH, Munich, Germany) was prepared fresh in H_2O.

4.4. Cell Viability, Cell Cycle Analysis and Apoptosis Assays

Cell viability upon small molecule inhibitors monotherapy, and combination treatment of Stattic and chemotherapy were performed after exposure to inhibitors for indicated time periods by Cell-Titer Blue® assay (Promega, Madison, WI, USA) according to manufacturer's protocol and absolute IC50 was calculated. For combination treatments of Stattic and Palbociclib and with adenovirus XVir-N-31, a Sulphorhodamine B (SRB) assay was performed. In brief, cells were fixed with 10% trichloroacetic acid, stained with 0.05% SRB and rinsed with 1% acetic acid and allowed to dry. Dried SRB was dissolved in 10 mM tris base and absorbance was measured at 590 nm. These assays were conducted in 12-well plates, seeding 1×10^4 cells/well. For Stattic and Palbociclib treatment, cells were incubated for 3 days post treatment.

The effect of virus induced cell killing in combination with small molecule inhibitors was analysed in 12-well plates. In total, 0.25–0.5×10^5 cells were seeded and infected with increasing concentrations (multiplicity of infection, MOI) of the adenovirus XVir-N-31 one day after treatment with Stattic in 200µl medium without FBS. At 1hpi, complete medium with or without Stattic was added to the cells. Cells were fixed 4 days post infection and cell viability was analysed by SRB assay.

Apoptosis (Caspase-Glo® 3/7 Assay-Promega) and cell cycle analysis (7-AAD, Thermo Fisher Scientific) were performed according to the manufacturer's protocol.

4.5. Combination Index Analysis and Bladder Cancer Molecular Alteration Analysis

For combination therapy with Stattic and chemotherapeutics, fixed ratio combinations were used. The fixed ratio combinations are as follows: For T24 cells: S:P (Stattic: Paclitaxel) at 122.2:1, S:C (Stattic and Cisplatin) at 1:2.1, S:G (Stattic and Gemcitabine) at 1:2.1 and S:D (Stattic: Docetaxel) at 1447.4:1; for J82 cells: S:P (Stattic: Paclitaxel) at 33.3:1, S:C (Stattic and Cisplatin) at 1:1, S:G (Stattic and Gemcitabin) at 25:1 and S:D (Stattic: Docetaxel) at 250:1; for HT1376 cells: S:P(Stattic:Paclitaxel) at 176:1, S:C (Stattic and Cisplatin) at 1:5.68, S:G (Stattic and Gemcitabine) at 149.15:1 and S:D (Stattic: Docetaxel) at 352:1; for RT112 cells: S:P(Stattic:Paclitaxel) at 500:1, S:C (Stattic and Cisplatin) at 1:1, S:G (Stattic and Gemcitabine) at 50:1 and S:D (Stattic: Docetaxel) at 2000:1; for SD cells: S:P(Stattic:Paclitaxel) at 444.4:1, S:C (Stattic and Cisplatin) at 1:1, S:G (Stattic and Gemcitabine) at 160:1 and S:D (Stattic: Docetaxel) at 4000:1. The combination index (CI) was assessed with the Chou–Talalay combination index (CI) theorem [51]. CI value of 1 was defined as additivity, CI < 1 as synergistic and CI >1 as antagonistic effects. The analysis was performed with CompuSyn software (Combosyn, NJ, USA). The Cancer Genome Atlas (TCGA) analysis was performed on cBioPortal (https://www.cbioportal.org/).

4.6. Immunoblot Analysis

Cells were seeded in 10 cm tissue culture plates and allowed to grow till 50–60% confluency. The medium was then changed with FBS-free medium overnight. Stattic was applied in indicated concentrations for 3 h and cells were stimulated by supplementing with IL-6 (25ng/mL) for 30 min. Then protein extraction (either total or compartmental) was performed. Cells were lysed on ice in protein lysis buffer comprising of 1% sodium dodecyl sulphate, 1 mM sodium orthovanadate and 10 mM tris, pH 7.4. Lysates were sheared using a 27-gauge needle (BD Biosciences®) until no viscosity was observed. The sheared lysates were then centrifuged at 30,000 RCF at 4 °C for total lysates. For compartmentalisation, cells were harvested by trypsin, pelleted then washed twice in phosphate-buffered saline, pelleted again by spinning at 600 RCF in microcentrifuge at 4 °C for 4 min. The pellet was resuspended in lysis buffer. After 5 min on ice, the lysates were spun at 600 RCF in microcentrifuge at 4 °C for 4 min. The supernatants were used as cytoplasmic extracts. The pelleted nuclei were briefly washed in lysis buffer without NP-40. The nuclear pellet was then resuspended in 50–100 μL nuclear extract buffer (20 mM Tris-HCl (pH 8.0), 420 mM NaCl, 1.5 mM $MgCl_2$, 0.2 mM EDTA, 25% glycerol) After a 10-min incubation at 4 °C, the nuclei were briefly vortexed and spun at 18300 RCF in microcentrifuge at 4 °C for 15 min. The supernatant was then removed and used as a nuclear extract. The primary antibodies used included: Stat3 (#9139), p-Stat3 (#9145), Jak1 (#3344), p-Jak1 (#3331), Jak2 (#3230), p-Jak2 (#3771), cyclin-D1(#2922) and GAPDH (#2118) from Cell Signaling Technology, Danvers, MA, USA. Actin (#A2066) from Sigma, Saint Louis, Missouri, USA and histone H1 (#05-457) from Millipore corporation, Temecula, CA, USA.

4.7. CAM Assay and Immunohistochemistry (IHC)

The CAM assay was performed as described previously [50]. In brief, 2 million cells were seeded on embryonic day 8 on the CAM. Topical treatment using 2 μM Stattic was performed daily from day 10 after the formation of visible xenografts. The control tumours were treated with PBS. On day 15, the tumours were harvested: embryos were transferred to a Styrofoam box containing dry ice and suffocated. Tumours were then removed from the CAM, immersed in a petri dish filled with ice-cold PBS and trimmed under a stereo microscope (Leica) with micro scissors to remove as much of the attached CAM as possible. The tumours were immersed in pre-weighed 1.5 mL reaction tubes containing PBS and weighed on a fine balance. IHC was done with Ki-67 (No. M7240, Dako Deutschland, Hamburg, Germany) using heat induced epitope retrieval with 0.01 M citrate buffer at pH 6.0.

4.8. Viral Replication and Particle Formation

Thus, 5×10^4 cells were seeded in 6-well plates and treated with specified concentrations of Stattic. Viral infection was performed a day after the inhibitor treatment in the same manner as described for cell viability assay. DNA lysates were made 4–48 h after infection for viral replication analysis and lysates and supernatant were collected at 72 h for viral particle formation analysis. Viral replication was analysed by real time PCR for fibre DNA using the ΔΔCT-method. Actin was used as the housekeeping gene. Viral titres in the lysates were measured in Hek293 cells seeded in 24-well plates by hexon staining. The protocols for viral replication analysis and hexon titre test were performed as described [37].

4.9. Statistical Analysis

All the cell error bars in cell viability assays, apoptosis assays are presented as mean ± standard error. Statistical analysis for patient's survival analysis and CAM assay was performed using SPSS software. $p < 0.05$ was considered as significant.

Supplementary Materials: Supplementary materials can be found at http://www.mdpi.com/1422-0067/21/3/1106/s1. Dose response curves for individual cell lines for Ruxolitinib (Figure S1), BSK-805 (Figure S2), SH-4-54 (Figure S3), Nifuroxazide (Figure S4) and Stattic (Figure S5) are generated 72 h after treatment. Dose response curves for the combination therapy of Stattic and chemotherapeutics are generated 72h after treatment (Figure S6).Molecular alterations in the JAK-STAT signalling pathway related genes in bladder cancer in TCGA (Table S1) and co-occurrence of altered genes (Table S2) are analysed using cBioPortal.

Author Contributions: Conceptualization: S.C.S. and R.N., Methodology: S.H., J.A.K., S.C.S., validation: J.S.-H., P.S.H., T.H. and R.N., formal analysis: S.C.S., A.Y., E.-M.B., D.W. and S.V.H., investigation: S.C.S., A.Y., E.-M.B., D.W. and S.V.H., resources: J.E.G., data curation: R.N., writing-original draft preparation: S.V.H. and R.N., writing review and editing: R.N., P.S.H., T.H. and J.E.G., supervision: R.N., funding acquisition: S.C.S, R.N. All authors have read and agreed to the published version of the manuscript.

Funding: This research was supported by the Deutsche Forschungsgemeinschaft, DFG, project number NA439/2-1, a fellowship for S.C.S. by the KKF-Curriculum, School of Medicine, TUM and the Reinhard-Nagel Foundation, Deutsche Gesellschaft für Urologie (DGU) and a fellowship for A.Y. by the Egyptian Mission Grant for Joint Supervision.

Acknowledgments: Not applicable.

Conflicts of Interest: The authors declare no conflict of interest. The funders had no role in the design of the study, in the collection, analyses, or interpretation of data; in the writing of the manuscript, or in the decision to publish the results.

Abbreviations

CAM	Chorioallantoic Membrane
FGFR	Fibroblast Growth Factor Receptor
JAK	Janus Kinase
STAT	Signal Transducer and Activator of Transcription
TCGA	The Cancer Genome Atlas

References

1. Bray, F.; Ferlay, J.; Soerjomataram, I.; Siegel, R.L.; Torre, L.A.; Jemal, A. Global cancer statistics 2018: GLOBOCAN estimates of incidence and mortality worldwide for 36 cancers in 185 countries. *CA Cancer J. Clin.* **2018**, *68*, 394–424. [CrossRef] [PubMed]

2. Apolo, A.B. Determining superior first-line therapy in metastatic bladder cancer. *Nat. Rev. Urol.* **2019**, *16*, 698–699. [CrossRef] [PubMed]

3. Boegemann, M.; Aydin, A.M.; Bagrodia, A.; Krabbe, L.M. Prospects and progress of immunotherapy for bladder cancer. *Expert Opin. Biol. Ther.* **2017**, *17*, 1417–1431. [CrossRef] [PubMed]

4. Koshkin, V.S.; Grivas, P. Emerging Role of Immunotherapy in Advanced Urothelial Carcinoma. *Curr. Oncol. Rep.* **2018**, *20*, 48. [CrossRef]

5. Duplisea, J.J.; Dinney, C.P.N. Should chemotherapy still be used to treat all muscle invasive bladder cancer in the "era of immunotherapy"? *Expert Rev. Anticancer Ther.* **2019**, *19*, 543–545. [CrossRef]

6. Grivas, P.; Yu, E.Y. Role of Targeted Therapies in Management of Metastatic Urothelial Cancer in the Era of Immunotherapy. *Curr. Treat Options Oncol.* **2019**, *20*, 67. [CrossRef]

7. Loriot, Y.; Necchi, A.; Park, S.H.; Garcia-Donas, J.; Huddart, R.; Burgess, E.; Fleming, M.; Rezazadeh, A.; Mellado, B.; Varlamov, S.; et al. Erdafitinib in Locally Advanced or Metastatic Urothelial Carcinoma. *N. Engl. J. Med.* **2019**, *381*, 338–348. [CrossRef]

8. Da Costa, J.B.; Gibb, E.A.; Nykopp, T.K.; Mannas, M.; Wyatt, A.W.; Black, P.C. Molecular tumor heterogeneity in muscle invasive bladder cancer: Biomarkers, subtypes, and implications for therapy. *Urol. Oncol.* **2018**, 1–8. [CrossRef]

9. Hammaren, H.M.; Virtanen, A.T.; Raivola, J.; Silvennoinen, O. The regulation of JAKs in cytokine signaling and its breakdown in disease. *Cytokine* **2019**, *118*, 48–63. [CrossRef]

10. Guo, C.; Yang, G.; Khun, K.; Kong, X.; Levy, D.; Lee, P.; Melamed, J. Activation of Stat3 in renal tumors. *Am. J. Transl. Res.* **2009**, *1*, 283.

11. Tong, M.; Wang, J.; Jiang, N.; Pan, H.; Li, D. Correlation between p-STAT3 overexpression and prognosis in lung cancer: A systematic review and meta-analysis. *PLoS ONE* **2017**, *12*, e0182282. [CrossRef] [PubMed]

12. Takemoto, S.; Ushijima, K.; Kawano, K.; Yamaguchi, T.; Terada, A.; Fujiyoshi, N.; Nishio, S.; Tsuda, N.; Ijichi, M.; Kakuma, T.; et al. Expression of activated signal transducer and activator of transcription-3 predicts poor prognosis in cervical squamous-cell carcinoma. *Br. J. Cancer* **2009**, *101*, 967–972. [CrossRef] [PubMed]

13. Chen, C.L.; Cen, L.; Kohout, J.; Hutzen, B.; Chan, C.; Hsieh, F.C.; Loy, A.; Huang, V.; Cheng, G.; Lin, J. Signal transducer and activator of transcription 3 activation is associated with bladder cancer cell growth and survival. *Mol. Cancer* **2008**, *7*, 78. [CrossRef] [PubMed]

14. Degoricija, M.; Situm, M.; Korac, J.; Miljkovic, A.; Matic, K.; Paradzik, M.; Marinovic Terzic, I.; Jeroncic, A.; Tomic, S.; Terzic, J. High NF-kappaB and STAT3 activity in human urothelial carcinoma: a pilot study. *World J. Urol.* **2014**, *32*, 1469–1475. [CrossRef] [PubMed]

15. Shen, H.B.; Gu, Z.Q.; Jian, K.; Qi, J. CXCR4-mediated Stat3 activation is essential for CXCL12-induced cell invasion in bladder cancer. *Tumor Biol.* **2013**, *34*, 1839–1845. [CrossRef] [PubMed]

16. Yang, X.; Ou, L.; Tang, M.; Wang, Y.; Wang, X.; Chen, E.; Diao, J.; Wu, X.; Luo, C. Knockdown of PLCepsilon inhibits inflammatory cytokine release via STAT3 phosphorylation in human bladder cancer cells. *Tumor Biol.* **2015**, *36*, 9723–9732. [CrossRef]

17. Gatta, L.B.; Melocchi, L.; Bugatti, M.; Missale, F.; Lonardi, S.; Zanetti, B.; Cristinelli, L.; Belotti, S.; Simeone, C.; Ronca, R.; et al. Hyper-Activation of STAT3 Sustains Progression of Non-Papillary Basal-Type Bladder Cancer via FOSL1 Regulome. *Cancers* **2019**, *11*, 1219. [CrossRef]

18. Ho, P.L.; Lay, E.J.; Jian, W.; Parra, D.; Chan, K.S. Stat3 activation in urothelial stem cells leads to direct progression to invasive bladder cancer. *Cancer Res.* **2012**, *72*, 3135–3142. [CrossRef]

19. Mitra, A.P.; Pagliarulo, V.; Yang, D.; Waldman, F.M.; Datar, R.H.; Skinner, D.G.; Groshen, S.; Cote, R.J. Generation of a concise gene panel for outcome prediction in urinary bladder cancer. *J. Clin. Oncol.* **2009**, *27*, 3929–3937. [CrossRef]

20. Sun, Y.; Cheng, M.K.; RL Griffiths, T.; Kilian Mellon, J.; Kai, B.; Kriajevska, M.; M Manson, M. Inhibition of STAT Signalling in Bladder Cancer by Diindolylmethane-Relevance to Cell Adhesion, Migration and Proliferation. *Curr. Cancer Drug Targets* **2013**, *13*, 57–68. [CrossRef]

21. Vlahou, A.; Gromova, I.; Svensson, S.; Gromov, P.; Moreira, J.M. Identification of BLCAP as a novel STAT3 interaction partner in bladder cancer. *PLoS ONE* **2017**, *12*. [CrossRef]

22. Groner, B.; von Manstein, V. Jak Stat signaling and cancer: Opportunities, benefits and side effects of targeted inhibition. *Mol. Cell. Endocrinol.* **2017**, *451*, 1–14. [CrossRef] [PubMed]

23. Kontzias, A.; Kotlyar, A.; Laurence, A.; Changelian, P.; O'Shea, J.J. Jakinibs: A new class of kinase inhibitors in cancer and autoimmune disease. *Curr. Opin. Pharmacol.* **2012**, *12*, 464–470. [CrossRef] [PubMed]

24. Wong, A.L.A.; Hirpara, J.L.; Pervaiz, S.; Eu, J.Q.; Sethi, G.; Goh, B.C. Do STAT3 inhibitors have potential in the future for cancer therapy? *Expert Opin. Investig. Drugs* **2017**, *26*, 883–887. [CrossRef] [PubMed]

25. Yang, L.; Lin, S.; Xu, L.; Lin, J.; Zhao, C.; Huang, X. Novel activators and small-molecule inhibitors of STAT3 in cancer. *Cytokine Growth Factor Rev.* **2019**, *49*, 10–22. [CrossRef]

26. Zhao, C.; Li, H.; Lin, H.J.; Yang, S.; Lin, J.; Liang, G. Feedback Activation of STAT3 as a Cancer Drug-Resistance Mechanism. *Trends Pharmacol. Sci.* **2016**, *37*, 47–61. [CrossRef]

27. Shao, D.; Ma, J.; Zhou, C.; Zhao, J.N.; Li, L.L.; Zhao, T.J.; Ai, X.L.; Jiao, P. STAT3 down-regulation induces mitochondria-dependent G2/M cell cycle arrest and apoptosis in oesophageal carcinoma cells. *Clin. Exp. Pharmacol. Physiol.* **2017**, *44*, 413–420. [CrossRef]

28. Zhou, C.; Ma, J.; Su, M.; Shao, D.; Zhao, J.; Zhao, T.; Song, Z.; Meng, Y.; Jiao, P. Down-regulation of STAT3 induces the apoptosis and G1 cell cycle arrest in esophageal carcinoma ECA109 cells. *Cancer Cell Int.* **2018**, *18*, 53. [CrossRef]

29. Sathe, A.; Koshy, N.; Schmid, S.C.; Thalgott, M.; Schwarzenbock, S.M.; Krause, B.J.; Holm, P.S.; Gschwend, J.E.; Retz, M.; Nawroth, R. CDK4/6 Inhibition Controls Proliferation of Bladder Cancer and Transcription of RB1. *J. Urol.* **2016**, *195*, 771–779. [CrossRef]

30. Sobhani, N.; D'Angelo, A.; Pittacolo, M.; Roviello, G.; Miccoli, A.; Corona, S.P.; Bernocchi, O.; Generali, D.; Otto, T. Updates on the CDK4/6 Inhibitory Strategy and Combinations in Breast Cancer. *Cells* **2019**, *8*, 321. [CrossRef]

31. McCartney, A.; Migliaccio, I.; Bonechi, M.; Biagioni, C.; Romagnoli, D.; De Luca, F.; Galardi, F.; Risi, E.; De Santo, I.; Benelli, M.; et al. Mechanisms of Resistance to CDK4/6 Inhibitors: Potential Implications and Biomarkers for Clinical Practice. *Front. Oncol.* **2019**, *9*, 666. [CrossRef] [PubMed]

32. Tong, Z.; Sathe, A.; Ebner, B.; Qi, P.; Veltkamp, C.; Gschwend, J.E.; Holm, P.S.; Nawroth, R. Functional genomics identifies predictive markers and clinically actionable resistance mechanisms to CDK4/6 inhibition in bladder cancer. *J. Exp. Clin. Cancer Res.* **2019**, *38*, 322. [CrossRef]

33. Harrington, K.; Freeman, D.J.; Kelly, B.; Harper, J.; Soria, J.C. Optimizing oncolytic virotherapy in cancer treatment. *Nat. Rev. Drug Discov.* **2019**, *18*, 689–706. [CrossRef] [PubMed]

34. Fukuhara, H.; Ino, Y.; Todo, T. Oncolytic virus therapy: A new era of cancer treatment at dawn. *Cancer Sci.* **2016**, *107*, 1373–1379. [CrossRef] [PubMed]

35. Conry, R.M.; Westbrook, B.; McKee, S.; Norwood, T.G. Talimogene laherparepvec: First in class oncolytic virotherapy. *Hum. Vaccines Immunother.* **2018**, *14*, 839–846. [CrossRef] [PubMed]

36. Matsuda, T.; Karube, H.; Aruga, A. A Comparative Safety Profile Assessment of Oncolytic Virus Therapy Based on Clinical Trials. *Ther. Innov. Regul. Sci.* **2018**, *52*, 430–437. [CrossRef] [PubMed]

37. Lichtenegger, E.; Koll, F.; Haas, H.; Mantwill, K.; Janssen, K.P.; Laschinger, M.; Gschwend, J.; Steiger, K.; Black, P.C.; Moskalev, I.; et al. The Oncolytic Adenovirus XVir-N-31 as a Novel Therapy in Muscle-Invasive Bladder Cancer. *Hum. Gene Ther.* **2019**, *30*, 44–56. [CrossRef]

38. Taguchi, S.; Fukuhara, H.; Homma, Y.; Todo, T. Current status of clinical trials assessing oncolytic virus therapy for urological cancers. *Int. J. Urol.* **2017**, *24*, 342–351. [CrossRef]

39. LaRocca, C.J.; Warner, S.G. Oncolytic viruses and checkpoint inhibitors: combination therapy in clinical trials. *Clin. Transl. Med.* **2018**, *7*, 35. [CrossRef]

40. Jiang, H.; Gomez-Manzano, C.; Rivera-Molina, Y.; Lang, F.F.; Conrad, C.A.; Fueyo, J. Oncolytic adenovirus research evolution: from cell-cycle checkpoints to immune checkpoints. *Curr. Opin. Virol.* **2015**, *13*, 33–39. [CrossRef]

41. Patel, M.R.; Dash, A.; Jacobson, B.A.; Ji, Y.; Baumann, D.; Ismail, K.; Kratzke, R.A. JAK/STAT inhibition with ruxolitinib enhances oncolytic virotherapy in non-small cell lung cancer models. *Cancer Gene Ther.* **2019**, *26*, 411–418. [CrossRef] [PubMed]

42. Ghonime, M.G.; Cassady, K.A. Combination Therapy Using Ruxolitinib and Oncolytic HSV Renders Resistant MPNSTs Susceptible to Virotherapy. *Cancer Immunol. Res.* **2018**, *6*, 1499–1510. [CrossRef] [PubMed]

43. Huang, W.T.; Yang, S.F.; Wu, C.C.; Chen, W.T.; Huang, Y.C.; Su, Y.C.; Chai, C.Y. Expression of signal transducer and activator of transcription 3 and suppressor of cytokine signaling in urothelial carcinoma. *Kaohsiung J. Med. Sci.* **2009**, *25*, 640–646. [CrossRef]

44. Chan, K.S.; Espinosa, I.; Chao, M.; Wong, D.; Ailles, L.; Diehn, M.; Gill, H.; Presti, J., Jr.; Chang, H.Y.; van de Rijn, M.; et al. Identification, molecular characterization, clinical prognosis, and therapeutic targeting of human bladder tumor-initiating cells. *Proc. Natl. Acad. Sci. USA* **2009**, *106*, 14016–14021. [CrossRef]

45. Robertson, A.G.; Kim, J.; Al-Ahmadie, H.; Bellmunt, J.; Guo, G.; Cherniack, A.D.; Hinoue, T.; Laird, P.W.; Hoadley, K.A.; Akbani, R.; et al. Comprehensive Molecular Characterization of Muscle-Invasive Bladder Cancer. *Cell* **2017**, *171*, 540–556. [CrossRef]

46. Horn, T.; Laus, J.; Seitz, A.K.; Maurer, T.; Schmid, S.C.; Wolf, P.; Haller, B.; Winkler, M.; Retz, M.; Nawroth, R.; et al. The prognostic effect of tumour-infiltrating lymphocytic subpopulations in bladder cancer. *World J. Urol.* **2016**, *34*, 181–187. [CrossRef]

47. Horiguchi, A.; Oya, M.; Shimada, T.; Uchida, A.; Marumo, K.; Murai, M. Activation of signal transducer and activator of transcription 3 in renal cell carcinoma—A study of incidence and its association with pathological features and clinical outcome. *J. Urol.* **2002**, *168*, 762–765. [CrossRef]

48. Igelmann, S.; Neubauer, H.A.; Ferbeyre, G. STAT3 and STAT5 Activation in Solid Cancers. *Cancers* **2019**, *11*, 1428. [CrossRef]

49. Fukada, T.; Ohtani, T.; Yoshida, Y.; Shirogane, T.; Nishida, K.; Nakajima, K.; Hibi, M.; Hirano, T. STAT3 orchestrates contradictory signals in cytokine-induced G1 to S cell-cycle transition. *EMBO J.* **1998**, *17*, 6670–6677. [CrossRef]

50. Skowron, M.A.; Sathe, A.; Romano, A.; Hoffmann, M.J.; Schulz, W.A.; van Koeveringe, G.A.; Albers, P.; Nawroth, R.; Niegisch, G. Applying the chicken embryo chorioallantoic membrane assay to study treatment approaches in urothelial carcinoma. *Urol. Oncol.* **2017**, *35*, 544.e11–544.e23. [CrossRef]

51. Chou, T.C. Drug combination studies and their synergy quantification using the Chou-Talalay method. *Cancer Res.* **2010**, *70*, 440–446. [CrossRef] [PubMed]

52. Joung, Y.H.; Na, Y.M.; Yoo, Y.B.; Darvin, P.; Sp, N.; Kang, D.Y.; Kim, S.Y.; Kim, H.S.; Choi, Y.H.; Lee, H.K.; et al. Combination of AG490, a Jak2 inhibitor, and methylsulfonylmethane synergistically suppresses bladder tumor growth via the Jak2/STAT3 pathway. *Int. J. Oncol.* **2014**, *44*, 883–895. [CrossRef] [PubMed]

53. Quintás-Cardama, A.; Vaddi, K.; Liu, P.; Manshouri, T.; Li, J.; Scherle, P.A.; Caulder, E.; Wen, X.; Li, Y.; Waeltz, P.; et al. Preclinical characterization of the selective JAK1/2 inhibitor INCB018424: therapeutic implications for the treatment of myeloproliferative neoplasms. *Blood* **2010**, *115*, 3109–3117. [CrossRef] [PubMed]

54. Baffert, F.; Régnier, C.H.; De Pover, A.; Pissot-Soldermann, C.; Tavares, G.A.; Blasco, F.; Brueggen, J.; Chène, P.; Drueckes, P.; Erdmann, D.; et al. Potent and Selective Inhibition of Polycythemia by the Quinoxaline JAK2 Inhibitor NVP-BSK805. *Mol. Cancer Ther.* **2010**, *9*, 1945–1955. [CrossRef]

55. Knudsen, E.S.; Witkiewicz, A.K. The Strange Case of CDK4/6 Inhibitors: Mechanisms, Resistance, and Combination Strategies. *Trends Cancer* **2017**, *3*, 39–55. [CrossRef] [PubMed]
56. Schust, J.; Sperl, B.; Hollis, A.; Mayer, T.U.; Berg, T. Stattic: A small-molecule inhibitor of STAT3 activation and dimerization. *Chem. Biol.* **2006**, *13*, 1235–1242. [CrossRef] [PubMed]
57. Haftchenary, S.; Luchman, H.A.; Jouk, A.O.; Veloso, A.J.; Page, B.D.; Cheng, X.R.; Dawson, S.S.; Grinshtein, N.; Shahani, V.M.; Kerman, K.; et al. Potent Targeting of the STAT3 Protein in Brain Cancer Stem Cells: A Promising Route for Treating Glioblastoma. *ACS Med. Chem. Lett.* **2013**, *4*, 1102–1107. [CrossRef]
58. Nelson, E.A.; Walker, S.R.; Kepich, A.; Gashin, L.B.; Hideshima, T.; Ikeda, H.; Chauhan, D.; Anderson, K.C.; Frank, D.A. Nifuroxazide inhibits survival of multiple myeloma cells by directly inhibiting STAT3. *Blood* **2008**, *112*, 5095–5102. [CrossRef]
59. Zhang, H.; Ye, Y.L.; Li, M.X.; Ye, S.B.; Huang, W.R.; Cai, T.T.; He, J.; Peng, J.Y.; Duan, T.H.; Cui, J.; et al. CXCL2/MIF-CXCR2 signaling promotes the recruitment of myeloid-derived suppressor cells and is correlated with prognosis in bladder cancer. *Oncogene* **2016**, *36*, 2095–2104. [CrossRef]
60. Tsujita, Y.; Horiguchi, A.; Tasaki, S.; Isono, M.; Asano, T.; Ito, K.; Asano, T.; Mayumi, Y.; Kushibiki, T. STAT3 inhibition by WP1066 suppresses the growth and invasiveness of bladder cancer cells. *Oncol. Rep.* **2017**, *38*, 2197–2204. [CrossRef]
61. Zhou, X.; Ren, Y.; Liu, A.; Jin, R.; Jiang, Q.; Huang, Y.; Kong, L.; Wang, X.; Zhang, L. WP1066 sensitizes oral squamous cell carcinoma cells to cisplatin by targeting STAT3/miR-21 axis. *Sci. Rep.* **2014**, *4*, 7461. [CrossRef]
62. Chiocca, E.A.; Rabkin, S.D. Oncolytic viruses and their application to cancer immunotherapy. *Cancer Immunol. Res.* **2014**, *2*, 295–300. [CrossRef] [PubMed]
63. Chahal, J.S.; Qi, J.; Flint, S.J. The human adenovirus type 5 E1B 55 kDa protein obstructs inhibition of viral replication by type I interferon in normal human cells. *PLoS Pathog.* **2012**, *8*, e1002853. [CrossRef] [PubMed]
64. Zheng, Y.; Stamminger, T.; Hearing, P. E2F/Rb Family Proteins Mediate Interferon Induced Repression of Adenovirus Immediate Early Transcription to Promote Persistent Viral Infection. *PLoS Pathog.* **2016**, *12*, e1005415. [CrossRef] [PubMed]
65. Toth, K.; Lee, S.R.; Ying, B.; Spencer, J.F.; Tollefson, A.E.; Sagartz, J.E.; Kong, I.K.; Wang, Z.; Wold, W.S. STAT2 Knockout Syrian Hamsters Support Enhanced Replication and Pathogenicity of Human Adenovirus, Revealing an Important Role of Type I Interferon Response in Viral Control. *PLoS Pathog.* **2015**, *11*, e1005084. [CrossRef]
66. Steinwaerder, D.S.; Carlson, C.A.; Lieber, A. DNA Replication of First-Generation Adenovirus Vectors in Tumor Cells. *Hum. Gene Ther.* **2000**, *11*, 1933–1948. [CrossRef]

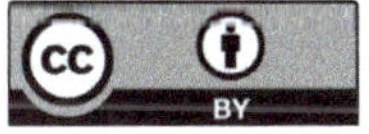

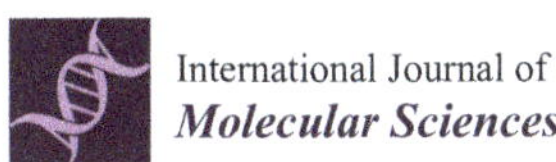

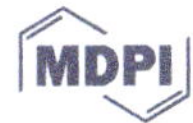

Article

TERT Promoter Mutation as a Potential Predictive Biomarker in BCG-Treated Bladder Cancer Patients

Rui Batista [1,2,3,†], Luís Lima [4,†], João Vinagre [1,2,3,†], Vasco Pinto [2,3], Joana Lyra [2,3], Valdemar Máximo [1,2,3], Lúcio Santos [4] and Paula Soares [1,2,3,*]

[1]   Instituto de Investigação e Inovação em Saúde (i3S), 4200-135 Porto, Portugal; rbatista@ipatimup.pt (R.B.); jvinagre@ipatimup.pt (J.V.); vmaximo@ipatimup.pt (V.M.)

[2]   Instituto de Patologia e Imunologia Molecular da Universidade do Porto (IPATIMUP), 4200-135 Porto, Portugal; vasco.sa.pinto@gmail.com (V.P.); joanaritalyra@gmail.com (J.L.)

[3]   Faculdade de Medicina da Universidade do Porto (FMUP), 4200-319 Porto, Portugal

[4]   Grupo de Patologia e Terapêutica Experimental, Instituto Português de Oncologia do Porto FG, EPE (IPO-Porto), 4200-072 Porto, Portugal; luis14lima@gmail.com (L.L.); llarasantos@gmail.com (L.S.)

*   Correspondence: psoares@ipatimup.pt; Tel.: +351-2255-70700

†   These authors contributed equally to this work.

Received: 28 December 2019; Accepted: 30 January 2020; Published: 31 January 2020

Abstract: Telomerase reverse transcriptase gene promoter (*TERTp*) mutations are recognized as one of the most frequent genetic events in bladder cancer (BC). No studies have focused on the relevance of TERTp mutations in the specific group of tumors treated with Bacillus Calmette–Guérin (BCG) intravesical therapy. Methods — 125 non muscle invasive BC treated with BCG therapy (BCG-NMIBC) were screened for *TERTp* mutations, *TERT* rs2853669 single nucleotide polymorphism, and Fibroblast Growth Factor Receptor 3 (*FGFR3*) hotspot mutations. Results — *TERTp* mutations were found in 56.0% of BCG-NMIBC and were not associated with tumor stage or grade. *FGFR3* mutations were found in 44.9% of the cases and were not associated with tumor stage or grade nor with *TERTp* mutations. The *TERT* rs2853669 single nucleotide polymorphism was associated with tumors of higher grade. The specific c.1-146G>A *TERTp* mutation was an independent predictor of nonrecurrence after BCG therapy (hazard ratio—0.382; 95% confidence interval—0.150–0.971, *p* = 0.048). Conclusions—*TERTp* mutations are frequent in BCG-NMIBC and -146G>A appears to be an independent predictive marker of response to BCG treatment with an impact in recurrence-free survival.

Keywords: *TERT* promoter mutations; *FGFR3*; non muscle invasive bladder cancer; BCG therapy

---

1. Introduction

Bladder cancer (BC) ranks as the fifth most common cancer in western society and the sixth most prevalent in the world, with an increasing incidence in the past years [1]. The increased incidence, along with the high costs in surveillance per BC patient, results in a high burden for public health systems [2,3]. BC can be divided in non muscle invasive (NMI) and muscle invasive (MI) tumors. NMI bladder cancer (NMIBC) accounts for 70% to 80% of all BC and is present as superficial and recurrent lesions that only seldom progress to an MI phenotype. Prompt treatment, usually with complete transurethral tumor resection, grants a 5-year survival rate that can surpass 90%. However, up to 70%-80% of them may relapse, making recurrence the main challenge in clinical management [3,4]. Present in approximately 70% of cases, Fibroblast Growth Factor Receptor 3 (FGFR3) activating mutations are the most frequent genetic event in the NMI phenotype [4]. MI bladder cancer (MIBC) accounts for the remaining 20% to 30% of BC cases and presents as an invasive tumor at diagnosis. Characterized by a high risk of distant metastasis, MIBC prognosis is considerably worse, with 5-year survival rates often described as lower than 40% [5]. MI tumors are genetically more heterogeneous than NMI tumours; present in approximately half of the cases, *TP53* mutations are identified as the most frequent genetic alteration in these tumors [4].

Cell immortalization is a classic hallmark of cancer cells and telomerase reactivation is proposed to be involved in the underlying process. In a large part of cancer models, the intervening mechanisms remained elusive, until in 2013, mutations of the promoter of the telomerase (*TERT*) were described in melanoma [6,7]. We and others reported for the first time the presence of recurrent somatic mutations in the *TERT* promoter (*TERTp*) in numerous types of cancer, including BC [8–15]. Studies focusing on BC have described a prevalence of *TERTp* mutations ranging from 52% to 85% of the cases [10,13,14,16–19]. Conflicting results have been obtained on the association between *TERTp* mutations and BC clinical outcome [13,14]. A common polymorphism in *TERTp* (rs2853669 single nucleotide polymorphism) is also accountable to act as a modifier of the promoter mutations' effect on survival and tumor recurrence in several cancers, such as glioblastoma, liver, and bladder cancer [18,20,21].

Clinicopathological features are the central determinants of recurrence, and according to the European Organization for Research and Treatment of Cancer (EORTC), the NMIBC high-risk group includes high-grade papillary tumors, carcinoma in situ, and those with multifocal or recurrent lesions [22]. Tumor resection followed by a schedule of intravesical instillations with Bacillus Calmette–Guérin (BCG) is the standard adjuvant therapy for this high-risk group (henceforth referred to as BCG-NMIBC) [22,23]. Nonetheless, 30% to 40% of patients present either intolerance or recurrence following BCG treatment, demanding a life-long follow-up and repeated courses of treatment [24]. This clinical relevance is recognized and there is a shortage of dedicated genetic markers predicting BCG-NMIBC subgroup outcomes, in particular, the now recognized two most common genetic events in NMIBC—*TERT* promoter and *FGFR3* mutations.

In this study, we screened a series comprising 125 BCG-NMIBCs resected before BCG therapy initiation for *TERTp* mutations, *FGFR3* mutations, and for the *TERTp* rs2853669 polymorphism. This represents a unique report of *TERTp* and *FGFR3* mutation genotyping dedicated to the BCG-NMI group of BC. To investigate the significance of *TERTp* mutations in the BCG-treated tumor response, we compared the obtained results with the available clinicopathological data, including recurrence-free survival following BCG therapy.

2. Results

2.1. TERTp and FGFR3 Mutation Analysis

In the 125 BCG-treated NMIBC (BCG-NMIBC) tumors screened for *TERTp* mutations, 56.0% (70/125) of the cases were mutated. The c.1-124G>A mutation was detected in 36.8% (46/125) and the c.1-146G>A in 17.6% (22/125). In two cases (1.6%), both c.-124G>A and c.1-146 G>A mutations were observed (Table 1). *FGFR3* mutations (exons 7, 10 and 15) were evaluated in 107 cases. In the tumors screened for *FGFR3* mutations, 44.9% (48/107) of the cases were mutated (Table 1). The large majority was mutated in exon 7 and less frequently in exons 10 and 15 (Table 1). When analyzing *FGFR3* cases with only mutations in exon 7 (45 cases), 42.2% (19/45) presented the p.R248C mutation whereas the p.S249C mutation was present in 55.6% (25/45). One case harbored both mutations (2.2%). A comparison between *TERTp* mutation status and *FGFR3* status revealed no significant association between the two genetic events in the BCG-NMI tumors. The rs2853669 SNP was evaluated in 98 cases; rs2853669 AA genotype accounted for 39.8% (39/98) of the cases, AG genotype for 48.0% (47/98) and GG genotype for 12.2% (12/98) (Table 1).

Table 1. Telomerase reverse transcriptase gene promoter (*TERTp*) mutations, Fibroblast Growth Factor Receptor 3 (*FGFR3*) mutations, and rs2853669 prevalence across BCG-treated cases of nonmuscle invasive bladder cancers (BCG-NMIBC).

	BCG-NMIBC, *n* (%)
TERTp	
Wild type	55 (44.0)
Mutated	70 (56.0)
Specific mutations	
c.1-124G>A	46 (36.8)
c.1-146G>A	22 (17.6)
c.1-124G>A/c.1-146G>A	2 (1.6)
FGFR3	
Wild type	59 (55.1)
Mutated	48 (44.9)
Specific mutations	
Exon 7 p.R248C	19 (39.6)
Exon 7 p.S249C	25 (52.0)
Exon 10 p.Y375C	1 (2.1)
Exon 7 p.R248C + p.S249C	1 (2.1)
Exon 7 p.R248C + Exon 10 p.Y375C	1 (2.1)
Exon 7 p.R248C + Exon 15 p.K652E	1 (2.1)
rs2853669	
AA	39 (39.8)
AG	47 (48.0)
GG	12 (12.2)

2.2. Clinicopathological Characteristics and Genetic Alterations

A comparison between the clinicopathological characteristics of *TERTp* wild type and mutated cases was performed (Table 2). An association was found between *TERTp* mutations and recurrence status prior to BCG therapy, where an over-representation of *TERTp* mutations in primary tumors when compared with recurrent tumors can be detected (61.4% vs. 38.6%, $p = 0.048$).

In the BCG-NMIBC cases a statistically significant association between tumor size and *FGFR3* p.R248C mutations was found ($p = 0.048$). There was an over-representation of the mutation presence among tumors larger than 3 cm in comparison with the smaller ones (27.9% vs. 11.5%), Table S2. However, multivariate analysis revealed that FGFR3 p.R248C is not independently associated with tumor size.

The stratification of tumors in two groups, those wild type for both *TERTp* and *FGFR3* and those mutated for any, did not present statistically significant differences in the clinicopathological characteristics. Regarding the relationship of the studied polymorphism and clinicopathological features, an over-representation of the rs2853669 AA genotype was found in high-grade tumors when compared with low-grade tumors (77.4% vs. 22.6%, $p = 0.018$) (Table 3).

Table 2. Relation between clinicopathological data and *TERTp* mutation status in BCG-NMIBC.

	TERTp		
	Wild Type, *n* **(%)**	**Mutated,** *n* **(%)**	***p*-value**
Age group			
<65 years	21 (38.2)	33 (47.1)	0.315
≥65 years	34 (61.8)	37 (52.9)	
Gender			
Female	11 (20.0)	8 (11.4)	0.185
Male	44 (80.0)	62 (88.6)	
Stage			
Ta	23 (41.8)	28 (40.0)	0.837
T1	32 (58.2)	42 (60.0)	
Grade			
Low	15 (27.3)	25 (35.7)	0.315
High	40 (72.7)	45 (64.3)	
Tumour size			
<3 cm	34 (63.0)	41 (58.6)	0.620
≥3 cm	20 (37.0)	29 (41.4)	
Multifocality			
No	28 (50.9)	32 (45.7)	0.564
Yes	27 (49.1)	38 (54.3)	
Recurrence status			
Primary	24 (43.6)	43 (61.4)	**0.048**
Recurrent	31 (56.4)	27 (38.6)	

p-Values obtained from Pearson's Chi-Square test for gender, stage, grade, tumor size, and multifocality and recurrence, bold values indicate $p < 0.05$.

Table 3. Relation between clinicopathological data and *rs2853669* single nucleotide polymorphism (SNP) status in BCG-NMIBC.

	rs2853669		
	AA, *n* **(%)**	**G Carrier,** *n* **(%)**	***p*-value**
Age group			
<65 years	17 (41.5)	22 (38.6)	0.775
≥65 years	24 (58.5)	35 (61.4)	
Gender			
Female	5 (37.5)	34 (40.5)	0.736
Male	9 (64.3)	50 (59.5)	
Stage			
Ta	15 (39.5)	24 (40.0)	0.959
T1	23 (60.5)	36 (60.0)	
Grade			
Low	7 (22.6)	32 (47.8)	**0.018**
High	24 (77.4)	35 (52.2)	
Tumour size			
<3 cm	22 (34.9)	17 (50.0)	0.148
≥3 cm	41 (65.1)	17 (50.0)	
Multifocality			
No	19 (43.2)	20 (37.0)	0.536
Yes	25 (56.8)	34 (63.0)	
Recurrence status			
Primary	22 (43.1)	17 (36.2)	0.481
Recurrent	29 (56.9)	30 (63.8)	

p-Values obtained from Pearson's Chi-Square test for gender, stage, grade, tumor size, and multifocality and recurrence, bold values indicate $p < 0.05$.

2.3. Clinicopathological and Molecular Characteristics with BCG Therapy Success

Prior to tumor sampling, the BCG-NMIBC patients were treated with a scheme of BCG intravesical therapy. We evaluated how the clinicopathological characteristics affected BCG therapy outcome. Success was defined as no recurrence detected until the last surveillance check-up. Failure was defined as any recurrence after BCG treatment. After a univariate analysis, the age group $\geq$65 years (hazard ratio (HR): 2.827; 95% CI: 1.481–5.398; $p = 0.002$), multifocality (HR: 2.000; 95% CI: 1.096-3.649; $p = 0.024$) and maintenance BCG (mBCG) schedule (HR: 0.505; 95% CI: 0.282-0.902; $p = 0.021$) were the only variables significantly associated with the outcome, Table S1.

Next, we evaluated if the molecular characteristics have an effect on BCG therapy success. We performed a univariate analysis considering *TERTp* and *FGFR3* mutations and BCG therapy success. No statistically significant association was found on univariate analysis. To adjust for the effect of age group, multifocality, and BCG schedule on treatment success, we then performed a multivariate Cox regression analysis. When adjusted, the effect of status (wild type vs. mutated) for *TERTp* and *FGFR3* remained nonsignificant (Tables 4 and 5). However, when we considered *TERTp* c.1-146G>A carriers against *TERTp* non c.1-146G>A carriers (either *TERTp* wild type or c.1-124G>A), the c.1-146G>A mutation was significantly associated with therapy success (HR: 0.382; 95% CI: 0.150-0.971; $p = 0.043$) (Tables 4 and 5). In our series, the *TERTp* mutation c.1-146G>A was an independent predictor of therapy sucess following BCG intravesical therapy.

We further investigated the possible role of *TERTp* genetic events in predicting BCG therapy success by evaluating the presence of the single nucleotide polymorphism rs2853669 in the BCG-NMIBC series. We characterized cases as either carrier or noncarrier. No significant association was found for rs2853669 *per se*, or for *TERTp* mutation effect after splitting for rs2853669.

Table 4. Univariate analysis of the relation between *TERTp* and *FGFR3* mutations and recurrence after BCG treatment.

	BCG Therapy			
	Success, *n* (%)	Failure, *n* (%)	HR (95% CI)	*p*-value
TERTp				
Wild type	34 (43.0)	21 (45.7)	1.0	0.580
Mutated	45 (57.0)	25 (54.3)	0.848 (0.473–1.520)	
TERTp genotype				
Wild type	34 (43.0)	21 (45.6)	1.0	
c.1-124G > A	26 (32.9)	20 (43.5)	1.158 (0.626–2.143)	0.639
c.1-146G > A	17 (21.5)	5 (10.9)	0.410 (0.152–1.108)	0.079
c.1-124G>A/c.1-146G>A	2 (2.5)	0 (0.0)	0.464 (0.040–5.327)	0.464
TERTp c.1-146G>A status				
c.1-146G>A carriers	60 (75.9)	41 (89.1)	1.0	**0.043**
non c.1-146G>A carriers	19 (24.1)	5 (10.9)	0.382 (0.150–0.971)	
FGFR3				
Wild type	39 (60.0)	20 (51.3)	1.0	0.367
Mutated	26 (40.0)	19 (48.7)	1.336 (0.712–2.507)	
FGFR3 status				
Wild type	39 (60.0)	20 (51.3)	1.0	
p.R248C	12 (18.5)	7 (17.9)	1.158 (0.524–3.015)	0.608
p.S249C	14 (21.5)	11 (28.2)	0.410 (0.650–2.842)	0.415
p.R248C/p.S249C	0 (0.0)	1 (2.6)	1.584 (0.804–3.120)	0.184

p-values obtained from Wald test; bold values indicate $p < 0.05$. HR, Hazard Ratio; CI, Confidence Interval.

Table 5. Multivariate analysis and risk estimation of TERT c.1-146G>A mutation influence on BCG therapy outcome.

TERTp c.1-146G>A Status	HR [a]	95% CI	*p*-value
c.1-146G>A carriers	1.0	Referent	
non c.1-146G>A carriers	0.256	0.098-0.667	0.005
Age ≥ 65 years	2.370	1.206-4.661	0.012
Multifocality	1.883	0.964-3.677	0.064
Recurrent tumor	1.352	0.703-2.600	0.367
iBCG schedule	2.225	1.211-4.088	0.010

HR, Hazard Ratio; CI, Confidence Interval. [a] adjusted for age, multifocality, recurrence status, and BCG schedule.

2.4. TERTp Mutations and Recurrence-Free Survival

The recurrence-free survival function of all 125 BCG-treated NMIBC patients, grouped according to the existence of a *TERTp* mutation, was evaluated and log-rank testing revealed no statistically significant difference for either group (Figure S1). When considering *TERTp* c.1-146G>A carriers against *TERTp* non c.1-146G>A carriers (either *TERTp* wild type or c.1-124G>A), the *TERTp* c.1-146G>A patients presented a longer recurrence-free survival in comparison with the noncarriers (mean 126 months vs. mean 100 months, log rank *p* = 0.035) (Figure 1).

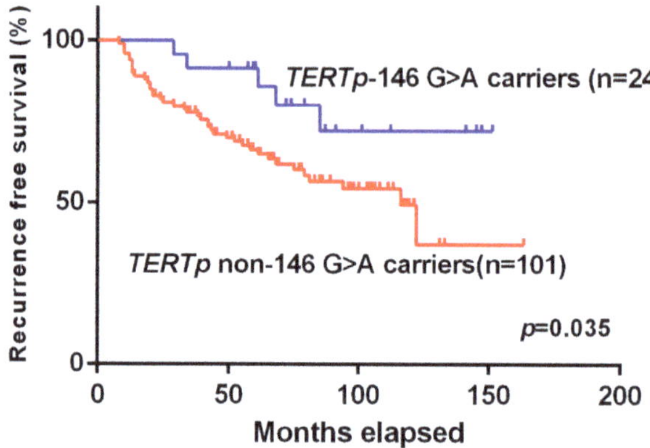

Figure 1. Kaplan–Meier recurrence-free survival function of BCG-NMIBC patients, grouped according to *TERTp* c.1-146G>A carriers against *TERTp* non c.1-146G>A carriers (either *TERTp* wild type or c.1-124G>A). Overall comparison of recurrence-free survival rates was performed using the log-rank test.

3. Discussion

TERTp mutations were reported in 52% to 85% of bladder cancer (BC) cases, depending on the series [10,13,14,16–19]. These results rank *TERTp* mutations as one of the most common genomic events observed in BC and possibly as the most frequent. Of all the *TERTp* mutations, c.1-124G>A has been consistently reported as the most frequent, detected in 88% to 95% of the positive cases [10,13,14,16–19]. In this study composed of BCG-treated NMIBC tumors, we report an overall *TERTp* mutation prevalence of 56.0%, in accordance with previously reported studies [10,13,14,16–19]. Conflicting results have been reported on the association between *TERTp* mutations and clinical stage and/or grade of bladder tumors. Wu et al. [19] found that *TERTp* mutations were more prevalent in MI tumors than in NMI tumors and in patients with advanced tumor stages. On the other hand, other studies reported no association between mutation status and stage or grade [13,14]. The results we present here support that *TERTp* mutations rates are not significantly different across grades or stages in this subset of BCG-treated NMIBC. However, it should be taken into account that this subset represents a group of particularly aggressive NMI tumors (BCG-NMIBC), and comparisons with NMIBC subseries in other studies must be made with caution.

Found in approximately 70% of tumors, *FGFR3* activating mutations are regarded as important genetic events in the NMI phenotype [4]. We found that 44.9% of the BCG-NMIBC cases were mutated for *FGFR3*. As *FGFR3* mutations are associated with low-grade and low-stage tumors and seem to predict a more favorable clinical outcome among patients with NMI tumors [3,25], it was expectable that the more aggressive BCG-NMIBC tumors presented lower mutation rates than those reported in other series [4]. Analyzing the specific *FGFR3* mutation distribution, a novel pattern emerges; previously, in NMIBC series, the most frequent mutations were at the exon 7 p.S249C (66.6% overall, 87.3% of the exon 7 mutations) and p.R248C (9.7% overall, 12.0% of the exon 7 mutations), and mutations in exon 10 and 15 were infrequent [26]. The *FGFR3* mutations detected in this study were mostly present on exon 7 (91.7%), but we observed a different prevalence of the specific mutations, with p.S249C accounting for 52.0%, and an enrichment for p.R248C, with 39.6%. In the BCG-NMIBC cases wild type and mutated for FGFR3, a statistically significant association between tumor size and FGFR3 p.R248C mutation was found ($p = 0.048$). However, multivariate analysis revealed that FGFR3 p.R248C is not independently associated with tumor size. One can discuss if FGFR3 p.R248C mutations are associated with more aggressive tumors, since it is particularly enriched in this subset of tumors and associated with larger tumor size in a univariate analysis. Loss of association in multivariate analysis may indicate that this association may be due to the influence of other clinicopathological features or, more likely, the analyzed cohort is too low to robustly perform this analysis. Further studies are required to elucidate these assumptions and findings. Finally, no significant association was found between the presence of *TERTp* and *FGFR3* mutations.

Intravesical BCG therapy is used as prophylaxis against NMIBC recurrences after tumor resection and it is in fact regarded as one of the first and most successful of all oncological immunotherapies [27,28]. BCG intravesical instillation results in multiple immune reactions. Although the precise immunological mechanism of BCG therapy is not clear, it appears to act through three main actions—infection of urothelial cells or bladder cancer cells, induction of immune responses, and induction of anti-tumour effects [27]. Although effective, 30% to 40% of the cases still show either intolerance or recurrence after BCG treatment, demanding life-long follow-up and repeated courses of treatment [24]. This results in extreme discomfort for the patients and exceedingly high financial costs, and ranks BC as the most expensive cancer per patient [3]. Biomarkers that could help identify which patients were more likely to respond to BCG versus those with risk of recurrence — those who would benefit the most from either a tighter surveillance or a different treatment — would be very useful in optimizing the clinical care offered to BC patients. In this study, we report the effects of *TERTp* and *FGFR3* mutations in BCG therapy success (recurrence or nonrecurrence) and recurrence-free survival. Age at BCG treatment, multifocality, and BCG schedule were independent predictors of BCG therapy success (defined as no recurrence), with the age group ≥65 years and multifocal tumours associated with a higher risk of recurrence, whereas mBCG schedule was associated with a lower risk of recurrence. These results are concordant with previous reports [29]. After adjusting for age, multifocality, and BCG schedule, we found no association between *FGFR3* mutations and BGC therapy success. Similarly, *TERTp*-mutated cases as a whole showed no difference when compared to wild type cases. However, when we compared carriers of the *TERTp* c.1-146G > A mutation against those without this mutation, we observed that this specific mutation was an independent predictor of better outcome (delayed or nonrecurrence).

Recently, Rachakonda et al. reported that a common polymorphism within a pre-existing Ets2 binding site in *TERTp*, rs2853669, acts as a modifier of the mutations' effect on survival and tumor recurrence [18]. The patients with the *TERTp* mutations presented a poorer survival in the absence, but not in the presence of the variant allele (G) of the polymorphism [18]. TERTp mutations in the absence of the variant allele were highly associated with disease recurrence in patients with Tis, Ta, and T1 tumors [18]. To further investigate this, we screened BCG-NMIBC tumors for this common

SNP. We found that rs2853669 carrier status did not modulate *TERTp* effect on BCG therapy success in our series, however, there was an association of rs2853669 AA carriers with tumors of higher grade. This association is in accordance with what Rachakonda and others described. In patients that harbor the germline rs2853669 AA genotype, the TERTp mutation effect is not reverted in the BC tumor. As Rachakonda described, patients with this combination (germline rs2853669 G absence, TERTp tumor positive) present poorer survival and increased disease recurrence, which are features compatible with the presence of more aggressive tumors, such as higher grade.

Finally, we analyzed recurrence-free survival after BCG treatment, comparing *TERTp* and *FGFR3* mutation status and specific mutations and rs2853669 carrier status. Kaplan–Meier survival analysis showed a promising recurrence-free survival advantage for those c.1-146G>A mutation carriers. Our results demonstrate that BCG-NMIBC c.1-146G>A mutation carriers are three time less likely to recur after BCG therapy and may have more favorable recurrence-free survival rates when compared to both *TERTp* wild type and c.1-124G>A cases. To interpret these findings, it is important to note that what we are evaluating is how *TERTp* mutations modulate the tumor response after BCG therapy. It has previously been suggested that the mechanism of BCG therapeutic effects on BC is related to its ability to reduce telomerase (*TERT*) activity [30] — we may speculate that c.1-146G>A mutated tumors might be more susceptible to the reduction of telomerase activity by BCG. As reported by Huang et al., *TERTp* mutations are associated with higher *TERT* transcription levels compared to wild type promoters but *TERTp* c.1-146G>A carriers have lower transcriptional capacity than those with the c.1-124G>A mutation [7]. We can speculate that the higher *TERT* expression induced by the c.1-124G>A mutation partially impairs BCG capability to sufficiently reduce telomeric activity to a therapeutic level — a level that could be achieved in a c.1-146G>A setting. Also, the lower frequency of *TERTp* mutations in BCG-treated recurrent tumors when compared to primary tumors could be explained by the enhanced BCG action on tumor cells harboring *TERTp* mutations, leading to clonal selection pressure towards cells harboring other alterations (such as *FGFR3* mutations) in recurrent tumors, hence shifting the prevalence of recurrent tumors towards TERTp-negative tumors. More studies comparing *TERT* expression and telomerase activity before and after BCG therapy with the different *TERTp* mutations are required to further interpret our results. To our knowledge, this study is one of the first studies addressing *TERTp* and *FGFR3* mutations in a BCG-NMI series of BC patients. We found no association between *TERTp* mutations, as a whole, and tumor grade or stage. However, we observed that the specific *TERTp* c.1-146G>A mutation was an independent predictor of nonrecurrence after BCG therapy in the BCG-NMI tumors. Our results suggest that it might be relevant to further study the role of *TERTp* mutations in tumor recurrence and as predictive markers of response to BCG therapy.

4. Materials and Methods

4.1. Human Cancer Samples and Clinicopathological Data

Formalin-fixed, paraffin-embedded (FFPE) tissues were obtained from 125 patients with NMI bladder urothelial cell carcinoma treated with intravesical BCG therapy, with samples being collected at the time of transurethral resection before any BCG therapy administration. Patients underwent resection of the tumors in the Portuguese Institute of Oncology — Francisco Gentil (IPO) Porto. Hematoxylin-eosin-stained sections were reviewed according to the standard histopathological examination by two independent pathologists. Staging and grading were conducted according to the American Joint Committee on Cancer [31], and the 2004 WHO classification system [32]. Clinicopathological and follow-up data were retrieved from the files of IPO databases. Age refers to age at BCG treatment initiation in the BCG-NMIBC group. Recurrence status characterizes the BCG-NMIBC cases as either a primary newly diagnosed tumor selected for BCG therapy or, alternatively, as a recurrence of a previously resected NMI tumor (that did not fill the criteria for being included in the BCG-NMIBC group before) that is only now selected for BCG therapy. BCG therapy selection was performed according to the EORTC criteria previously described [22]. BCG schedule characterizes the treatment regimen used as maintenance (mBCG) or induction-only (iBCG) intravesical BCG instillation. BCG therapy success was defined as no recurrence and failure was defined as any recurrence after BCG treatment. Analysis of patients' age by age groups (<65 years and ≥65 years) was recognized as an informative analysis and has been used previously [33]. All the procedures described in this study were in accordance with national and institutional ethical standards and previously approved by Local Ethical Review Committees (Ethics Committee of the Portuguese Institute of Oncology of Porto with the number CES IPOPFG-EPE 586/08 in 25 of September of 2008). According to Portuguese law, informed consent is not required for retrospective studies.

4.2. DNA Extraction, PCR, and Sanger Sequencing

DNA was obtained from FFPE (10-micron sections) after careful microdissection. DNA extraction was performed using an Ultraprep Tissue DNA Kit (AHN Biotechnologie, Nordhaussen, Germany) following manufacturer's instructions.

To screen for *TERTp* mutations, we analyzed by PCR followed by Sanger sequencing of the hotspots previously identified [10]. *TERTp* mutation analysis was performed with the pair of primers Fw *TERT*—5′-CAGCGCTGCCTGAAACTC-3′ and Rv *TERT*—5′-GTCCTGCCCCTTCACCTT-3′. Amplification of genomic DNA (25–100ng) was performed by PCR using the Qiagen Multiplex PCR kit (Qiagen, Hilden, Germany) according to the manufacturer's instructions. Sequencing reaction was performed with the ABI Prism BigDye Terminator Kit (Perkin Elmer, Foster City, CA, USA), and the fragments were run in an ABI prism 3100 Genetic Analyzer (Perkin-Elmer). The sequencing reaction was performed in a forward direction, and an independent PCR amplification/sequencing, both in a forward and reverse direction, was performed in positive samples or samples that were inconclusive. To screen for *FGFR3*, we analyzed the hotspots previously identified in exon 7, 10, and 15 in 107 BCG-NMIBC cases (18 cases have been excluded due to insufficient DNA for the analysis) by PCR followed by Sanger sequencing. *FGFR3* exon 7, 10, and 15 mutation analysis was performed with the respective pairs of primers Fw Exon 7—5′-AGTGGCGGTGGTGGTGAGGGAG-3′ and Rv Exon 7—5′-GCACCGCCGTCTGGTTGG-3′; Fw Exon 10—5′-CAACGCCCATGTCTTTGCAG-3′ and Rv Exon 10—5′-AGGCGGCAGAGCGTCACAG-3′; Fw Exon 15—5′-GACCGAGGACAACGTGATG-3′ and Rv Exon 15—5′-GTGTGGGAAGGCGGTGTTG-3′. Subsequent steps followed the same methodology as outlined for the *TERT* promoter mutation screening.

4.3. Single Nucleotide Polymorphism Assay

Screening for the rs2853669 polymorphism was performed in 98 BCG-NMIBC cases (27 cases were excluded due to insufficient DNA for the analysis) using the rs2853669 TaqMan® SNP Genotyping Assay (Applied Biosystems, Foster City, USA). Peripheral blood DNA was extracted using a genomic DNA extraction kit (Qiagen). The purified genomic DNA was used for the assay. The procedure was performed according to manufacturer's instructions.

4.4. Uromonitor Real-Time PCR screening Assay

Screening of 125 nonmuscle invasive BC tumors treated with BCG therapy (BCG-NMIBC) for *TERTp* mutations and *FGFR3* hotspot mutations were confirmed by using a specific IVD commercial kit Uromonitor®—Real-Time PCR kit for the amplification and detection of *TERTp* and *FGFR3* hotspot mutations (U-Monitor, Porto, Portugal), according to manufacturer's instructions.

4.5. Statistical Analysis

The statistical analysis was performed using IBM SPSS statistics software version 25.0. For the analysis of the relationship between patients' age, we used the independent-samples *t*-test. Pearson's Chi-square and Fisher's exact test were used in the statistical analysis of the other parameters, according to sample size. Cox proportional hazard ratios were estimated to obtain risks of recurrence for cases in each molecular factor stratum before and after adjusting for other confounding variables. Kaplan–Meier survival curves were computed by each category of the potential prognostic factors and the log-rank and Breslow tests were applied to compare curves. Means were used instead of medians because some survival curves did not fall under 50%. Results were considered statistically significant if $p < 0.05$.

Supplementary Materials: Supplementary Materials can be found at http://www.mdpi.com/1422-0067/21/3/947/s1.

Author Contributions: Conceptualization, R.B., J.V., V.M., L.S. and P.S.; data curation, L.L.; formal analysis, R.B. and L.L.; funding acquisition, J.V., V.M., L.S. and P.S.; investigation, R.B., L.L., J.V., V.P., J.L. and P.S.; methodology, R.B., V.P. and J.L.; project administration, L.S. and P.S.; resources, J.V. and P.S.; supervision, V.M., L.S. and P.S.; validation, R.B. and J.V.; writing—original draft, R.B., L.L., J.V., V.P. and J.L.; writing—review and editing, R.B., L.L., J.V., V.M., L.S. and P.S. All authors have read and agreed to the published version of the manuscript.

Funding: This research was funded by FCT—Fundação para a Ciência e a Tecnologia, Ministério da Ciência, Tecnologia e Ensino Superior by a research contract to João Vinagre (CEECIND/00201/2017) and a PhD grant to Rui Batista (SFRH/BD/111321/2015). Further funding was obtained from the project "Advancing cancer research: from basic knowledge to application" NORTE-01- 0145-FEDER-000029: "Projetos Estruturados de I & D & I", funded by Norte 2020—Programa Operacional Regional do Norte. Additional funding was obtained from the project PTDC/MED-ONC/31438/2017 (The other faces of Telomerase: Looking beyond tumor immortalization), supported by Norte Portugal Regional Operational Programme (NORTE 2020), under the PORTUGAL 2020 Partnership Agreement, through the European Regional Development Fund (ERDF), COMPETE 2020 - Operational Programme for Competitiveness and Internationalization (POCI) and by Portuguese funds through FCT under project POCI-01-0145-FEDER-016390: CANCEL STEM".

Conflicts of Interest: The authors declare no conflict of interest.

Abbreviations

BC	Bladder cancer
BCG	Bacillus Calmette–Guérin
BCG-NMI	BCG-treated nonmuscle invasive
NMI	Nonmuscle invasive

References

1. Ferlay, J.; Colombet, M.; Soerjomataram, I.; Mathers, C.; Parkin, D.M.; Pineros, M.; Znaor, A.; Bray, F. Estimating the global cancer incidence and mortality in 2018: GLOBOCAN sources and methods. *J. Int. Cancer* **2019**, *144*, 1941–1953. [CrossRef]

2. Ploeg, M.; Aben, K.K.; Kiemeney, L.A. The present and future burden of urinary bladder cancer in the world. *World J. Urol.* **2009**, *27*, 289–293. [CrossRef] [PubMed]

3. van Rhijn, B.W.; Burger, M.; Lotan, Y.; Solsona, E.; Stief, C.G.; Sylvester, R.J.; Witjes, J.A.; Zlotta, A.R. Recurrence and progression of disease in non-muscle-invasive bladder cancer: from epidemiology to treatment strategy. *Eur. Urol.* **2009**, *56*, 430–442. [CrossRef] [PubMed]

4. Netto, G.J. Molecular biomarkers in urothelial carcinoma of the bladder: are we there yet? *Nat. Rev. Urol.* **2011**, *9*, 41–51. [CrossRef] [PubMed]

5. Northrup, H.; Krueger, D.A.; International Tuberous Sclerosis Complex Consensus, G. Tuberous sclerosis complex diagnostic criteria update: recommendations of the 2012 Iinternational Tuberous Sclerosis Complex Consensus Conference. *Pediatr. Neurol.* **2013**, *49*, 243–254. [CrossRef]

6. Horn, S.; Figl, A.; Rachakonda, P.S.; Fischer, C.; Sucker, A.; Gast, A.; Kadel, S.; Moll, I.; Nagore, E.; Hemminki, K.; et al. TERT promoter mutations in familial and sporadic melanoma. *Science* **2013**, *339*, 959–961. [CrossRef]

7. Huang, F.W.; Hodis, E.; Xu, M.J.; Kryukov, G.V.; Chin, L.; Garraway, L.A. Highly recurrent TERT promoter mutations in human melanoma. *Science* **2013**, *339*, 957–959. [CrossRef]

8. Killela, P.J.; Reitman, Z.J.; Jiao, Y.; Bettegowda, C.; Agrawal, N.; Diaz, L.A., Jr.; Friedman, A.H.; Friedman, H.; Gallia, G.L.; Giovanella, B.C.; et al. TERT promoter mutations occur frequently in gliomas and a subset of tumors derived from cells with low rates of self-renewal. *Proc. Natl. Acad. Sci. USA* **2013**, *110*, 6021–6026. [CrossRef]

9. Liu, X.; Bishop, J.; Shan, Y.; Pai, S.; Liu, D.; Murugan, A.K.; Sun, H.; El-Naggar, A.K.; Xing, M. Highly prevalent TERT promoter mutations in aggressive thyroid cancers. *Endocr. Relat. Cancer* **2013**, *20*, 603–610. [CrossRef]

10. Vinagre, J.; Almeida, A.; Populo, H.; Batista, R.; Lyra, J.; Pinto, V.; Coelho, R.; Celestino, R.; Prazeres, H.; Lima, L.; et al. Frequency of TERT promoter mutations in human cancers. *Nat. Commun.* **2013**, *4*, 2185. [CrossRef]

11. Nault, J.C.; Mallet, M.; Pilati, C.; Calderaro, J.; Bioulac-Sage, P.; Laurent, C.; Laurent, A.; Cherqui, D.; Balabaud, C.; Zucman-Rossi, J. High frequency of telomerase reverse-transcriptase promoter somatic mutations in hepatocellular carcinoma and preneoplastic lesions. *Nat. Commun.* **2013**, *4*, 2218. [CrossRef] [PubMed]

12. Griewank, K.G.; Schilling, B.; Murali, R.; Bielefeld, N.; Schwamborn, M.; Sucker, A.; Zimmer, L.; Hillen, U.; Schaller, J.; Brenn, T.; et al. TERT promoter mutations are frequent in atypical fibroxanthomas and pleomorphic dermal sarcomas. *Mod. Pathol.: Off. J. US Can. Acad. Pathol. Inc.* **2014**, *27*, 502–508. [CrossRef] [PubMed]

13. Allory, Y.; Beukers, W.; Sagrera, A.; Flandez, M.; Marques, M.; Marquez, M.; van der Keur, K.A.; Dyrskjot, L.; Lurkin, I.; Vermeij, M.; et al. Telomerase reverse transcriptase promoter mutations in bladder cancer: high frequency across stages, detection in urine, and lack of association with outcome. *Eur. Urol.* **2014**, *65*, 360–366. [CrossRef] [PubMed]

14. Hurst, C.D.; Platt, F.M.; Knowles, M.A. Comprehensive mutation analysis of the TERT promoter in bladder cancer and detection of mutations in voided urine. *Eur. Urol.* **2014**, *65*, 367–369. [CrossRef]

15. Scott, G.A.; Laughlin, T.S.; Rothberg, P.G. Mutations of the TERT promoter are common in basal cell carcinoma and squamous cell carcinoma. *Mod. Pathol.: Off. J. US Can. Acad. Pathol. Inc.* **2014**, *27*, 516–523. [CrossRef]

16. Liu, X.; Wu, G.; Shan, Y.; Hartmann, C.; von Deimling, A.; Xing, M. Highly prevalent TERT promoter mutations in bladder cancer and glioblastoma. *Cell Cycle* **2013**, *12*, 1637–1638. [CrossRef]

17. Kinde, I.; Munari, E.; Faraj, S.F.; Hruban, R.H.; Schoenberg, M.; Bivalacqua, T.; Allaf, M.; Springer, S.; Wang, Y.; Diaz, L.A., Jr.; et al. TERT promoter mutations occur early in urothelial neoplasia and are biomarkers of early disease and disease recurrence in urine. *Cancer Res.* **2013**, *73*, 7162–7167. [CrossRef]

18. Rachakonda, P.S.; Hosen, I.; de Verdier, P.J.; Fallah, M.; Heidenreich, B.; Ryk, C.; Wiklund, N.P.; Steineck, G.; Schadendorf, D.; Hemminki, K.; et al. TERT promoter mutations in bladder cancer affect patient survival and disease recurrence through modification by a common polymorphism. *Proc. Natl. Acad. Sci. USA* **2013**, *110*, 17426–17431. [CrossRef]

19. Wu, S.; Huang, P.; Li, C.; Huang, Y.; Li, X.; Wang, Y.; Chen, C.; Lv, Z.; Tang, A.; Sun, X.; et al. Telomerase reverse transcriptase gene promoter mutations help discern the origin of urogenital tumors: a genomic and molecular study. *Eur. Urol.* **2014**, *65*, 274–277. [CrossRef]

20. Ko, E.; Seo, H.W.; Jung, E.S.; Kim, B.H.; Jung, G. The TERT promoter SNP rs2853669 decreases E2F1 transcription factor binding and increases mortality and recurrence risks in liver cancer. *Oncotarget* **2016**, *7*, 684–699. [CrossRef]

21. Batista, R.; Cruvinel-Carloni, A.; Vinagre, J.; Peixoto, J.; Catarino, T.A.; Campanella, N.C.; Menezes, W.; Becker, A.P.; de Almeida, G.C.; Matsushita, M.M.; et al. The prognostic impact of TERT promoter mutations in glioblastomas is modified by the rs2853669 single nucleotide polymorphism. *Int. J. Cancer* **2016**, *139*, 414–423. [CrossRef] [PubMed]

22. Babjuk, M.; Oosterlinck, W.; Sylvester, R.; Kaasinen, E.; Bohle, A.; Palou-Redorta, J.; Roupret, M.; European Association of U. EAU guidelines on non-muscle-invasive urothelial carcinoma of the bladder, the 2011 update. *Eur. Urol.* **2011**, *59*, 997–1008. [CrossRef] [PubMed]

23. Askeland, E.J.; Newton, M.R.; O'Donnell, M.A.; Luo, Y. Bladder Cancer Immunotherapy: BCG and Beyond. *Adv. Urol.* **2012**, *2012*, 181987. [CrossRef] [PubMed]

24. Yates, D.R.; Roupret, M. Contemporary management of patients with high-risk non-muscle-invasive bladder cancer who fail intravesical BCG therapy. *World J. Urol.* **2011**, *29*, 415–422. [CrossRef] [PubMed]

25. Billerey, C.; Chopin, D.; Aubriot-Lorton, M.H.; Ricol, D.; Gil Diez de Medina, S.; Van Rhijn, B.; Bralet, M.P.; Lefrere-Belda, M.A.; Lahaye, J.B.; Abbou, C.C.; et al. Frequent FGFR3 mutations in papillary non-invasive bladder (pTa) tumors. *Am. J. Pathol.* **2001**, *158*, 1955–1959. [CrossRef]

26. Roe, J.S.; Kim, H.; Lee, S.M.; Kim, S.T.; Cho, E.J.; Youn, H.D. p53 Stabilization and Transactivation by a von Hippel-Lindau Protein. *Mol. Cell* **2006**, *22*, 395–405. [CrossRef]

27. Kawai, K.; Miyazaki, J.; Joraku, A.; Nishiyama, H.; Akaza, H. Bacillus Calmette-Guerin (BCG) immunotherapy for bladder cancer: current understanding and perspectives on engineered BCG vaccine. *Cancer Sci.* **2013**, *104*, 22–27. [CrossRef]

28. Herr, H.W.; Morales, A. History of bacillus Calmette-Guerin and bladder cancer: an immunotherapy success story. *J. Urol.* **2008**, *179*, 53–56. [CrossRef]

29. Dabora, S.L.; Jozwiak, S.; Franz, D.N.; Roberts, P.S.; Nieto, A.; Chung, J.; Choy, Y.-S.; Reeve, M.P.; Thiele, E.; Egelhoff, J.C.; et al. Mutational Analysis in a Cohort of 224 Tuberous Sclerosis Patients Indicates Increased Severity of TSC2, Compared with TSC1, Disease in Multiple Organs. *Am. J. Hum. Genet.* **2001**, *68*, 64–80. [CrossRef]

30. Saitoh, H.; Mori, K.; Kudoh, S.; Itoh, H.; Takahashi, N.; Suzuki, T. BCG effects on telomerase activity in bladder cancer cell lines. *Int. J. Clin. Oncol.* **2002**, *7*, 165–170. [CrossRef]

31. Edge, S.B.; Compton, C.C. The American Joint Committee on Cancer: the 7th edition of the AJCC cancer staging manual and the future of TNM. *Ann. Surg. Oncol.* **2010**, *17*, 1471–1474. [CrossRef] [PubMed]

32. Davis, C.J.; Woodward, P.J.; Dehner, L.P.; Eble, J.N.; Sauter, G.; Epstein, J.I. WHO Classification of Tumors. Pathology and Genetics of Tumors of the Urinary System and Male Genital Organs. *IARC Press* **2004**, 267–276.

33. Lima, L.; Oliveira, D.; Tavares, A.; Amaro, T.; Cruz, R.; Oliveira, M.J.; Ferreira, J.A.; Santos, L. The predominance of M2-polarized macrophages in the stroma of low-hypoxic bladder tumors is associated with BCG immunotherapy failure. *Urol. Oncol.* **2014**, *32*, 449–457. [CrossRef] [PubMed]

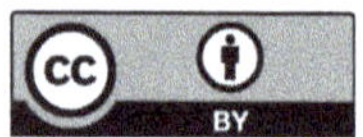

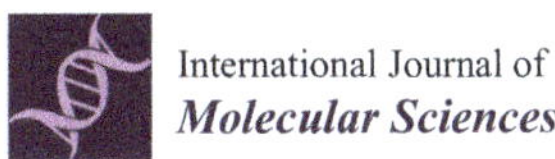

International Journal of
Molecular Sciences

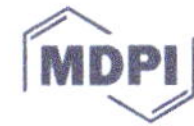

Article

Transgelin, a p53 and PTEN-Upregulated Gene, Inhibits the Cell Proliferation and Invasion of Human Bladder Carcinoma Cells In Vitro and In Vivo

Ke-Hung Tsui [1,†], Yu-Hsiang Lin [1,2,†], Kang-Shuo Chang [3,4], Chen-Pang Hou [1,2],
Pin-Jung Chen [3,4], Tsui-Hsia Feng [5] and Horng-Heng Juang [1,3,4,*]

[1]   Department of Urology, Chang Gung Memorial Hospital-Linkou, Kwei-Shan, Tao-Yuan 33302, Taiwan;
      t2130@cgmh.org.tw (K.-H.T.); linyh@doctorvoice.org (Y.-H.L.); glucose1979@gmail.com (C.-P.H.)
[2]   Graduate Institute of Clinical Medical Science, College of Medicine, Chang Gung University, Kwei-Shan,
      Tao-Yuan 33302, Taiwan
[3]   Department of Anatomy, College of Medicine, Chang Gung University, Kwei-Shan, Tao-Yuan 33302, Taiwan;
      D0501301@stmail.cgu.edu.tw (K.-S.C.); lulu581623@gmail.com (P.-J.C.)
[4]   Graduate Institute of Biomedical Sciences, College of Medicine, Chang Gung University, Kwei-Shan,
      Tao-Yuan 33302, Taiwan
[5]   School of Nursing, College of Medicine, Chang Gung University, Kwei-Shan, Tao-Yuan 33302, Taiwan;
      thf@mail.cgu.edu.tw
*   Correspondence: hhj143@mail.cgu.edu.tw; Tel.: +886-3-2118800; Fax: +886-3-2118112
†   These authors contributed equally to this work.

Received: 8 August 2019; Accepted: 3 October 2019; Published: 7 October 2019

Abstract: Transgelin (TAGLN/SM22-α) is a regulator of the actin cytoskeleton, affecting the survival, migration, and apoptosis of various cancer cells divergently; however, the roles of TAGLN in bladder carcinoma cells remain inconclusive. We compared expressions of TAGLN in human bladder carcinoma cells to the normal human bladder tissues to determine the potential biological functions and regulatory mechanisms of TAGLN in bladder carcinoma cells. Results of RT-qPCR and immunoblot assays indicated that TAGLN expressions were higher in bladder smooth muscle cells, fibroblast cells, and normal epithelial cells than in carcinoma cells (RT-4, HT1376, TSGH-8301, and T24) in vitro. Besides, the results of RT-qPCR revealed that TAGLN expressions were higher in normal tissues than the paired tumor tissues. In vitro, TAGLN knockdown enhanced cell proliferation and invasion, while overexpression of TAGLN had the inverse effects in bladder carcinoma cells. Meanwhile, ectopic overexpression of TAGLN attenuated tumorigenesis in vivo. Immunofluorescence and immunoblot assays showed that TAGLN was predominantly in the cytosol and colocalized with F-actin. Ectopic overexpression of either p53 or PTEN induced TAGLN expression, while p53 knockdown downregulated TAGLN expression in bladder carcinoma cells. Our results indicate that TAGLN is a p53 and PTEN-upregulated gene, expressing higher levels in normal bladder epithelial cells than carcinoma cells. Further, TAGLN inhibited cell proliferation and invasion in vitro and blocked tumorigenesis in vivo. Collectively, it can be concluded that TAGLN is an antitumor gene in the human bladder.

Keywords: bladder; TAGLN; F-actin; PTEN; p53; tumorigenesis; proliferation; invasion

1. Introduction

Transglin/SM22-α/WS3-10/mp27 (TAGLN), a kind of 22-kDa protein, presents primarily in smooth muscle-containing tissues of vertebrates. Cytogenetically, the human TAGLN gene is located to the chromosome 11 q23.2 [1]. When using the TAGLN-deficient mouse embryo model, TAGLN may not be required for the development of the embryo, but plays roles in the morphological transformation of the smooth muscle cell (SMC) [2]. A study has found that decreased levels of TAGLN disrupted normal actin organization leading to the changes in the motile behavior of REF52 fibroblast cells [3]. The depletion of TAGLN resulted in an increase in the capacity of cells to go initiate spontaneous podosome formation, with a concomitant increase in the ability of invasion from Matrigel assays; therefore, TAGLN seemed to be a marker of active stromal remodeling in vicinity of invasive carcinomas [4].

The reduction in the expressions of TAGLN are often found in tumor cell lines, and the TAGLN depletion increases actin dynamics and enhances tumorigenic phenotypes of the cells [3]. Early study indicated that abolition of TAGLN expression is an important early event in tumor progression and a diagnostic marker for breast and colon cancer development [5]. However, issues concerning the tumorigenesis of TAGLN in different tissues are still in controversy. Studies have reported that TAGLN is an antitumor gene in esophageal squamous cell carcinoma and regarded as an oncogene for gastric cancer [6–8]. Other studies indicated that TAGLN exerts an anti-metastasis effect in colon and colorectal cancers [9–13]. However, contrary results from different independent laboratories showed that overexpression of TAGLN causes a poor prognosis in colon cancer in vivo and contributes to colorectal cancer progression and metastasis [14,15]. Similar, contrary reports are also found in studies of lung cancer [16,17].

An early study of rabbit bladders suggested that TAGLN is an SMC-lineage marker [18]. However, previous studies indicated that *TAGLN* is one of the common differentially-expressed genes which is significantly decreased in bladder cancer compared with normal bladder tissues [19,20]. The precise functions and the regulatory mechanisms of *TAGLN* in the bladder carcinoma cells are still not illustrated and explored.

In this study, we determined the expressions of *TAGLN* in both bladder carcinoma cells and bladder tissues, and examined the regulatory mechanisms and potential functions of *TAGLN* in bladder carcinoma cells.

2. Results

2.1. Expressions of TAGLN in Bladder Smooth Muscle Cells, Fibroblast Cells, Normal Epithelial Cells, and Carcinoma Cells

To understand the expression of TAGLN in human bladder cells, we compared levels of TAGLN in human normal primary bladder epithelial cells (HBdEC), bladder smooth muscle cells (HBdSMC), bladder stromal fibroblasts (HBdSF), and four lines of cultured bladder carcinoma cells (RT4, HT1376, T24, and TSGH-8301). Results of RT-qPCR assays revealed that levels of *TAGLN* were higher in both HBdSMC and HBdEC cells than the bladder carcinoma cells (Figure 1A). Further immunoblot assays showed that T24 cells expressed the highest TAGLN protein levels among the four carcinoma cell lines (Figure 1B) which were similar to the results of RT-qPCR assays presented in the Figure 1A. The immunoblot assays also revealed that HBdSMC cells expressed higher protein levels of alpha-smooth muscle actin (α-SMA), and HBdEC cells exhibited higher protein levels of uroplakin-2 (UPK-2), a marker of bladder transitional cells (Figure 1C). The normal primary bladder epithelial cells (HBdEC) presented far higher TAGLN protein levels in comparison to the bladder carcinoma T24 cells (Figure 1D).

2.2. Expressions of TAGLN in Paired Human Bladder Tissues

The RT-qPCR analysis of paired human bladder tissues showed that means of $\Delta\Delta C_t$ between normal and cancer tissues were 3.77 ± 0.67 using *β-actin* as internal control (Figure 1E) and 4.33 ± 0.72 using *18S* as internal control (Figure 1F), respectively, suggesting significantly higher expressions of *TAGLN* mRNA levels in normal bladder tissues than that in bladder cancer tissues.

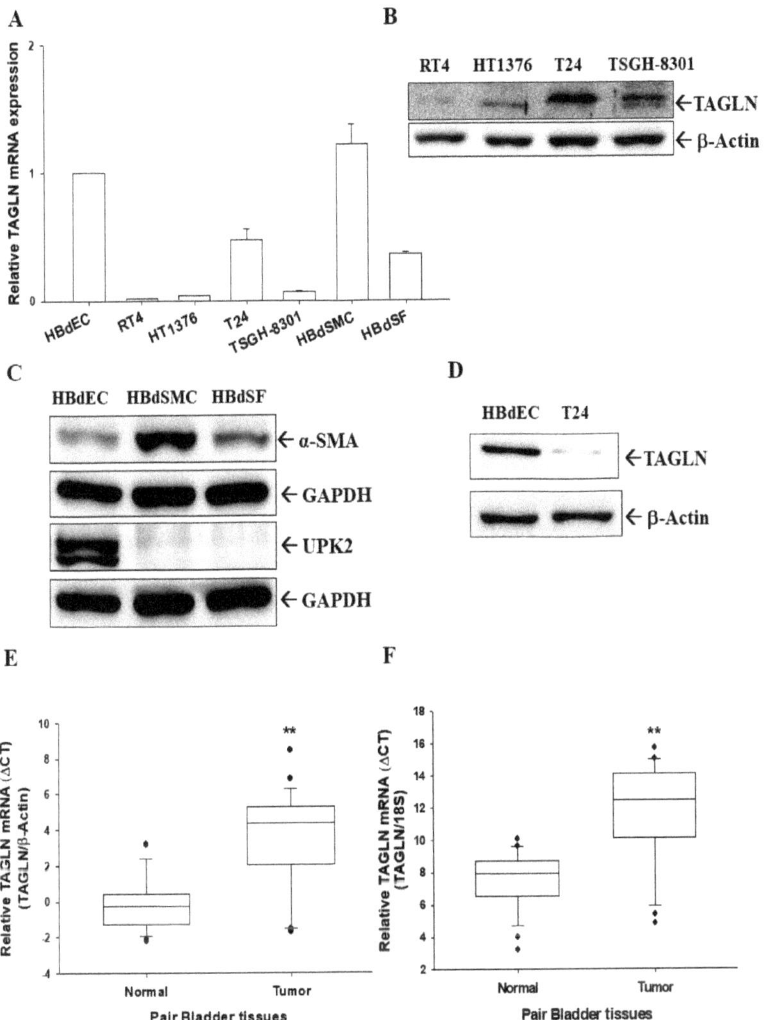

Figure 1. Gene expression of *TAGLN* in human bladder cells and tissues. (**A**) Total RNA from bladder smooth muscle cells (HBdSMC), fibroblast cells (HBdSF), normal epithelial cells (HBdEC), and carcinoma cell lines (RT4, HT1376, T24, and TSGH-8301) were extracted for RT-qPCR ($\pm$ SE; $n = 3$) assays. (**B**) Bladder carcinoma cell lines (RT4, HT1376, T24, and TSGH-8301) were lysed, and TAGLN and β-actin were determined by immunoblotting. (**C**) HBdEC, HBdSMC, and HBdSF cells were lysed and α-SMA, UPK2, and GAPDH were determined by immunoblotting. (**D**) HBdEC and T24 cells were lysed and TAGLN and β-actin were determined by immunoblotting. Quantitative analysis of TAGLN expression in paired bladder cancerous and normal tissues was determined by RT-qPCR using the β-actin (**E**) or 18S (**F**) as the internal control. Box plot analysis was used to compare the TAGLN expressions in cancerous and normal bladder tissues ($n = 25$). ** represented the $p < 0.01$.

2.3. TAGLN's Localization is Predominantly Cytosolic and with F-actin

In order to understand the subcellular location of TAGLN in the bladder carcinoma cells, we transiently overexpressed TAGLN in HT1376 cells. Results of immunofluorescence staining indicated that HT-TAGLN cells expressed higher protein levels of TAGLN, located predominantly in the cytosol, in comparison to HT-DNA cells (Figure 2A,E). The cells were also stained with Texas Red X-Phalloidin to determine the F-actin (Figure 2B,F), and DAPI to highlight the nuclei of HT-DNA and HT-TAGLN cells (Figure 2C,G). Results of immunofluorescence indicated that TAGLN expression colocalized with F-actin (Figure 2D,H). Further study of immunoblot assays with subcellular extraction confirmed the ectopic-TAGLN expression in HT1376 cells (HT-TAGLN). Expression was predominantly present in the cytoplasm, with a little expression in the membrane. TAGLN did not express in the nuclei of HT-DNA and HT-TAGLN cells (Figure 2I).

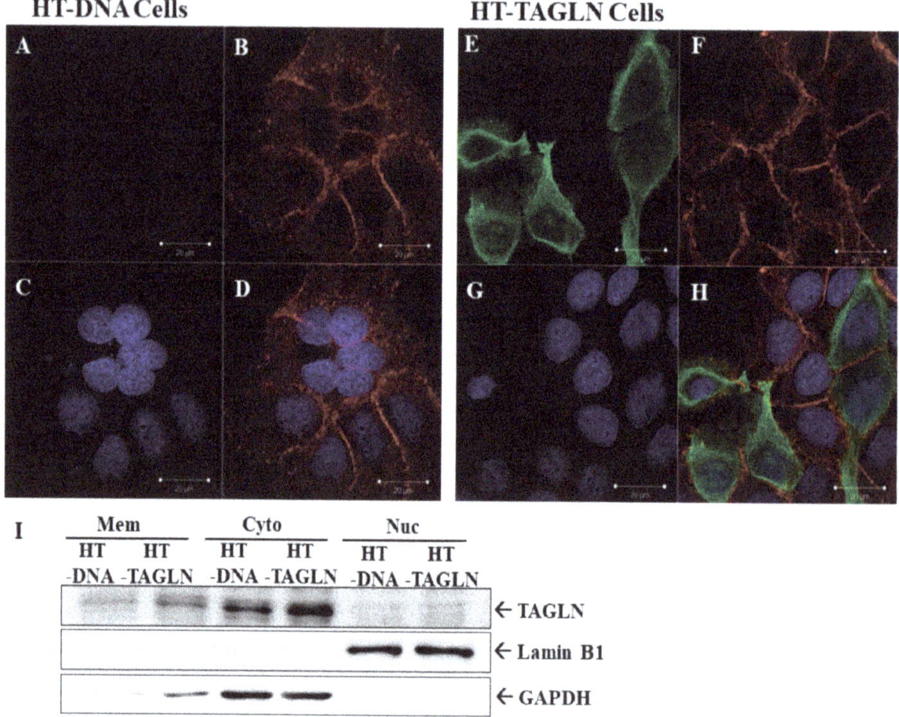

Figure 2. Immunofluorescence staining of TAGLN in TAGLN-overexpressed-HT1376 cells. Immunofluorescence detection of TAGLN in mock-transfected HT1376 (HT-DNA) (**A**) and TAGLN-overexpressed HT1376 (HT-TAGLN) (**E**) cells. The red-stained with Texas Red X-Phalloidin represents the F-actin (**B,F**). The blue-stained by DAPI represents nuclei of cells (**C,G**). All images were observed and recorded under the same settings with a confocal microscope. Immunofluorescence results indicated that TAGLN expression colocalized with F-actin (**D,H**). (**I**) Cells were subcellularly extracted into the membrane (Mem), cytosol (Cyto), and nuclei (Nuc). The protein levels of TAGLN, Lamin B, and GAPDH were determined using immunoblot assays.

2.4. The Effects of TAGLN on Cell Proliferation in Bladder Carcinoma Cells

Using immunoblot and RT-qPCR assays, we confirmed that expression of *TAGLN* was about 50% in the TAGLN-knockdown T24 cells compared to mock-knockdown (T24_shCOL) cells (Figure 3A). The results of EdU flow cytometry (Figure 3C) and EdU staining proliferation (Figure 3D) assays showed that knockdown of TAGLN (T24_shTAGLN) increased 10% and 9% of cells with EdU-staining compared to mock-transduced (T24_shCOL) cells, respectively. Opposite results were found for ectopic overexpression of TAGLN in HT1376 cells. Figure 3B confirmed the ectopic overexpression of TAGLN in HT1376 (HT-TAGLN) cells compared to mock-transfected HT1376 (HT-DNA) cells, as determined by immunoblot and RT-qPCR assays. When cells were overexpressed the TAGLN, the percentage of positive cells with EdU incorporation were decreased, which was determined by flow cytometry (Figure 3E) and EdU staining proliferation (Figure 3F) assays. Decreasing cell proliferation after ectopic overexpression of TAGLN was also found in the TAGLN-overexpressed HT1376 and TSGH-8301 cells, respectively, determined by Ki67 proliferation assays (Figure S1).

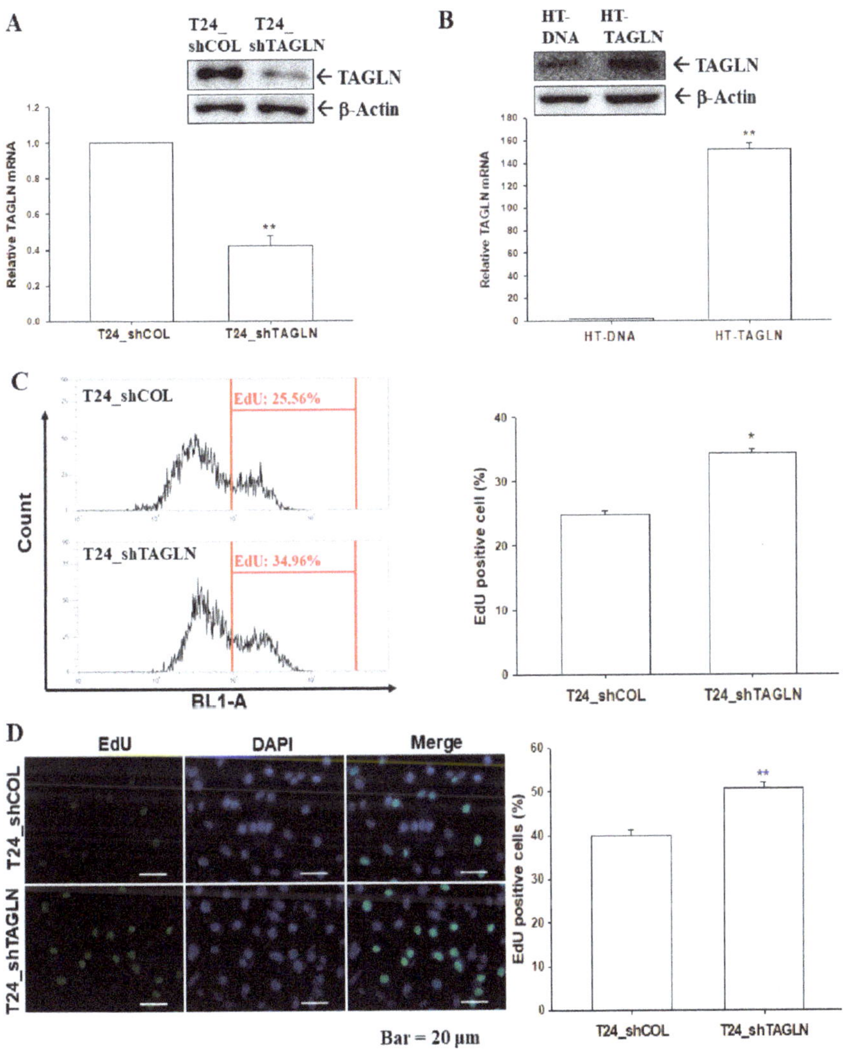

Figure 3. *Cont.*

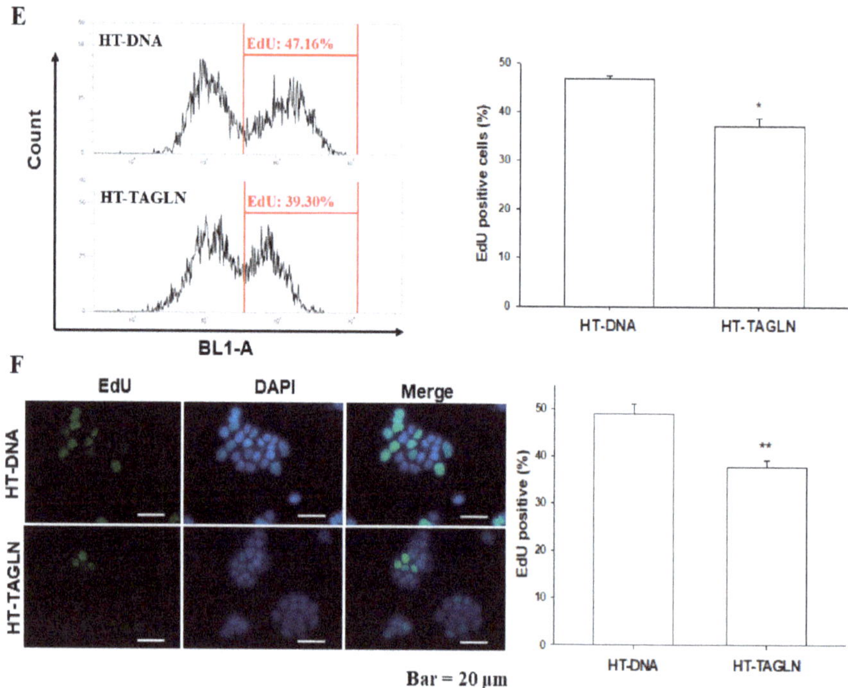

Figure 3. The effects of TAGLN on the cell proliferation of bladder carcinoma cells. The expressions of TAGLN in T24-knockdown T24 (T24_shTAGLN) cells (**A**) and ectopic TAGLN-overexpressed HT1376 (HT-TAGLN) cells (**B**) in comparison to mock-transfected control cells (T24_shCOL and HT-DNA) were determined by immunoblot (top) and RT-qPCR (bottom) assays (± SE; $n = 3$). The proliferation abilities of T24_shCOL and T24_shTAGLN cells were determined by flow cytometry with Click-iT EdU flow cytometry assays (**C**) and EdU cell immunofluorescence staining (± SE; $n = 4$) (**D**). The proliferation abilities of HT-DNA and HT-TAGLN cells were determined by flow cytometry with (**E**) Click-iT EdU flow cytometry assays and (**F**) EdU cell immunofluorescence staining (± SE; $n = 4$). * represented the $p < 0.05$ and the ** represented the $p < 0.01$.

2.5. The Effects of TAGLN on Cell Invasion in Bladder Carcinoma Cells

The results of Matrigel invasion assays indicated that the knockdown of TAGLN resulted in a two-fold increase in invasion capacity compared to T24_shCOL cells (Figure 4A). On the contrary, the invasion capacity was downregulated 45% in HT-TAGLN cell compared to HT-DNA cells (Figure 4B). We further cloned the TAGLN-overexpressed TSGH-8301 (8301-TAGLN) cells (Figure 4C) and the TAGLN-knockdown TSGH-8301 (8301_shTAGLN) cells (Figure 4D) to confirm the expression of TAGLN by immunoblot and RT-qPCR assays. The Matrigel invasion assays showed that 8301-TAGLN cells expressed markedly lower invasive capacity than 8301-DNA cells (Figure 4E), while the knockdown of TAGLN in bladder carcinoma TSGH-8301 cells enhanced cell invasion (Figure 4F). Results of wound healing assays also revealed the decreased migration ability of HT1376 cell after the ectopic overexpression of TAGLN (Figure S2).

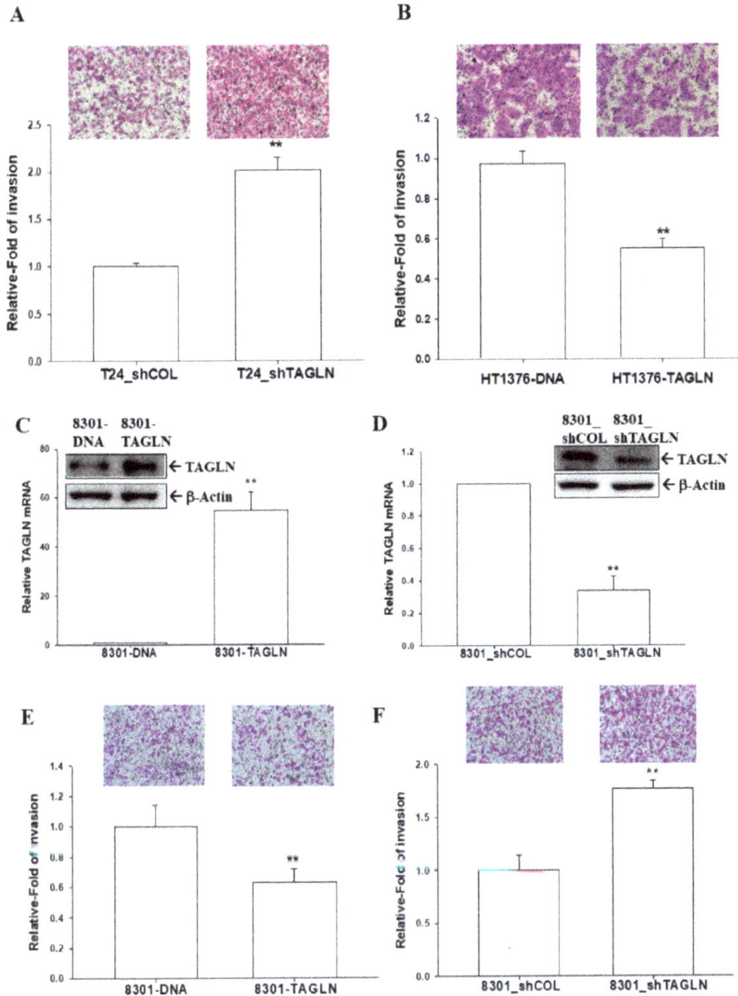

Figure 4. Modulation of TAGLN on cell invasion in bladder carcinoma cells. The invasion abilities of cells were determined by in vitro Matrigel invasion assays. Data are presented as mean percentages (± SE; n = 3) in relation to those of the T24_shCOL (**A**) or HT-DNA (**B**) groups. (**C**) Expressions of TAGLN in mock-transfected TSGH-8301 (8301-DNA) and ectopic TAGLN overexpression TSGH-8301 (8301-TAGLN) cells were determined by immunoblotting (top) and RT-qPCR (bottom) assays (± SE; n = 3). (**D**) Expressions of TAGLN in mock-knockdown TSGH-8301 (8301_shCOL) and TAGLN-knockdown TSGH-8301 (8301_shTAGLN) cells were determined using immunoblot (top) and RT-qPCR (bottom) assays (± SE; n = 3). The invasion abilities of cells were determined by in vitro Matrigel invasion assays. Data are presented as mean percentages (± SE; n = 3) in relation to those of the 8301-DNA (**E**) or (**F**) 8301_shCOL groups. ** represented the $p < 0.01$.

2.6. The Effect of the Ectopic Overexpression of TAGLN on the Tumorigenesis of Bladder Carcinoma HT1376 Cells

The effect of TAGLN on tumor growth in vivo was evaluated by using xenografts in BALB/cAnN-Foxn1^{NU} mice. Tumors generated from HT-DNA cells (Figure 5A) grew faster than those derived from HT-TAGLN cells (Figure 5B). There were no significant differences in the mean body weights of animals between the two groups (Figure 5C). Additionally, tumors generated from HT-TAGLN cells were approximately 26% smaller than the tumors generated from HT-DNA (93.11 ± 19.73 versus 364.13 ± 60.83 mm^3) after 46 days of growth (Figure 5D). The weight of tumors derived from HT-DNA cells was about four times that from the group of HT-TAGLN cells (0.40 ± 0.07 versus 0.11 ± 0.02; Figure 5E). We randomly selected five tissues from each group to perform RT-qPCR assays, and the results confirmed that TAGLN was overexpressed in the xenograft tumors derived from HT-TAGLN cells (Figure 5F).

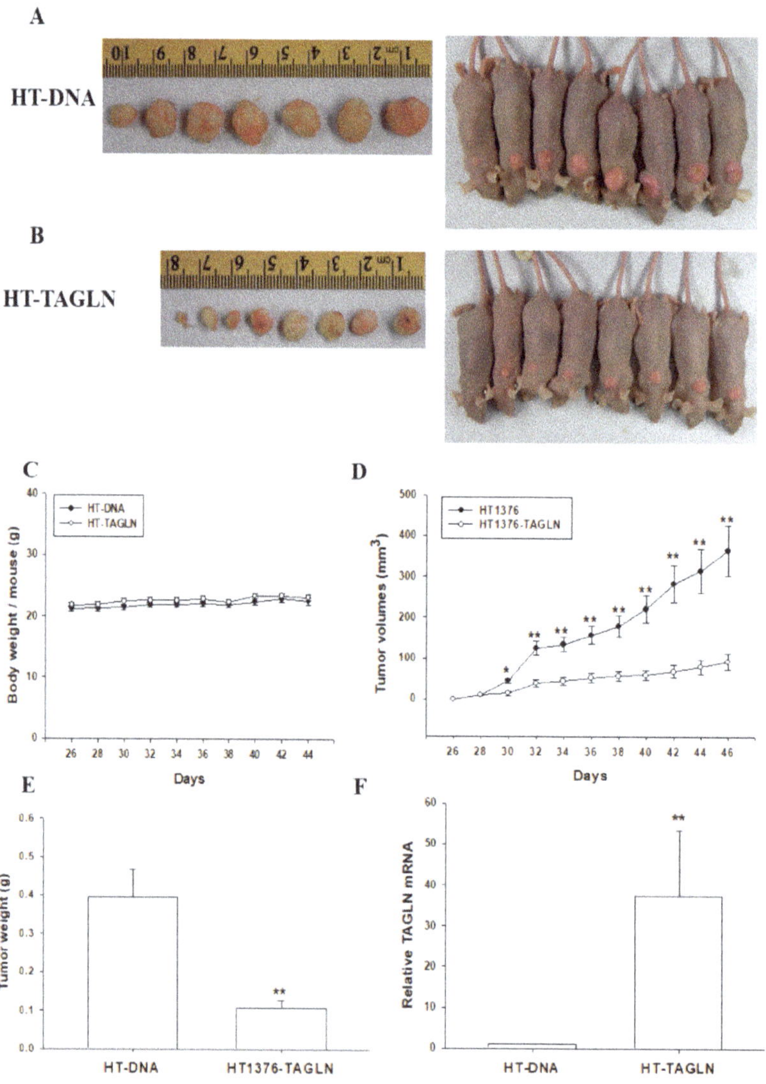

Figure 5. The ectopic overexpression of TAGLN attenuates tumorigenesis, in vivo, for bladder carcinoma HT1376 cells. Four-week-old male athymic nude (nu/nu) mice were randomized into two

groups: HT-DNA (*n* = 7; **A**) and HT-TAGLN (*n* = 7; **B**). HT-DNA cells and HT-TAGLN cells (1×10^6) were injected subcutaneously in the dorsal area of the mice, respectively. The animal body weights (**C**) and tumor growth rates (**D**) were measured every 2 days, starting at the 3-weeks-of-growth point (day 26), at which the tumors became perceptible under the skin after inoculation. The tumor weights (**E**) and levels of TAGLN mRNA (**F**) were determined after the animals were sacrificed ($\pm$ SE; *n* =7). * represented the *p* < 0.05 and the ** represented the *p* < 0.01.

2.7. p53 and PTEN Upregulated TAGLN Expression in Bladder Carcinoma Cells

The immunoblot (Figure 6A) and RT-qPCR (Figure 6B) assays confirmed that the overexpression of p53 induced TAGLN expression in HT1376 cells. Further, the immunoblot assays showed that camptothecin, a topoisomerase inhibitor, induced not only p53 but also TAGLN expressions, while p53-knockdown attenuated these effects in p53-wild type RT-4 cells (Figure 6C). Similar results found in the reporter assays indicated that a transiently cotransfected-p53 expression vector induced the reporter activity of *TAGLN* reporter vector containing the 5′-flanking region of the human *TAGLN* gene in HT1376 cells (Figure 6D). Further immunoblot assays revealed that the ectopic overexpression of PTEN in T24 cells blocked AKT phosphorylation but enhanced TAGLN expression, whereas PTEN knockdown in RT-4 cells reversed those effects (Figure 6E). Results of RT-qPCR assays showed that ectopic overexpression of PTEN induced *TAGLN* gene expression in T24 cells (Figure 6F), while PTEN-knockdown downregulated *TAGLN* expression in RT-4 cells (Figure 6G). Further reporter assays revealed that a transiently cotransfected-PTEN expression vector upregulated the reporter activity of human *TAGLN* reporter vector in HT1376 cells (Figure 6H). Collectively, TAGLN is upregulated by p53 and PTEN in bladder carcinoma cells.

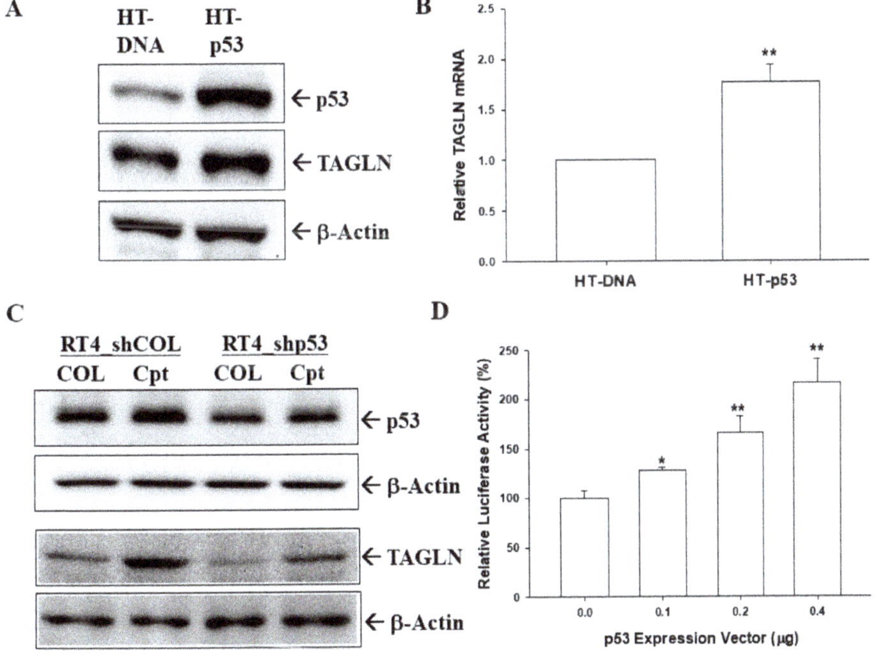

Figure 6. *Cont.*

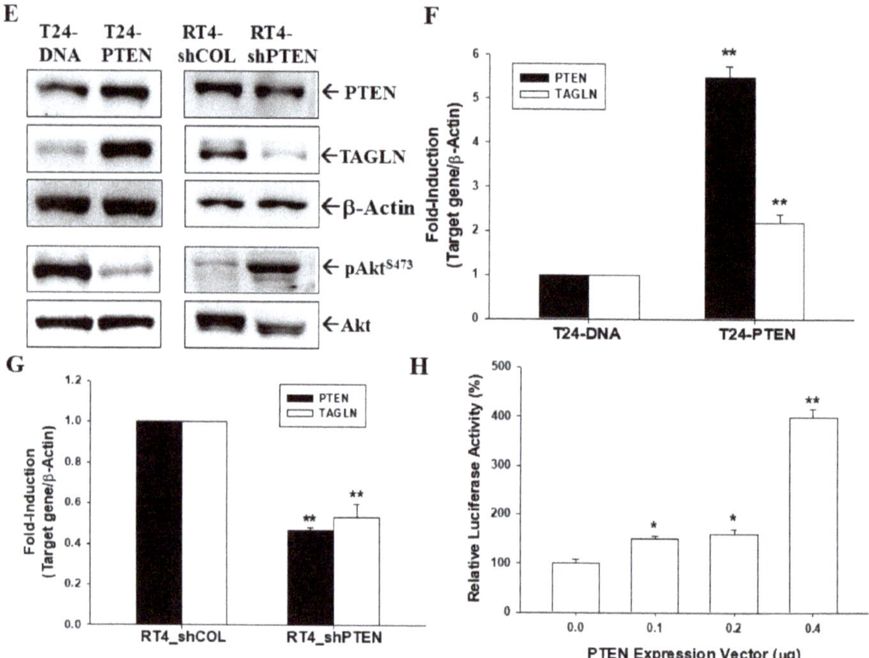

Figure 6. Modulation of p53 and PTEN on TAGLN expression in bladder carcinoma cells. The mock-transfected HT1376 (HT-DNA) and p53-overexpressed HT1376 (HT-p53) cells were lysed, and then TAGLN, p53, and β-actin were determined by immunoblotting (**A**) and RT-qPCR (**B**) assays ($\pm$ SE; $n = 3$). The mock-knockdown RT4 (RT4_shCOL) and p53-knockdown RT4 (RT4_shp53) cells were treated with camptothecin (1 µM) for 16 h. The cells were lysed, and then TAGLN, p53, and β-actin were determined by immunoblotting (**C**). (**D**) The reporter activity of TAGLN reporter vector cotrasnfected with various dosages of p53, as indicated in HT1376 cells. Data are expressed as the mean percentages $\pm$ SEs ($n = 6$) of luciferase activity relative to the mock-transfected group. The mock-transfected T24 (T24-DNA), PTEN-overexpressed T24 (T24-PTEN), mock-knockdown RT4 (RT4_shCOL), and PTEN-knockdown RT4 (RT4_shpPTEN) cells were lysed, and then TAGLN, PTEN, Akt, pAkt^S473, and β-actin were determined by immunoblotting (**E**). Expressions of PTEN and TAGLN in T24-DNA, T24-PTEN (**F**), RT4_shCOL, and RT4_shPTEN (**G**) cells were determined by RT-qPCR assays ($\pm$ SE; $n = 3$). (**H**) The reporter activity of TAGLN reporter vector cotrasnfected with various dosages of PTEN, as indicated in HT1376 cells. Data are expressed as the mean percentages $\pm$ SEs ($n = 6$) of luciferase activity relative to the mock-transfected group. * represented the $p < 0.05$ and the ** represented the $p < 0.01$.

3. Discussion

Bladder cancer is the ninth most common cancer and ranks 13th in terms of deaths worldwide, with the highest incidence rates observed in men around the world [21]. In the United States, bladder cancer is the sixth most common cancer with an estimated 79,030 new cases and 16,870 deaths in 2017 [22]. It seems critical nowadays to explore a new therapeutic molecular target for patients with bladder cancer, since multiple factors are associated with bladder cancer [23,24].

TAGLN may play roles in the morphologic transform process in smooth muscle cells, although TAGLN is not required for the normal development of mouse embryos [2]. Overexpression of TAGLN was strictly limited to the regulation of the tumor-induced, reactive, myofibroblastic stromal tissue, compartment-specific cell type's expression in tumoral stroma compared to neoplastic epithelial cells [4]. The TAGLN depletion increased the capacity of cells to form podosomes spontaneously with a concomitant increase in the ability to invade Matrigel, suggesting that TAGLN may relate to the tumorigenic properties of cells [3]. A prior study indicated that an early loss of *TAGLN* gene expression is important for tumor progression and viewed that as a diagnostic marker for breast and colon cancer development [5]. However, results from the functional assays of TAGLN in different cancers are still inconclusive. Although studies in bladder cancer suggested that *TAGLN* was one of common differentially-expressed genes, significantly decreased in cancer compared with normal tissues [19,20], the precise functions and regulatory mechanisms of *TAGLN* in bladder carcinoma cells are still unexplored.

This study illustrated that protein and mRNA levels of *TAGLN* are higher in human normal primary bladder epithelial cells (HBdEC) than in bladder carcinoma cells. Meanwhile, a recent study showed that *TAGLN* was expressed in bladder carcinoma T24 and SW780 cells at the transcription and translation levels [25]. Although our study suggested that TAGLN expressions among the bladder carcinoma cell lines could be dependent on the cell type but not relevant to the extent of neoplasia in vitro, the RT-qPCR analysis of paired human bladder tissues further demonstrated a significantly lower expression of *TAGLN* mRNA levels in bladder tumors than adjacent normal bladder tissues (Figure 1). These results are in agreement to other studies of badder cancer in vivo [19,20,26], suggesting that *TAGLN* is a tumor suppressor gene in the bladder. The family of transgelins consists of three homologs (TAGLN, transgelin-2, and transgelin-3) in human tissues. A prior study has suggested that TAGLN and trangelin-2 act as cancer biomarkers and are differentially expressed in the tumor and stroma cells [27]. Further studies implied that transgelin-2 has a potentially oncogenic function in bladder cancer, both in vitro and in vivo [28,29]. Our study presents the tumor suppressor characteristics of TAGLN in bladder cancer, both in vitro and in vivo, and agrees with the concept of that the role of transgelin-2 in tumor development might be contradictory to the role of TAGLN [27].

This study also found high levels of TAGLN expressed in the bladder's smooth muscle cells (HBdSMC) and stromal fibroblasts (HBdSF) in vitro (Figure 1). Earlier study indicated that TAGLN is an SMC-lineage marker in rabbit bladders [18]; however, TAGLN was regarded as a marker of active stromal remodeling in the vicinity of invasive carcinomas as well [4]. In the prostate study, TAGLN levels were found to be elevated in the stroma but decreased in the carcinomic epithelial cells during cancer progression [30,31]. However, further investigation into the function of TAGLN in the stroma of bladders is still necessary.

Our finding indicated that the expression of TAGLN was predominant in the cytosol and associated with F-actin during the ectopic overexpression of bladder carcinoma HT1376 cells. Further immunoblot assays with subcellular extraction confirmed that TAGLN did not express in the nuclei but in the cytoplasm, mostly with a little expression in the membrane (Figure 2). These results are in agreement with previous studies, which implied that TAGLN is localized to the cytosol where it binds to F-actin [32].

Early studies suggested that *TAGLN* was a tumor suppressor gene in various cancers, while some cancers possessed the oncogenic characteristic of *TAGLN*. The overexpression of TAGLN potentially contributed to the progression and metastasis of colorectal cancer; meanwhile, high levels of TAGLN related to a poor prognosis of colon cancer in vivo [14,15]. TAGLN was upregulated in cell lines from the human lung adenocarcinoma under hypoxic conditions that caused the migration ability of the tumor cells; moreover, a high TAGLN expression correlated with an advanced TNM stage, lymph node metastasis, and greater differentiation in lung adenocarcinoma [16]. However, other studies concluded that *TAGLN* is a tumor suppressor gene associated with a poor prognosis in colorectal carcinoma patients [9,10]. An in vitro study declared that apigenin upregulated the expression of TAGLN in mitochondria to exert its anti-tumor growth and anti-metastasis effects in colorectal cancer [11]. The restoration of the TAGLN-induced inhibition of colon carcinogenesis in vivo and in vitro suggested that TAGLN might potentially function as a novel tumor suppressor [12,13]. A previous study of prostates also identified *TAGLN* as a tumor suppressor gene in vivo and in vitro [31], and others found the same in bladder cancer, based on a gene profile analysis [19,20,26]. Our study is the first study providing direct evidence to demonstrate that *TAGLN* is an antitumor gene in the bladder carcinoma cells. Results from this study revealed that the ectopic overexpression of TAGLN decreased cell proliferation, invasion, and migration in bladder carcinoma cells in vitro, while the knockdown of *TAGLN* reversed the effects (Figure 3, Figure 4, Figures S1 and S2). The anti-tumorigenesis characteristics of *TAGLN* in bladder carcinoma cells was also demonstrated by an in vivo xenograft animal study (Figure 5).

Previous studies have indicated that *TAGLN* is a TGFβ-inducible gene of human skeletal stem cells, prostate carcinoma cells, and prostate fibroblast cells [31,33,34]. Steroid receptor coactivatior and mir-145 also modulated *TAGLN* expression in different cells [35,36]. Interestingly, *TAGLN* was regarded as an ARA54-associated AR inhibitor that suppressed AR function, and induced the apoptosis of human prostate LNCaP cells through its interaction with p53 [37]. Our study is the first to reveal that *TAGLN* is the downstream gene of *p53* and *PTEN* in bladder carcinoma cells. *p53* is a well-known tumor suppressor gene and *p53* mutations correlate with a variety of human cancers [38]. The overexpression of p53 in p53-mutant HT1376 cells, or with camptothecin (a topoisomerase I inhibitor) treatment in p53-wild type RT-4 cells, induced TAGLN expression, while p53-knockdown attenuated this effect. It was found that camptothecin induced p53 expression in RT-4 cells in a previous study that used bladder carcinoma cells [39]. Two putative p53 response elements (5′-AGGCAAGTTCTGTGTTAGTCATGCAC-3′, −2151 to −2126; and 5′-AAACTTGTTTTTATAGCTCTG CTTGAAG-3′, −1956 to −1929), which are similar to the p53 response element consensus sequence (RRRCWWGYYYN$_{0-13}$RRRCWWGYYY), as previously reported [40], were found in the promoter region of the human *TAGLN* gene—determined by in silico analysis. The precise mechanisms of the modulation *TAGLN* gene expression by p53 still need to be further investigated.

Phosphatase and tensin homolog deleted on chromosome 10 (*PTEN*) has been widely known as a tumor suppressor gene, and *PTEN* mutation or deletion is frequently noted in a lot of cancers, including bladder [39,41,42]. The most known function of PTEN is as the negative regulator of the PI3K/Akt/mTOR pathway, which is a crucial signal transduction pathway for cancer cell growth [39,43]. For bladder cancer, a loss of PTEN expression has been correlated with the cell growth and the invasion of bladder carcinoma [39,41]. In this study, we found that ectopic overexpression of PTEN in PTEN-mutant T24 cells blocked Akt phosphorylation but induced *TAGLN* expression, while knockdown of *PTEN* in PTEN-wildtype RT-4 cells reversed those effect (Figure 6). Conclusively, our study confirmed that *TAGLN* is a target gene of p53 and PTEN, and should be referred to as a tumor suppressor in bladder carcinoma cells, both in vitro and in vivo.

4. Materials and Methods

4.1. Cell Cultures and Chemicals

The four bladder-transitional carcinoma cell lines, RT-4, HT1376, TSGH-8301, and T24 cells, were purchased from the Bioresource Collection and Research Center (BCRC, Hsinchu, Taiwan) as described previously [44]. Human bladder smooth muscle cells (HBdSMC), bladder stromal fibroblasts (HBdSF), smooth muscle cell medium, and fibroblast medium were purchased from ScienCell Research Laboratories Inc. (Carlsbad, CA, USA). Human normal primary bladder epithelial cells (HBdEC; ATCC PCS-420-010) were purchased from American Type Culture Collection (ATCC; Manassas, VA, USA) and maintained in the prostate epithelial cells' basal mediums (ATCC PCS 440-030). DAPI (4,6-diamino-2-phenylindole) and camptothecin were obtained from Sigma-Aldrich Co. (St. Louis, MO, USA). Fetal calf serum (FCS) was from HyClone (Logan, UT, USA), and RPMI 1640 media was obtained from Invitrogen (Carlsbad, CA, USA).

4.2. Tissue Collection and Analysis

The specimens of the human paired bladder tissue biopsies were obtained from patients admitted to the Department of Urology, Chang Gung Memorial Hospital-Linkou (Tao-Yuan, Taiwan). Bladder tissues were classified based on the pathological examinations of the parallel preparations from respective samples by attending pathologists. The Institutional Review Board of the Chang Gung Memorial Hospital approved the protocol for tissue collection and analysis (IRB 201800981B0, 1 September 2018).

4.3. Expression Vector and Stable Transfection

The full-length human *TAGLN* cDNA (HG14991-UT) was purchased from Sino Biologic Inc. (Beijing, China). Electroporation was conducted using an ECM 830 Square Wave Electroporation System (BTX, San Diego, CA, USA), set at 180 V (for TSGH-8301 cells) or 190 V (for HT1376 cells), with a 70-msec pulse length and one pulse setting. Transfected cells (8301-TAGLN and HT-TAGLN) were selected by 100 μg/mL of hygromycin (Sigma-Aldrich Co.). For construction of the mock-transfected cells (8301-DNA and HT1376-DNA), cells were transfected with a controlled pCMV3 expression vector (Sino Biologic Inc.) and were clonally selected in the same manner as described above. The *p53* and *PTEN* expression vectors were constructed and p53-overexpressed HT1376 (HT-p53) cells and PTEN-overexpression T24 (T24-PTEN) cells were cloned as described previously [39].

4.4. Knock-Down TAGLN, p53, and PTEN

TSGH-8301 and T24 cells were transduced with control shRNA lentiviral particles-A (Sc-108080) or transgelin shRNA (h) Lentiviral Particles (sc-44163-V) that were purchased from Santa Cruz Biotechnology, Inc. (Santa Cruz, CA, USA). Two days after transduction, the cells (8301_shCOL, 8301_shTAGLN, T24_shCOL, and T24_shTAGLN) were selected by incubation with 10 μg/mL puromycin dihydrochloride for at least another 5 generations. The p53-knockdown RT-4 (RT4_shp53), PTEN-knockdown RT-4 (RT4_shPTEN), and mock-knockdown RT-4 (RT4_shCOL) cells were cloned as previously described [39].

4.5. Immunoblot Assays

Cells were cultured in RPMI-1640 medium with 10% FCS for 48 h. The nuclear and cytoplasmic fractions were separated using the subcellular protein fractionation kit (Thermo Fisher Scientific Inc., Rockford, NJ, USA) as described previously [44]. Equal amounts of whole cell, membrane, nuclear, or cytoplasmic lysates were separated on a 10%–12% SDS-polyacrylamide gel and assayed by the Western lightning plus-ECL detection system, as instructed by the manufacturer (PerkinElmer Inc, Waltham, MA, USA). The blotting membranes were probed with the antisera of p53 (DO-1, Santa Cruz Biotechnology), PTEN (#9552, Cell Signaling Technology, Danvers, MA, USA), Akt (#4691, Cell Signaling Technology), phopsho-Akt^{S473} (#9271, Cell Signaling Technology), or β-actin antiserum (MAB1501, Merck Millipore, Burlington, MA, USA). The intensities of different bands were recorded using the LuminoGraph II (Atto corporation, Tokyo, Japan).

4.6. Real-Time Reverse Transcriptase-Polymerase Chain Reaction (RT-qPCR)

Total RNA from tissues or cells was isolated using Trizol reagent (Ambion, Life Technologies, Carlsbad, CA, USA). The cDNA was synthesized using Superscript III pre-amplification system (Invitrogen), as described previously [45]. The PCR probes for human *p53* (Hs01034249_m1), *PTEN* (Hs02621230_Sl), *TAGLN* (Hs01038777_g1), *β-actin* (Hs01060665_g1), and *18S* (Hs03003631_g1) were purchased from Applied Biosystems (Foster City, CA, USA). Real-time polymerase chain reactions (qPCR) were performed using an CFX Connect Real-Time PCR system (Bio-Rad Laboratories, Foster city, CA, USA) and the mean cycle threshold (C_t) values were calculated for internal control and target genes, as described previously [44].

4.7. Cell Immunofluorescence and F-Actin Staining

Cells were seeded onto the glass bottom culture dishes (MatTek, Ashland, MD, USA) which were precoated with 50 μL fibronectin. Cells were fixed at room temperature in 4% paraformaldehyde in phosphate buffered saline (PBS) for 20 min after 24 h of attachment. After that, cells were permeabilized for 10 min in a 0.2% solution of Triton X-100 and blocked in 1% BSA for 1 h after being washed with PBS. The coverslips were incubated with 1:100 diluted anti-TAGLN antiserum overnight at 4 °C and then incubated with donkey anti-rabbit secondary antibody (A21206, Invitrogen) for 1 h. The F-actin protein expression was revealed by incubation with Texas Red X-Phalloidin (Invitrogen). The coverslips were mounted with the Prolong Gold antifade reagent with DAPI (Thermo Fisher Scientific Inc.). The immunofluorescence was examined using a confocal microscope (LSM510 Meta, Zeiss, Oberkochen, Germany) as described previously [46].

4.8. EdU Staining Proliferation Assay

Cells were seeded onto the sterile glass coverslips. After 48 h of attachment, EdU was added to the culture medium to a final concentration of 50 μM for another 2 h. Cells were washed and fixed in 3.7% paraformaldehyde in phosphate buffered saline (PBS) at room temperature for 15 min, and then washed twice with 200 μL of 3% BSA in PBS. Cells were permeabilized with saponin-based permeabilization and washing reagent for 20 min, and then incubated for 30 min with Click-iT reaction cocktail, containing fluorescent dye azide, $CuSO_4$, PBS, and reaction buffer (Thermo Fisher Scientific Inc.). Cells were washed twice with 200 μL of 3% BSA in PBS, and the coverslip was mounted with Prolong Gold antifade reagent with DAPI. The EdU fluorescence was recorded and photographed under a microscope (BX43, OLYMPUS, Tokyo, Japan).

4.9. EdU Flow Cytometry Assay

Cells (5×10^5) were serum starved for 24 h, and then incubated with RPMI1640 medium with 10% serum for another 48 h. EdU (5-ethynyl-2′-deoxyuridine; 10 μM) was added to the culture medium for further 2 h. Cells were collected, fixed, and permeabilized with saponin-based permeabilization and washing reagent for 20 min, and then incubated for 30 min with Click-iT reaction cocktail (Thermo Fisher Scientific Inc.), as described by the manufacturer. The EdU fluorescence of cells was detected using Attune NxT acoustic focusing cytometer (Thermo Fisher Scientific Inc.).

4.10. Ki67 Proliferation Assay

Cells were serum-starvated for 24 h, and then incubated with RPMI1640 medium with 10% serum for further 48 h. Cells were stained with PE Mouse Anti-Ki-67 kit (catalogue number 556027; BD Biosciences, Bedford, MA, USA) as described by the manufacturer. Briefly, cells were washed, pelleted, and fixed with cold, 70% ethanol at −20 °C overnight. The PE-conjugated anti-Ki-67 antibody and PE-conjugated mouse IgG1 were added to the cells and the mixture was incubated at room temperature for further 30 min in the dark, after the cells had been washed twice with washing buffer (PBS with 1% FBS, 0.09% NaN_3). The cells were washed with washing buffer and re-suspended in PBS, and then the Ki67 fluorescence of cells were detected using Attune NxT acoustic focusing cytometer.

4.11. Cell Migration Assay

The cell migration analysis was determined by a wound healing assay, as described previously [46]. In brief, the cell sheets were wounded with a plastic pipette tip when they attained a confluent monolayer. The wound closure (the gap width) was photographed microscopically (IX71, Olympus, Tokyo, Japan) with a digital camera during the indicated times. The quantification of cell migration was determined within a defined area using the Image J program.

4.12. Matrigel Invasion Assay

The in vitro invasion ability of cells was determined by the Matrigel invasion assay (BD Biosciences). Cells that invaded into other side of the membrane were fixed using 4% paraformaldehyde and then stained with 0.1% crystal violet solution for 10 min. The quantity of cells that invaded the Matrigel was recorded microscopically (IX71, Olympus, Tokyo, Japan) and the images were analyzed as described previously [44].

4.13. Xenograft Animal Model

The performance of animal studies was approved by the Chang Gung University Animal Research Committee (Approval No.: CGU107-092, 1 September 2018). The male nude mice (BALB/cAnN-Foxn1) were obtained from the animal center of National Science Council, Taiwan, at 4 weeks old. In all the procedures, every effort was made to minimize the suffering of the laboratory animals in accordance with the United States' National Institutes of Health Guide for the Care and Use of Laboratory Animals. The cells were detached with Gibco^{Tm} Versene solution and washed with RPMI 1640 medium with 10% FCS, and then were re-suspended in a PBS solution. The mice were anesthetized intraperitoneally and 1×10^6 cell/100 µL cells were injected subcutaneously on the right or left lateral back wall in close proximity to the shoulder of each mouse. The growth of the xenografts was measured by vernier caliper measurements on the days indicated. The tumor volume was determined by the formula volume = $\pi/6 \times W \times D^2$, as described previously [47].

4.14. TAGLN Reporter Vector and Reporter Assays

The 5′-DNA fragment (-1 to -4573) of the human *TAGLN* gene, according to the sequence from GenBank (AP005018.1), was synthesized by Invitrogen. The human *TAGLN* reporter vector was constructed by cloning the DNA fragment into the pbGL3 reporter vector (Promega Biosciences, Madison, WI, USA) with *Hind III* sites. Proper ligation was confirmed by extensive restriction mapping and sequencing. The cells were plated onto 24-well plates at 1×10^4 cells/well for 1 day prior to transfection. Cells were transiently cotransfected with reporter vectors and expression vectors as indicated, using the X-tremeGene HP DNA transfection reagent (Roche Diagnostics GmbH, Mannheim, Germany), as described previously [48]. The luciferase activity was adjusted for transfection efficiency using the normalization control plasmid pCMVSPORTβgal.

4.15. Statistical Analysis

All the results are expressed as the means ± S.Es. Statistical significance was determined by one-way ANOVA and Student's *t* tests using the SigmaPlot 10.0 (SPSS Inc., Chicago, IL, USA). The * represented the $p < 0.05$ and the ** represented the $p < 0.01$.

5. Conclusions

Our results indicated that the expression of transgelin, a regulator of the actin cytoskeleton, is higher in bladder normal epithelial cells than in carcinoma cells. Our experiments provided evidence suggesting that *TAGLN* is a p53 and PTEN-downstream gene, which attenuates cell proliferation and invasion in vitro, and tumorigenesis in vivo. *TAGLN* seems to function as a tumor suppressor gene in bladder carcinoma cells.

Supplementary Materials: Supplementary materials can be found at http://www.mdpi.com/1422-0067/20/19/4946/s1. Figure S1: Effect of TAGLN on cell proliferation of bladder carcinoma HT1376 and TSGH-8301 cells determined by Ki-67 assays. Proliferation rates between (A) mock-transfected HT1376 (HT-DNA) and ectopic TAGLN overexpressed HT1376 (HT-TAGLN), and (B) between mock-transfected TSGH-8301 (8301-DNA) and ectopic TAGLN overexpressed TSGH-8301 (8301-TAGLN) cells were determined by Ki-67 assays (± SE; $n = 3$). ** is represented the $p < 0.01$. Figure S2: Effect of TAGLN on cell migration of bladder carcinoma HT1376 cells. The migration ability of HT-DNA and HT-TAGLN cells was determined by wound healing assays during the indicated times. ** is represented the $p < 0.01$.

Author Contributions: Funding acquisition, K.-H.T. and H.-H.J.; investigation, K.-H.T. and Y.-H.L.; Methodology, K.-S.C., C.-P.H. and P.-J.C.; writing–original draft, T.-H.F.; writing–review and editing, T.-H.F. and H.-H.J.

Funding: This research was supported by grants from the Taiwan Ministry of Science and Technology (MOST-107-2314-B-182A-017-MY3 and MOST-105-2320-B-182-020-MY3), and Chang Gung Memorial Hospital (CRRPD1F0041-3, CMRPD1I0111-3, CMRPG3G0821-2, CMRPG3F081-3, and CMRP-G3H1321-3).

Conflicts of Interest: The authors declare no conflict of interest.

References

1. Camoretti-Mercado, B.; Forsythe, S.M.; LeBeau, M.M.; Espiosa, R.; Vieira, J.E.; Halayko, A.J.; Willadsen, S.; Kurtz, B.; Ober, C.; Evans, G.A.; et al. Expression and cytogenetic localization of the human SM22 gene (TAGLN). *Genomics* **1998**, *49*, 452–457. [CrossRef] [PubMed]

2. Yang, X.Y.; Yao, J.H.; Cheng, L.; Wei, D.W.; Xue, J.L.; Lu, D.R. Molecular cloning and expression of a smooth muscle-specific gene SM22alpha in zebrafish. *Biochem. Biophys. Res. Comm.* **2003**, *312*, 741–746. [CrossRef] [PubMed]

3. Thompson, O.; Moghraby, J.S.; Ayscough, K.R.; Winder, S.J. Depletion of the actin bundling protein SM22/transgelin increases actin dynamics and enhances the tumourigenic phenotypes of cells. *BMC Cell Biol.* **2012**, *13*, 1. [CrossRef] [PubMed]

4. Rho, J.H.; Roehrl, M.H.; Wang, J.Y. Tissue proteomics reveals differential and compartment-specific expression of the homologs transgelin and transgelin-2 in lung adenocarcinoma and its stroma. *J. Proteome Res.* **2009**, *8*, 5610–5618. [CrossRef] [PubMed]

5. Shields, J.M.; Rogers-Graham, K.; Der, C.J. Loss of transgelin in breast and colon tumors and in RIE-1 cells by Ras deregulation of gene expression through Raf-independent pathways. *J. Biol. Chem.* **2002**, *277*, 9790–9799. [CrossRef] [PubMed]

6. Zhang, J.; Wang, K.; Zhang, J.; Liu, S.S.; Dai, L.; Zhang, J.Y. Using proteomic approach to identify tumor-associated proteins as biomarkers in human esophageal squamous cell carcinoma. *J. Proteome Res.* **2011**, *10*, 2863–2872. [CrossRef]

7. Li, N.; Zhang, J.; Liang, Y.; Shao, J.; Peng, F.; Sun, M.; Xu, N.; Li, X.; Wang, R.; Liu, S.; et al. A controversial tumor marker: Is SM22 a proper biomarker for gastric cancer cells? *J. Proteome Res.* **2007**, *6*, 3304–3312. [CrossRef]

8. Yu, B.; Chen, X.; Li, J.; Qu, Y.; Su, L.; Peng, Y.; Huang, J.; Yan, J.; Yu, Y.; Gu, Q.; et al. Stromal fibroblasts in the microenvironment of gastric carcinomas promote tumor metastasis via upregulating TAGLN expression. *BMC Cell Biol.* **2013**, *14*, 17. [CrossRef]

9. Zhao, L.; Wang, H.; Deng, Y.J.; Wang, S.; Liu, C.; Jin, H.; Ding, Y.Q. Transgelin as a suppressor is associated with poor prognosis in colorectal carcinoma patients. *Modern Pathol.* **2009**, *22*, 786–796. [CrossRef]

10. Xie, X.L.; Liu, Y.B.; Liu, Y.P.; Du, B.L.; Li, Y.; Han, M.; Li, B.H. Reduced expression of SM22 is correlated with low autophagy activity in human colorectal cancer. *Pathol. Res. Prac.* **2013**, *209*, 237–243. [CrossRef]

11. Chunhua, L.; Donglan, L.; Xiuqiong, F.; Lihua, Z.; Qin, F.; Yawei, L.; Liang, Z.; Ge, W.; Linlin, J.; Ping, Z.; et al. Apigenin up-regulates transgelin and inhibits invasion and migration of colorectal cancer through decreased phosphorylation of AKT. *J. Nutr. Biochem.* **2013**, *24*, 1766–1775. [CrossRef]

12. Pang, J.; Liu, W.P.; Liu, X.P.; Li, L.Y.; Fang, Y.Q.; Sun, Q.P.; Liu, S.J.; Li, M.T.; Su, Z.L.; Gao, X. Profiling protein markers associated with lymph node metastasis in prostate cancer by DIGE-based proteomics analysis. *J. Proteome Res.* **2010**, *9*, 216–226. [CrossRef] [PubMed]

13. Yeo, M.; Park, H.J.; Kim, D.K.; Kim, Y.B.; Cheong, J.Y.; Lee, K.J.; Cho, S.W. Loss of SM22 is a characteristic signature of colon carcinogenesis and its restoration suppresses colon tumorigenicity in vivo and in vitro. *Cancer* **2010**, *116*, 2581–2589. [CrossRef] [PubMed]

14. Yokota, M.; Kojima, M.; Higuchi, Y.; Nishizawa, Y.; Kobayashi, A.; Ito, M.; Saito, N.; Ochiai, A. Gene expression profile in the activation of subperitoneal fibroblasts reflects prognosis of patients with colon cancer. *Int. J. Cancer* **2016**, *138*, 1422–1431. [CrossRef] [PubMed]

15. Zhou, H.; Zhang, Y.; Chen, Q.; Lin, Y. AKT and JNK Signaling pathways increase the metastatic potential of colorectal cancer cells by altering transgelin expression. *Dig. Dis. Sci.* **2016**, *61*, 1091–1097. [CrossRef] [PubMed]

16. Wu, X.; Dong, L.; Zhang, R.; Ying, K.; Shen, H. Transgelin overexpression in lung adenocarcinoma is associated with tumor progression. *Int. J. Mol. Med.* **2014**, *34*, 585–591. [CrossRef]

17. Li, L.S.; Kim, H.; Rhee, H.; Kim, S.H.; Shin, D.H.; Chung, K.Y.; Park, K.S.; Paik, Y.K.; Chang, J.; Kim, H. Proteomic analysis distinguishes basaloid carcinoma as a distinct subtype of nonsmall cell lung carcinoma. *Proteomics* **2004**, *4*, 3394–3400. [CrossRef]

18. Chiavegato, A.; Roelofs, M.; Franch, R.; Castellucci, E.; Sarinella, F.; Sartore, S. Differential expression of SM22 isoforms in myofibroblasts and smooth muscle cells from rabbit bladder. *J. Muscle Res. Cell Motil.* **1999**, *20*, 133–146. [CrossRef]

19. Zaravinos, A.; Lambrou, G.I.; Boulalas, I.; Delakas, D.; Spandidos, D.A. Identification of common differentially expressed genes in urinary bladder cancer. *PLoS ONE* **2011**, *6*, e18135. [CrossRef]

20. Chen, R.; Feng, C.; Xu, Y. Cyclin-dependent kinase-associated protein Cks2 is associated with bladder cancer progression. *J. Int. Med. Res.* **2011**, *39*, 533–540. [CrossRef]

21. Antomi, S.; Ferlay, J.; Soerjomataram, I.; Znaor, A.; Jemal, A.; Bray, F. Bladder cancer incidence and mortality: A global overview and recent trends. *Eur. Urol.* **2017**, *71*, 96–108. [CrossRef] [PubMed]

22. Siegel, R.L.; Miller, K.D.; Jemal, A. Cancer statistics, 2017. *CA Cancer J. Clin.* **2017**, *67*, 7–30. [CrossRef]

23. Goodison, S.; Rosser, C.J.; Urquidi, V. Bladder cancer detection and monitoring: Assessment of urine- and blood based marker tests. *Mol. Diag. Ther.* **2013**, *17*, 71–84. [CrossRef] [PubMed]

24. Narayan, V.M.; Adejoro, O.; Schwartz, I.; Ziegelmann, M.; Elliott, S.; Konety, B.R. The prevalence and impact of urinary marker testing in patients with bladder cancer. *J. Urol.* **2018**, *199*, 74–80. [CrossRef] [PubMed]

25. Chen, Z.; He, S.; Zhan, Y.; He, A.; Fang, D.; Gong, Y.; Li, X.; Zhou, L. TGF-β-induced transgelin promotes bladder cancer metastasis by upregulating epithelial-mesenchymal transition and invadopodia formation. *EBioMedicine* **2019**, *47*, 208–220. [CrossRef]

26. Ning, X.; Deng, Y. Identification of key pathways and genes influencing prognosis in bladder urothelial carcinoma. *Onco. Targets Ther.* **2017**, *10*, 1673–1686. [CrossRef] [PubMed]

27. Dvorakova, M.; Nenutil, R.; Bouchal, P. Transgelins, cytoskeletal proteins implicated in different aspects of cancer development. *Expert. Rev. Proteomics* **2014**, *11*, 149–165. [CrossRef]

28. Yoshino, H.; Chiyomaru, T.; Enokida, H.; Kawakami, K.; Tatarano, S.; Nishiyama, K.; Nohata, N.; Seki, N.; Nakagawa, M. The tumour-suppressive function of miR-1 and miR-133a targeting TAGLN2 in bladder cancer. *Br. J. Cancer* **2011**, *104*, 808–818. [CrossRef] [PubMed]

29. Zhang, H.; Jiang, M.; Liu, Q.; Han, Z.; Zhao, Y.; Ji, S. miR-145-5p inhibits the proliferation and migration of bladder cancer cells by targeting TAGLN2. *Oncol. Lett.* **2018**, *16*, 6355–6360. [CrossRef]

30. Webber, J.P.; Spary, L.K.; Mason, M.D.; Tabi, Z.; Bewis, I.A.; Clayton, A. Prostate stromal cell proteomic analysis discriminates normal from tumour reactive stroma phenotypes. *Oncotarget* **2016**, *7*, 20124–20139. [CrossRef]

31. Prasad, P.D.; Stanton, J.A.; Assinder, S.J. Expression of the actin-associated protein transgelin (SM22) is decreased in prostate cancer. *Cell Tissue Res.* **2010**, *339*, 337–347. [CrossRef] [PubMed]

32. Matsui, T.S.; Ishikawa, A.; Deguchi, S. Transgelin-1 (SM22α) interacts with actin stress fibers and podosomes in smooth muscle cells without using its actin binding site. *Biochem. Biophys. Res. Commun.* **2018**, *505*, 879–884. [CrossRef] [PubMed]

33. Elsafadi, M.; Manikandan, M.; Dawud, R.A.; Alajez, N.M.; Hamam, R.; Alfayez, M.; Kassem, M.; Aldahmash, A.; Mahmood, A. Transgelin is a TGFβ-inducible gene that regulates osteoblastic and adipogenic differentiation of human skeletal stem cells through actin cytoskeleston organization. *Cell Death Dis.* **2016**, *7*, e2321. [CrossRef] [PubMed]

34. Untergasser, G.; Gander, R.; Lilg, C.; Lepperdinger, G.; Plas, E.; Berger, P. Profiling molecular targets of TGF-beta1 in prostate fibroblast-to-myofibroblast transdifferentiation. *Mech. Ageing Dev.* **2005**, *126*, 59–69. [CrossRef] [PubMed]

35. Fenne, I.S.; Helland, T.; Flageng, M.H.; Dankel, S.N.; Mellgren, G.; Sagen, J.V. Downregulation of steroid receptor coactivator-2 modulates estrogen-responsive genes and stimulates proliferation of mcf-7 breast cancer cells. *PLoS ONE* **2013**, *8*, e70096. [CrossRef] [PubMed]

36. Pashaie, E.; Guzel, E.; Ozgurses, M.E.; Demirel, G.; Aydin, N.; Ozen, M. A meta-analysis: Identification of common mir-145 target gens that have similar behavior in different GEO datasets. *PLoS ONE* **2016**, *11*, e0161491. [CrossRef] [PubMed]

37. Zhang, Z.W.; Yang, Z.M.; Zheng, Y.C.; Chen, Z.D. Transgelin induces apoptosis of human prostate LNCaP cells through its interaction with p53. *Asian J. Androl.* **2010**, *12*, 186–195. [CrossRef] [PubMed]

38. Osman, I.; Drobnjak, M.; Fazzari, M.; Ferrara, J.; Scher, H.I.; Cordon-Cardo, C. Inactivation of the p53 pathway in prostate cancer: Impact on tumor progression. *Clin. Cancer Res.* **1999**, *5*, 2082–2088. [PubMed]

39. Tsui, K.H.; Chiang, K.C.; Feng, T.H.; Chang, K.S.; Lin, Y.H.; Juang, H.H. BTG2 is a tumor suppressor gene and upregulated by p53 and PTEN in human bladder carcinoma cells. *Cancer Med.* **2018**, *7*, 184–195. [CrossRef]

40. El-Deiry, W.S. Regulation of p53 downstream genes. *Semin. Cancer Biol.* **1998**, *8*, 345–357. [CrossRef]

41. Lee, H.; Choi, S.K.; Ro, J.Y. Overexpression of DJ-1 and HSP90alpha, and loss of PTEN associated with invasive urothelial carcinoma of urinary bladder: Possible prognostic markers. *Oncol. Lett.* **2012**, *3*, 507–512. [PubMed]

42. Boosani, C.S.; Agrawal, D.K. PTEN modulators: A patent review. *Expert. Opin. Ther. Pat.* **2013**, *23*, 569–580. [CrossRef] [PubMed]

43. Morgensztern, D.; McLeod, H.L. PI3K/Akt/mTOR pathway as a target for cancer therapy. *Anti-cancer Drugs* **2005**, *16*, 797–803. [CrossRef] [PubMed]

44. Tsui, K.H.; Hou, C.P.; Chang, K.S.; Lin, Y.H.; Feng, T.H.; Chen, C.C.; Shin, Y.S.; Juang, H.H. Metallothionein 3 is a hypoxia-upregulated oncogene enhancing cell invasion and tumorigenesis in human bladder carcinoma cells. *Int. J. Mol. Sci.* **2019**, *20*, 980. [CrossRef] [PubMed]

45. Tsui, K.H.; Hsu, S.Y.; Chung, L.C.; Lin, Y.H.; Feng, T.H.; Lee, T.Y.; Chang, P.L.; Juang, H.H. Growth differentiation factor-15: A p53- and demethylation-upregulating gene represses cell proliferation, invasion, and tumorigenesis in bladder carcinoma cells. *Sci. Rep.* **2015**, *5*, 12870. [CrossRef] [PubMed]

46. Tsui, K.H.; Chang, Y.L.; Yang, P.S.; Hou, C.P.; Lin, Y.H.; Lee, B.W.; Feng, T.H.; Juang, H.H. The inhibitory effects of capillarisin on cell proliferation and invasion of prostate carcinoma cells. *Cell Prolif.* **2018**, *51*, e12419. [CrossRef] [PubMed]

47. Chang, K.S.; Tsui, K.H.; Lin, Y.H.; Hou, C.P.; Feng, T.H.; Juang, H.H. Migration and invasion enhancer 1 is an NF-κB-inducing gene enhancing the cell proliferation and invasion ability of human prostate carcinoma cells in vitro and in vivo. *Cancers* **2019**, *11*, 1486. [CrossRef] [PubMed]

48. Tsui, K.H.; Lin, Y.H.; Chung, L.C.; Chuang, S.T.; Feng, T.H.; Chiang, K.C.; Chang, P.L.; Yen, C.L.; Juang, H.H. Prostate-derived ets factor represses tumorigenesis and modulates epithelial-to-mesenchymal transition in bladder carcinoma cells. *Cancer Lett.* **2016**, *375*, 142–151. [CrossRef]

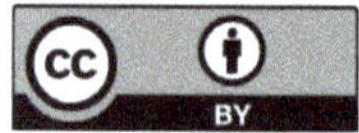

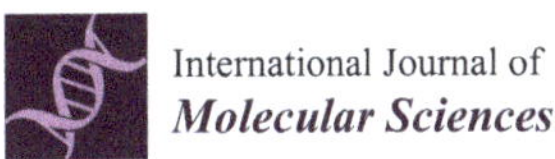 International Journal of
Molecular Sciences

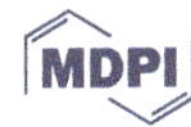

Article

Specificity of the Metallothionein-1 Response by Cadmium-Exposed Normal Human Urothelial Cells

Rhiannon V. McNeill [1,†], **Andrew S. Mason** [1], **Mark E. Hodson** [2], **James W.F. Catto** [3] and **Jennifer Southgate** [1,*]

[1]   Jack Birch Unit for Molecular Carcinogenesis, Department of Biology, York Biomedical Research Institute, University of York, York YO10 5DD, UK; rvm8828@gmail.com (R.V.M.); andrew.mason@york.ac.uk (A.S.M.)
[2]   Department of Environment and Geography, University of York, York YO10 5DD, UK; mark.hodson@york.ac.uk
[3]   Academic Urology Unit, University of Sheffield, Sheffield S10 2TN, UK; j.catto@sheffield.ac.uk
*   Correspondence: j.southgate@york.ac.uk
†   Current address: Department of Psychiatry, Psychosomatic Medicine, and Psychotherapy, University Hospital of Frankfurt, 60590 Frankfurt, Germany.

Received: 29 January 2019; Accepted: 13 March 2019; Published: 17 March 2019

Abstract: Occupational and environmental exposure to cadmium is associated with the development of urothelial cancer. The metallothionein (MT) family of genes encodes proteins that sequester metal ions and modulate physiological processes, including zinc homeostasis. Little is known about the selectivity of expression of the different MT isoforms. Here, we examined the effect of cadmium exposure on MT gene and isoform expression by normal human urothelial (NHU) cell cultures. Baseline and cadmium-induced MT gene expression was characterized by next-generation sequencing and RT-PCR; protein expression was assessed by Western blotting using isoform-specific antibodies. Expression of the zinc transporter-1 (*SLC30A1*) gene was also assessed. NHU cells displayed transcription of *MT-2A*, but neither *MT-3* nor *MT-4* genes. Most striking was a highly inducer-specific expression of MT-1 genes, with cadmium inducing transcription of *MT-1A*, *MT-1G*, *MT-1H*, and *MT-1M*. Whereas *MT-1G* was also induced by zinc and nickel ions and *MT-1H* by iron, both *MT-1A* and *MT-1M* were highly cadmium-specific, which was confirmed for protein using isoform-specific antibodies. Protein but not transcript endured post-exposure, probably reflecting sequestration. *SLC30A1* transcription was also affected by cadmium ion exposure, potentially reflecting perturbation of intracellular zinc homeostasis. We conclude that human urothelium displays a highly inductive profile of MT-1 gene expression, with two isoforms identified as highly specific to cadmium, providing candidate transcript and long-lived protein biomarkers of cadmium exposure.

Keywords: Metallothionein; urothelium; urothelial cancer; cadmium exposure; zinc transporter

---

1. Introduction

Occupational and environmental exposure to cadmium has increased as a result of the burning of fossil fuels and widespread use of the "heavy" metal in anthropological activities, such as battery production, electroplating, smelting, and soldering (reviewed [1]). Cadmium ions accumulate in the body in an almost irreversible manner [2], as the metal cannot be metabolized to a less toxic species [3] and has a low excretion rate [4]. This low excretion rate is thought to be due to intracellular sequestration of cadmium ions by metal-binding proteins [5–7]. An association between cadmium exposure and bladder (urothelial) carcinogenesis has been reported, with higher cadmium concentrations demonstrated in the blood [8] and urine [9–11] of patients with bladder cancer. In vitro research supports these correlative studies, with malignant transformation of the immortalized RWPE-1, TLR1215, 16HBE, and UROtsa cell lines reported after extended chronic cadmium exposure [12–15]. The bladder stores concentrated urine prior to voiding, meaning that the urothelial lining of the bladder (which functions as one of the tightest epithelial barriers [16]) is potentially exposed to excreted xenobiotics [16–18]. It is currently not known whether exposure to urinary cadmium is limited by the presence of an intact urinary barrier.

The metallothioneins (MTs) are a superfamily of low-molecular weight (~6 kDa), cysteine-rich proteins that are induced by and bind a range of metal ions, including cadmium [19,20]. Through this sequestration of metal ions MTs are considered to play a primary role in metal detoxification [21,22], but also metal (e.g., zinc) homeostasis [23–25] and the scavenging of reactive oxygen species (ROS) [26,27]. MT involvement in the bodily response to cadmium exposure has been well-documented, with numerous studies demonstrating cadmium-induced MT expression both in vitro [28–34] and in vivo [35,36].

Direct binding of MT protein to cadmium ions [37,38] results in a MT-cadmium complex that is highly resistant to degradation [5–7]. In humans, four main MT subfamilies exist (MT-1, MT-2/2A, MT-3, and MT-4), with MT-1 consisting of nine isoforms (-A, -B, -E, -F, -G, -H, -L, -M, and -X) [39] each encoded on individual genes. It is predicted that the individual MT isoforms have distinct properties including structure [40,41], tissue- and inducer-specific expression [22,34,42–47], induction rate [48], translational efficiency [41], and degradation rate [49,50]. Cadmium is reported to be the most potent inducer of MT expression [51]. This offers the potential that individual MT isoforms may be utilized as specific biomarkers of human exposure to cadmium, although it remains unclear which isoform(s) are responsible for cadmium sequestration. This lack of discrimination is largely due to the high homology between isoforms and the lack of discriminatory reagents, with no validated antibodies able to distinguish MT-1 and MT-2 subfamilies, nor the different MT-1 isoforms [41,52].

MTs are reported to work cooperatively with zinc transporters to regulate cellular zinc homeostasis, potentially by modulating cellular zinc ion concentration [39], although the exact mechanisms are unknown. Thus, a possible consequence of exposure to cadmium ions may be altered cellular zinc homeostasis. Cadmium and zinc possess highly similar properties, and it has been shown that cadmium can substitute for zinc in biological systems [53]. This can disrupt the normal functioning of various biological pathways [54,55], thus indirectly influencing processes involved in carcinogenesis such as cell proliferation and metastasis [56].

Our aims were to investigate MT isoform expression and specificity of induction in human urothelium under baseline and cadmium-exposed conditions, using a well-characterized normal human urothelial (NHU) cell culture system that includes polarized differentiated NHU cell sheets possessing tight barrier function [57,58]. Prior to cadmium exposure, cellular growth assays were performed to assess cytotoxicity. Next, we exposed NHU cells to a variety of potential MT inducers, including reactive oxygen species (ROS) [59,60], essential metals [44,61–66], and heavy metals [67–70] to define the specificity of response. Previously unpublished MT-1 isoform-specific antibodies were used to discriminate between MT-1 isoform proteins. Lastly, we determined whether transcription of the free zinc efflux regulator zinc transporter-1 (*SLC30A1*) [71] was altered as a consequence of cadmium exposure. The results revealed that MT isoform expression was inducer-specific, and that abundance of both *MT-1A* and *MT-1M* transcript and protein was highly cadmium-specific, highlighting their potential as biomarkers of exposure. Cadmium was able to penetrate an intact urothelial barrier and effected transcriptional upregulation of *SLC30A1*, indicating a potential route for cadmium uptake and possible subsequent substitution in zinc homeostatic mechanisms.

2. Results

2.1. Influence of Cadmium on NHU Cell Culture Growth and Uptake of Cadmium across an Intact Urothelial Barrier

Exposure of nondifferentiated NHU cells to cadmium revealed that cell growth was unaffected by concentrations $\leq 10\ \mu M$ CdCl$_2$ whilst exposure to 20 μM CdCl$_2$ resulted in distinct cytotoxicity (Figure 1A). Replication in a second independent cell line confirmed that exposure to 10 μM CdCl$_2$

did not affect NHU cell growth (Figure 1B); this concentration was therefore selected for further experiments. When differentiated NHU cell cultures (three independent cell lines) were grown on permeable membranes in triplicate and exposed apically to 10 µM CdCl$_2$ for 72 h, no effect was seen on barrier function (control versus cadmium-exposed transepithelial electrical resistance (TEER) of 3.24 ± 0.48 kΩ.cm^2 versus 3.17 ± 0.52 kΩ.cm^2, mean ± SEM; p = 0.93; Table S1). The barrier was retained during CdCl$_2$ exposures of at least seven days, over which time the TEER increased in the cadmium-exposed culture to 1.8-fold over control. Analysis of cell lysates by inductively coupled plasma optical emission spectroscopy (ICP-OES) revealed an intracellular cadmium concentration of 0.94 µM in lysates from cadmium-exposed cultures compared to 0.08 µM for control cultures.

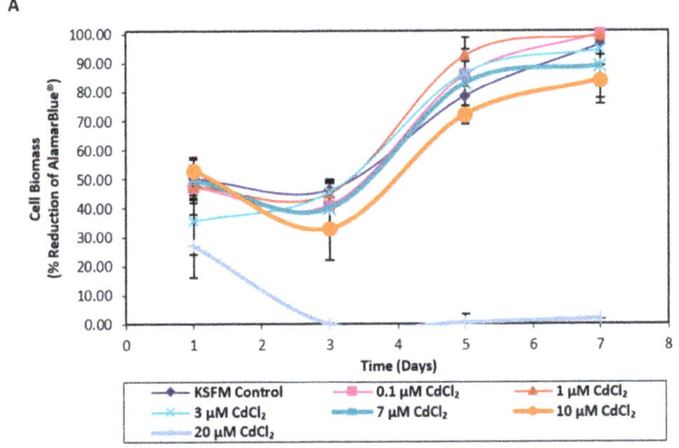

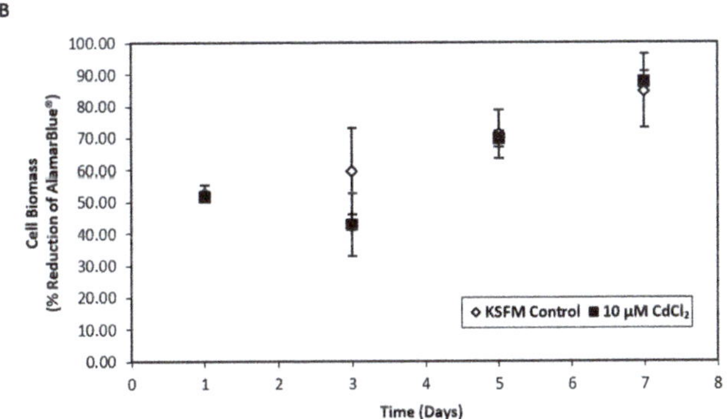

Figure 1. Biomass growth assays for in vitro normal human urothelial (NHU) cell cultures exposed to cadmium. AlamarBlue® assays were performed over 7 days on NHU cell cultures seeded at 6 × 10^4 cells/cm^2. (**A**) NHU cells were exposed to a range of cadmium concentrations from 0 to 20 µM (n = 1 independent cell line). Each data point represents mean percentage reduction in AlamarBlue® ± S.D. from three replicate cultures. (**B**) NHU cells were exposed to 10 µM CdCl$_2$ for up to 7 days. Data points represent mean percentage reduction in AlamarBlue® ± S.D. from two independent NHU cell lines, each performed in triplicate.

2.2. Baseline and Cadmium-Induced MT Transcription in NHU Cells

NHU cells maintained in culture in nondifferentiated and differentiated states were examined for baseline expression of MT genes. Analysis by mRNA-seq of nondifferentiated NHU cells revealed high expression of *MT-1E* and *MT-1X* and low expression of *MT-1A*, *MT-1B*, *MT-1F*, and *MT-1G*; there was no detection of *MT-1H* or *MT-1M* transcripts (Figure 2A). *MT-2A* expression was three times greater than all the MT-1 genes combined. No expression was detected for *MT-3* or *MT-4*. In almost all cases where MT gene expression was detected in nondifferentiated NHU cells, the expression was reduced in the differentiated state. This was most striking for *MT-2A* ($\log_2$FC = 4.2; q = 4.08 $\times$ 10^{-3}) and *MT-1E* ($\log_2$FC = 1.5; q = 4.0 $\times$ 10^{-4}), although between-donor variation prohibited statistical significance for many genes with lower expression. The apparent exception was *MT-1X*, where the average expression increased in the differentiated state. However, this was inconsistent between donors, and the differential expression was nonsignificant. Interestingly, *MT-1L* (which generates a transcript with a premature stop codon [72]) was expressed at similar abundance to *MT-1E* in the nondifferentiated cells, but with a much greater downregulation in the differentiated state ($\log_2$FC = 5.4; q = 8.4 $\times$ 10^{-4}). Previous reports of a truncation-rescuing polymorphism [73] was not identified in these donors, so while *MT-1L* is unlikely to form a functional protein, it may play a role in MT-1 transcript regulation. Expression was detected for *SLC30A1* in both nondifferentiated and differentiated states (Figure 2A), but there was no significant differentiation-associated change in expression.

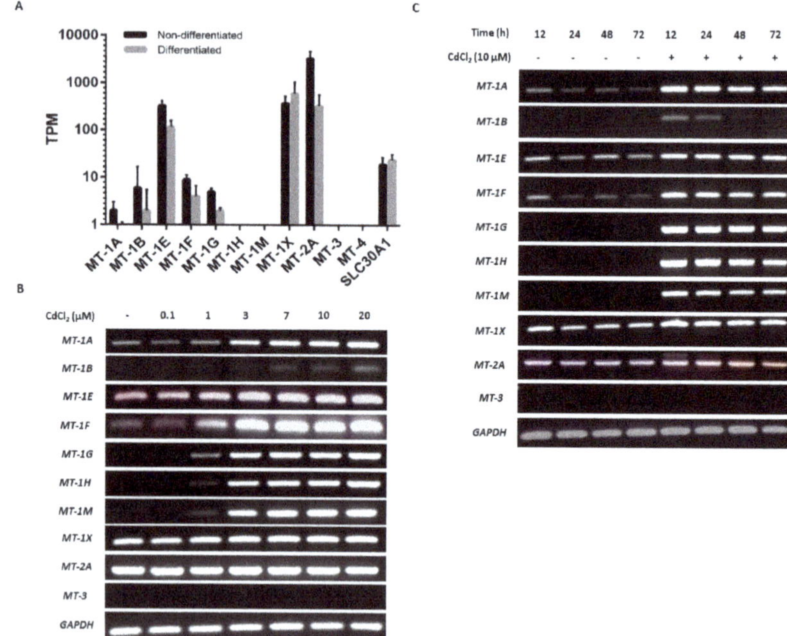

Figure 2. Baseline and cadmium-induced MT transcript expression by NHU cells in vitro. (**A**) Next-generation sequencing data showing baseline MT isoform transcription in nondifferentiated and differentiated NHU cells (*n* = 3 independent cell lines; standard deviation is shown). (**B,C**) MT gene expression in NHU cells assessed by RT-PCR. The total cDNA input was 1 µg and PCR reaction products were removed after 25 cycles; *GAPDH* was included as input control. See Table 1 for primer sequences and product sizes. Note that medium was changed at time T = 0 only and there was no renewal of cadmium over the period. The figure shows results representative of *n* = 3 independent NHU cell lines. Additional PCR controls included genomic DNA as a positive control and a no-template (H$_2$O) negative control; RT negative samples confirmed absence of genomic contamination. In (**B**), the result of exposing nondifferentiated NHU cells to different concentrations of cadmium (0–20 µM) for 72 h on MT gene expression is shown. In (**C**), MT gene expression is shown in differentiated NHU cell cultures following exposure to 10 µM CdCl$_2$ for up to 72 h.

RT-PCR results supported the NGS data, although the variability in transcript detection in nondifferentiated NHU cells indicated a potentially inducible state (Figure 2B). Differentiated NHU cell cultures revealed a more consistent baseline expression of several MT-1 genes, particularly *MT-1X* (Figure 2C).

Exposure to cadmium ions caused a massive induction of all eight MT-1 genes (*MT-1A*, *MT-1B*, *MT-1E*, *MT-1F*, *MT-1G*, *MT-1H*, *MT-1M*, and *MT-1X*) within 12 h of initial exposure, as demonstrated by the RT-PCR results, with expression receding over time (Figure 2B,C). Whereas expression of *MT-1* transcripts was mostly lost after 48 h of continuous cadmium exposure in nondifferentiated cell cultures (Figure 2B with independent cell line repeats in supplementary Figures S1 and S2), MT-1 subfamily transcript expression was still detectable in differentiated cell cultures after 72 h exposure (Figure 2C; with independent repeats in supplementary Figures S3 and S4).

Irrespective of differentiation state and the presence or absence of cadmium, *MT-2A* transcript expression was constitutively high, whilst *MT-3* and *MT-4* transcripts were invariably absent. Based on this, the *MT-2A*, *MT-3*, and *MT-4* genes were not further studied. By contrast, the strong induction of the *MT-1A, -1G, -1H,* and *-1M* paralogs, which was consistent following cadmium exposure in three independent NHU cell lines, was further investigated for specificity. As the RT-PCR results demonstrated a striking on/off transcriptional response of these MT-1 isoforms to cadmium exposure, it was decided to continue with this approach, as quantitative PCR would not have added anything to the data.

2.3. Specificity of Cadmium-Induced MT Transcription

NHU cell cultures were exposed to a variety of candidate MT inducers identified from the literature.

ROS is reported as a by-product of cadmium exposure [59], and therefore we sought to determine the effects of ROS on transcription of MT-1 genes. The ROS-inducing agent sulforaphane ($C_6H_{11}NOS_2$) and ROS-inhibitor ascorbic acid ($C_6H_8O_6$) were titrated against transcription of the ROS-sensitive heme oxygenase-1 (*HMOX1*) gene [74,75] to infer intracellular ROS activity (Figure 3A,B, respectively). Induction of expression of the four MT-1 genes in response to cadmium exposure was unaffected by 25 µg/mL ascorbic acid used to inhibit ROS, suggesting that ROS was not responsible (Figure 3C). This conclusion was supported by the failure of 5 µM sulforaphane to induce MT-1 expression (replicate in supplementary material, Figure S5).

Differential induction of MT-1 paralogs was examined in response to other metal ions, both essential and carcinogenic (replicates in supplementary material, Figures S6 and S7). Both zinc and nickel exposure induced *MT-1G* transcription, whereas *MT-1H* transcript expression was only minimally induced by zinc, and nickel had no effect. *MT-1A* transcription was constitutively low under all conditions apart from cadmium exposure, which increased expression, and *MT-1M* transcription was highly induced by exposure to cadmium alone.

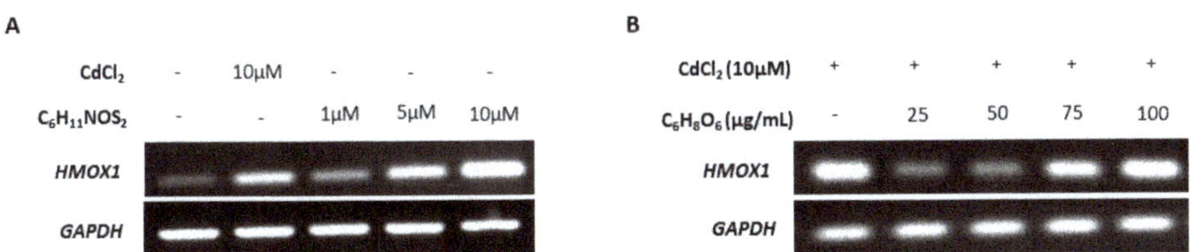

Figure 3. *Cont.*

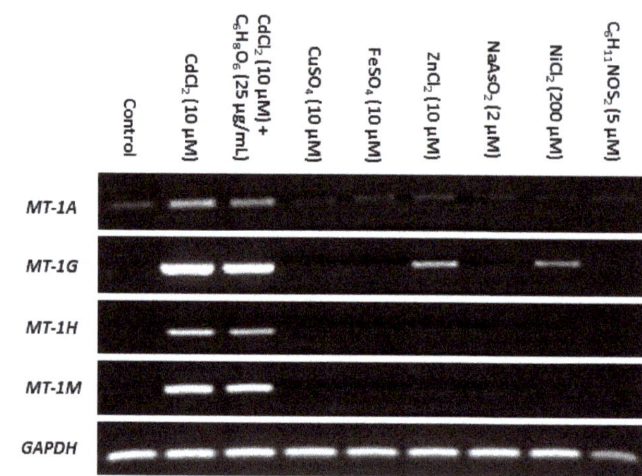

Figure 3. Specificity of metallothionein (MT) transcription induction by cadmium. MT gene expression was assessed by RT-PCR in NHU cells exposed to a variety of candidate inducers. The total cDNA input was 1 μg and PCR reaction products were removed after 25 cycles; *GAPDH* was included as input control. Note that medium was changed at time T = 0 only and there was no renewal of treatments over the period. Additional PCR controls included genomic DNA as a positive control and a no-template (H$_2$O) negative control; RT negative samples confirmed absence of genomic contamination. In (**A**), nondifferentiated NHU cell cultures were treated with a range of concentrations of sulforaphane (C$_6$H$_{11}$NOS$_2$) for 12 h, and the effect on transcription of the ROS-sensitive gene *HMOX1* assessed in comparison to exposure to 10 μM CdCl$_2$ (*n* = 1 independent cell line). The concentration of C$_6$H$_{11}$NOS$_2$ that induced transcription of *HMOX1* to a comparable extent to cadmium was selected. In (**B**), nondifferentiated NHU cell cultures were treated with a range of concentrations of ascorbic acid (C$_6$H$_8$O$_6$) for 12 h in combination with 10 μM CdCl$_2$ and the effect on *HMOX1* transcription assessed. The concentration of C$_6$H$_8$O$_6$ that caused the biggest decrease in *HMOX1* transcription was selected. In (**C**), NHU cell cultures (*n* = 2 independent cell lines) were exposed to a range of candidate regulators and transcript expression was assessed for the MT-1 genes shown above to be most sensitive to cadmium induction (from Figure 2B,C). Candidate inducers tested were cadmium (10 μM CdCl$_2$), cadmium combined with ascorbic acid (10 μM CdCl$_2$ + 25 μg/mL C$_6$H$_8$O$_6$), copper (10 μM CuSO$_4$), iron (10 μM FeSO$_4$), zinc (10 μM ZnCl$_2$), arsenite (2 μM NaAsO$_2$), nickel (200 μM NiCl$_2$), and sulforaphane (5 μM C$_6$H$_{11}$NOS$_2$). Essential metals were applied at equivalent concentrations to cadmium. Arsenite and nickel were both used at their highest noncytotoxic concentrations based on initial titration experiments (not shown).

2.4. Immunoblotting With Isoform-Specific Antibodies

To examine if the observed induction of MT-1 gene expression translated to protein, antibodies specific to the MT-1A and MT-1M isoforms were used to perform Western blotting. Control nondifferentiated NHU cells lacked MT-1A and MT-1M protein expression (Figure 4A). Cadmium exposure caused induction of both MT-1A and MT-1M proteins after 72 h (replicate in supplementary material, Figure S8). Both proteins were also induced in cadmium-exposed differentiated NHU cells (Figure 4B; replicated in supplementary material, Figure S9).

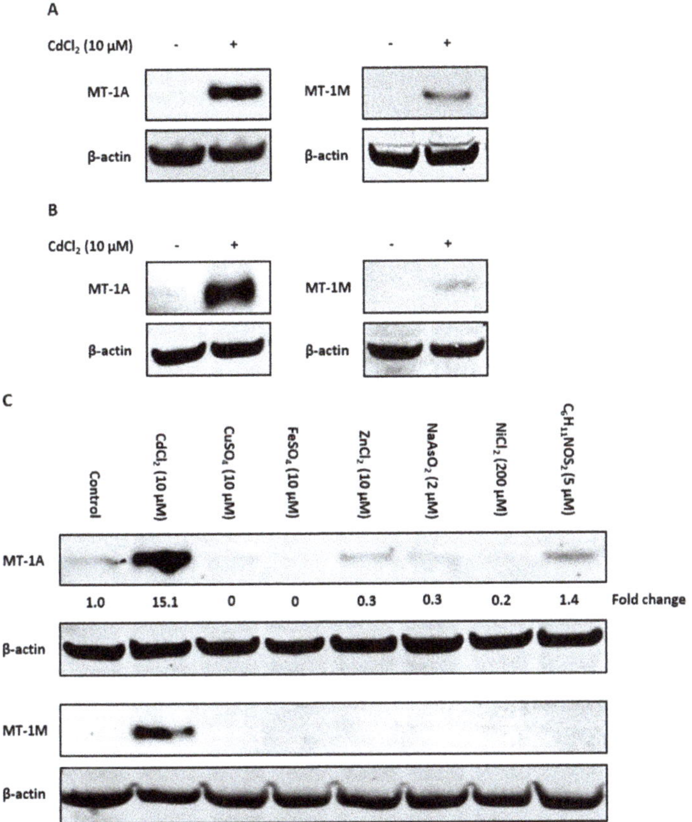

Figure 4. Western blot detection of cadmium-induced MT-1A and MT-1M expression in NHU cells using subtype-specific antibodies. MT-1A and MT-1M protein induction was observed by Western blotting of NHU cells exposed to 10 µM CdCl$_2$ for 72 h. Total protein input was 20 µg per track, with β-actin expression used to verify equal protein loading. Figures show western blots probed with MT-1A and MT-1M isoform-specific antibodies in (**A**) nondifferentiated and (**B**) differentiated NHU cell cultures exposed to cadmium for 72 h (representative blots shown from *n* = 3 independent cell lines). In (B), differentiated barrier formation was confirmed by TEER (see Figure 3B). (**C**) Western blot showing specificity of MT-1A and MT-1M protein induction (representative of *n* = 2 independent cell lines tested). Proliferating NHU cells were exposed to a range of potential inducers for 72 h and protein expression assessed. The candidate inducers tested were cadmium (10 µM CdCl$_2$), copper (10 µM CuSO$_4$), iron (10 µM FeSO$_4$), zinc (10 µM ZnCl$_2$), arsenite (2 µM NaAsO$_2$), nickel (200 µM NiCl$_2$), and sulforaphane (5 µM C$_6$H$_{11}$NOS$_2$). MT-1A protein expression is reported as fold-change relative to unexposed control cells.

The specificity of MT-1A and MT-1M protein induction was examined in response to the wider range of candidate inducers. Western blotting revealed that the MT-1M isoform was induced only by cadmium exposure, supporting the RT-PCR results (Figure 4C; replicated in supplementary material, Figure S10). MT-1A protein expression was highly induced by cadmium exposure, although low protein expression was observed under other conditions. As assessed by densitometry, only cadmium was capable of increasing MT-1A protein expression over control, resulting in a ~6-fold increase in MT-1A protein expression (Figure 4D).

2.5. Upregulation of Zinc Transporter-1 (SLC30A1) Transcription in Cadmium-Exposed NHU Cells

RT-PCR of both nondifferentiated and differentiated NHU cells revealed that cadmium exposure resulted in increased *SLC30A1* gene transcription compared to unexposed controls (Figure 5A; replicated in supplementary material, Figure S11). After cessation of exposure, *SLC30A1* transcript expression receded over time, and this decrease was observed to occur most rapidly in nondifferentiated (after 24 h; Figure 3B) compared to differentiated (after 11 days; Figure 5C) cell cultures.

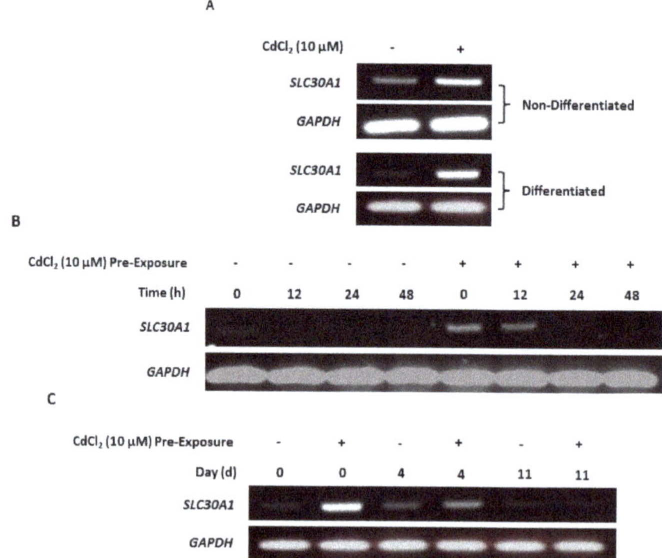

Figure 5. Cadmium induction of zinc transporter-1 (*SLC30A1*) gene transcription. *SLC30A1* gene transcript expression was assessed by RT-PCR, with PCR reaction products removed after 25 cycles. PCR controls included genomic DNA as a positive control and a no-template (H_2O) negative control. Total cDNA input was 1 µg with *GAPDH* used as an input loading control; RT-ve samples confirmed the absence of genomic contamination. For differentiated NHU cells, differentiation was confirmed by assessment of TEER as >1000 $\Omega.cm^2$ (see supplementary materials, Table S1). (**A**) NHU cells in nondifferentiated and differentiated states were maintained in control medium or with 10 µM $CdCl_2$ for up to 72 h. Note that medium was changed at time T = 0 and there was no renewal of the cadmium over the period. The figure shows representative results from $n = 3$ (nondifferentiated) and $n = 1$ (differentiated) independent NHU cell lines. (**B**) RT-PCR of NHU cells in a nondifferentiated state maintained in standard medium (control) or with 10 µM $CdCl_2$ for up to 24 h prior to the experiment ('pre-exposure'), whereupon cadmium was removed from the medium (time point 0) and culture continued for a further 48 h. (**C**) RT-PCR of NHU cells in a differentiated state maintained in standard medium (control) or with 10 µM $CdCl_2$ for up to 3 days prior to the experiment ('pre-exposure'), whereupon cadmium was removed from the medium (time point 0) and culture continued for up to 11 days.

3. Discussion

To the best of the authors' knowledge, this is the first study to investigate if cadmium exposure affects urothelial tight barrier function. Previous studies have examined the effect of cadmium exposure on renal [76] and bronchial [77] epithelia, with both studies reporting a decrease or complete collapse of barrier function. By contrast, the results from this study showed that urothelial barrier function was retained and even tightened. This may reflect the type of epithelium being tested, as urothelial cells are known to form one of the tightest epithelial barriers in the human body and thus may be unique in their resistance to cadmium. Although cadmium did not compromise urothelial barrier function, our results found that apical exposure induced expression of MT-1 isoforms in underlying NHU cells and using ICP-OES, cadmium was directly detected in differentiated urothelial cell sheets. Taken together, these results indicate that the urothelium remains intact and may even mount a protective response to cadmium in terms of tight junction tightening, yet the heavy metal is still able to penetrate the urothelial barrier.

Also for the first time, we describe specific MT gene expression by normal human urothelium. Our results are consistent with previous reports in other tissues that MT-1 is the inducible subfamily [22,40,78] whereas *MT-2A* is the most widely expressed isoform, accounting for up to 50 % total MT expression in humans [6,79]. In agreement with the consensus that MT-3 is neural-restricted [80], we found no baseline expression and no agents that could induce *MT-3* transcription in urothelial cells. As an anomaly, one group has previously suggested a link between heavy metal exposure, MT-3 induction, and urothelial carcinogenesis based on high MT-3 expression in malignant bladder cancer [81]. This group further supported their findings using in vitro studies in cadmium-transformed UROtsa cells [82,83]. However, we were not able to replicate those findings in our normal cell system.

Of the MT-1 gene family, transcription of *MT-1F* and *MT-1G* has previously been described as constitutive in human umbilical vein epithelial cells (HUVEC) under baseline conditions [42]. Both these genes exhibited low basal but inducible expression in NHU cells, therefore it cannot be certain whether the expression differences between tissues are constitutive, or perhaps due to inducers present in the culture medium. Whereas we found the majority of MT-1 gene paralogs to be inducible by cadmium exposure, transcript expression was transient, presumably due to sequestration leaving fewer free cadmium ions to maintain induction. By contrast, expression of MT-1 proteins was more stable and in line with the sequestering nature of the formed MT-cadmium complex. Previously, MT-1 protein isoform detection has been performed using mass spectrometry [41], but the demonstrated availability of specific antibodies now opens the door to detection using immunochemical approaches.

Exposure of proliferating NHU cell cultures to a range of divalent metal ions revealed differential and inducer-specific induction of MT-1 isoforms. For example, zinc ions induced strong transcription of *MT-1G*, but not *MT-1A* genes, whereas nickel ions caused *MT-1G* expression exclusively. Inducer-specific expression of MT-1 genes has been noted in other cell types [34,44–47], supporting the hypothesis that individual isoforms have very selective metal ion sequestering functions [5,6,22,39,40,84]. Western blotting revealed that cadmium was the most potent inducer of MT-1A protein expression, whereas MT-1M protein expression was highly specific to cadmium, revealing the potential of both as biomarkers of cadmium exposure. Neither arsenic nor nickel induced MT-1A or MT-1M protein expression, further demonstrating the specificity of MT-1 isoforms to differentiate between different nongenotoxic carcinogenic metals [85,86].

Alongside a pathophysiological role in sequestering carcinogenic metals, the MTs are considered to contribute to the normal homeostasis of zinc, which as a cofactor involved in many key cellular processes [56] is under tight control. MT sequestration and zinc transporter efflux coordinated by a common transcription factor *MTF-1* [87] is thought to regulate the availability of zinc [88–91]. Changes in intracellular zinc concentration have been associated with tumor growth and progression [92]. The displacement of zinc from the proteome by cadmium may affect the intracellular concentration and/or availability of zinc ions and can substitute and destabilize the functional sites of zinc-containing proteins, such as zinc-finger transcription factors, changing the character and/or rendering them nonfunctional [54,55].

Preliminary investigation into the effect of cadmium exposure on zinc homeostasis in normal urothelial cells revealed an upregulation of the zinc transporter-1 (*SLC30A1*) gene transcript in nondifferentiated NHU cells. *SLC30A1* upregulation was also observed in cadmium-exposed differentiated NHU cell sheets possessing a functional barrier, further suggesting that cadmium can penetrate an intact urothelial barrier. Our results agree with a previous study using the human hepatic HepG2 cell line, which demonstrated increased *SLC30A1* protein expression and localization at the cell membrane after acute cadmium exposure [93]. A later study showed cadmium exposure resulted in a 93% increase in the intracellular labile zinc concentration, suggesting a large displacement of zinc ions from the proteome, possibly due to substitution by cadmium [94].

MT expression is often seen as a 'double-edged sword', as on the one hand it functions to protect the cell, but by the same mechanisms can also facilitate malignant events [6,22,95,96]. MTs may contribute to cell survival by increasing resistance to ROS-induced apoptosis [97] and increasing cellular proliferation [32]. Cadmium exposure can result in inhibition of DNA repair [98], which coupled with increased cellular protection via cadmium-induced MT expression, increases the probability of deleterious cells surviving and passing on defects to their progeny [96]. The ability of MT to counteract ROS could also play a role in chemotherapy resistance, and high expression of MT has been correlated with treatment resistance in bladder cancer [99,100]. Specifically, after radical surgery and adjuvant chemotherapy 100% patients with high tumor MT expression progressed within nine months, whereas in patients with low MT expression only 65% had progressed after five years [101].

Our study supports a concordant induction of MT isoforms and *SLC30A1* transcription in response to cadmium exposure. Whereas this does not directly contradict hypotheses that cadmium exposure increases cellular zinc concentration or that cellular zinc homeostasis is maintained through the cooperative regulation of MT and zinc transporters [39], it does proffer a more direct relationship with cadmium responsible for regulating *SLC30A1* expression. This may reveal new insight as to the role of cadmium in (bladder) cancer, where previously reported *SLC30A1* and MT changes may reflect increased concentrations of intracellular cadmium rather than zinc. Our demonstration of differential MT-1 gene paralog induction by zinc and cadmium should help design future (e.g., knockout) experiments to clarify the respective roles. Further experiments might also directly quantify intracellular zinc in NHU cells after cadmium exposure and determine the consequences of cadmium on zinc homeostasis and dysregulated cadmium-substituted proteins.

4. Materials and Methods

4.1. NHU Cell Culture and Exposure to Cadmium and Other Agents

Normal human urothelial (NHU) cells were obtained from the ureter/renal pelvis of patients undergoing urological surgery, and maintained in vitro as nonimmortalized cell lines, as detailed elsewhere [57,102]. For routine culture, NHU cells were grown as adherent monolayers on Primaria™ plasticware (BD Biosciences, Wokingham, UK) in low calcium [0.09 mM] keratinocyte serum-free medium (KSFM) containing bovine pituitary extract and recombinant epidermal growth factor (Fisher Scientific UK Ltd, Loughborough, UK) supplemented with 30 ng/mL cholera toxin (KSFMc). NHU cell lines were subcultured by trypsinization at just-confluence and used in experiments between passages 3–5.

For cadmium exposure, medium was replaced with fresh medium containing 10 μM cadmium chloride ($CdCl_2$). This concentration was selected after preliminary titration for toxicity (Figure 1A,B). For other treatment agents, concentrations were selected following initial titration and target gene expression assessment (Figure 3A,B).

Nonimmortalized NHU cell lines retain the capacity to differentiate to form a functional tight barrier epithelium [58]. Differentiation was induced by switching NHU cells into medium supplemented with 5% adult bovine serum for 5 days before subculture onto semipermeable ThinCert™ (Greiner Bio-One Ltd., Stonehouse, UK) membranes with 0.4-μm pore size. After 24 h, the exogenous calcium (Ca^{2+}) concentration was increased to 2 mM (near physiological) and cultures were maintained for a further 7–9 days to develop a tight barrier. For cadmium exposure of differentiated NHU cell cultures, medium was removed from the apical chamber after establishment of a barrier >1000 $\Omega.cm^2$

(see below) and replaced with fresh medium supplemented with 10 μM CdCl$_2$, in order to mimic apical exposure. RNA and protein were then harvested from these membranes for further analysis.

4.2. Measurement of Transepithelial Electrical Resistance

The barrier function of differentiated NHU cell sheets was assessed in triplicate cultures by measuring the transepithelial electrical resistance (TEER) using an EVOM™ voltohmmeter (World Precision Instruments, Hertfordshire, UK), as described [103]. A blank (no cell) membrane measurement was subtracted from each TEER reading.

4.3. MT Transcript Abundance Quantification by Next-Generation Sequencing

mRNA-seq data for three donor-matched NHU cultured nondifferentiated and differentiated samples were previously generated by our group [104]. Sequencing reads were 'pseudoaligned' to the Ensembl v.91 human transcriptome (GRCh38.p10) using kallisto v0.44.0 [105] and relative gene abundance was calculated as transcripts per million (TPM) following gene-level aggregation with tximport v1.8.0 [106]. Differentiation-associated expression changes in the MT gene family were detected by a differential expression analysis conducted by sleuth [107] accounting for matched-donor samples. Differentially-expressed genes are reported with their log$_2$ transformed fold change (log$_2$FC) and 'q' value (Benjamini–Hochberg correction).

4.4. Reverse Transcriptase-Polymerase Chain Reaction (RT-PCR)

RT-PCR was performed to observe actual patterns of MT isoform induction (rather than relative change). RNA was extracted from cells using TRIzol® (Fisher Scientific UK Ltd., Loughborough, UK) and treated with a DNA-free™ kit (Ambion, supplied by Fisher Scientific UK Ltd., Loughborough, UK). cDNA synthesis was performed on 1 μg RNA with random hexamers and the SuperScript®II First-Strand Synthesis System (Fisher Scientific UK Ltd., Loughborough, UK). PCR primers were designed specifically to detect all known splice variants for each MT-1 isoform gene, with GAPDH used as the internal transcript control [108]. Primer sequences and optimized PCR conditions are provided in Table 1. PCR was carried out in a T100 thermal cycler (Bio-Rad Services UK Ltd., Hemel Hempstead Hertfordshire, UK) using 25 reaction cycles. Controls consisted of genomic DNA (gDNA as template positive control), water (no template control), and no reverse transcriptase (gDNA negative control). PCR products were separated on 2 % (*w/v*) agarose gels, stained using SYBR® Safe DNA gel stain (Invitrogen supplied by Fisher Scientific UK Ltd., Loughborough, UK) and visualized on a Gene Genius Gel Imaging System (Syngene, Cambridge, UK).

Table 1. Details of primers used for experiments.

Target Gene	Forward or Reverse	Sequence (5′–3′)	Product Size (bp)
GAPDH	Forward	CAAGGTCATCCATGACAACTTTG	90
GAPDH	Reverse	GGGCCATCCACAGTCTTCTG	90
HMOX1	Forward	CCAGCAACAAAGTGCAAGATTC	102
HMOX1	Reverse	GTGTAAGGACCCATCGGAGAAG	102
MT-1A	Forward	CTCGAAATGGACCCCAACT	219
MT-1A	Reverse	ATATCTTCGAGCAGGGCTGTC	219
MT-1B	Forward	GGAACTCCAGGCTTGTCTTGG	77
MT-1B	Reverse	TTGCAGGAGGTACATTTG	77
MT-1E	Forward	TGCGCCGGCTCCTGCAAGTC	118
MT-1E	Reverse	ATGCCCCTTTGCAGACGCAGC	118

Table 1. *Cont.*

Target Gene	Forward or Reverse	Sequence (5′–3′)	Product Size (bp)
MT-1F	Forward	CCTGCACCTGCGCTGGTTCC	110
MT-1F	Reverse	ACAGCCCTGGGCACACTTGC	110
MT-1G	Forward	CTTCTCGCTTGGGAACTCTA	309
MT-1G	Reverse	AGGGGTCAAGATTGTAGCAAA	309
MT-1H	Forward	CCTCTTCTCTTCTCGCTTGG	317
MT-1H	Reverse	GCAAATGAGTCGGAGTTGTAG	317
MT-1M	Forward	CTAGCAGTCGCTCCATTTATCG	180
MT-1M	Reverse	CAGCTGCAGTTCTCCAACGT	180
MT-1X	Forward	GGACCCAACTGCTCCTGCTC	151
MT-1X	Reverse	TTTGCAGATGCAGCCCTGGGC	151
MT-2A	Forward	CCGACTCTAGCCGCCTCTT	259
MT-2A	Reverse	GTGGAAGTCGCGTTCTTTACA	259
MT-3	Forward	AGTGCGAGGGATGCAAATG	98
MT-3	Reverse	GCCTTTGCACACACAGTCCTT	98
SLC30A1	Forward	GCATCAGTTTATGAGGCTGGTCCT	352
SLC30A1	Reverse	CAGGCTGAATGGTAGTAGCGTGAA	352

4.5. Western Blotting

NHU cell cultures were lysed into electrophoresis sample buffer containing protease inhibitors and sonicated. Twenty micrograms of protein was resolved on 4–12% Bis-Tris NuPage™ polyacrylamide gels (Invitrogen) in 2-(N-morphilino) ethanesulfonic acid (MES) buffer and electro-transferred onto polyvinylfluoride membranes (Millipore). Membranes were blocked with Odyssey® blocking buffer (LI-COR Biotechnology OK Ltd., Cambridge, UK), incubated with primary antibodies for 16 h at 4 °C and bound antibody detected using Alexa Fluor® 680-conjugated anti-mouse secondary antibody (Invitrogen, Invitrogen supplied by Fisher Scientific UK Ltd., Loughborough, UK) or an IRDye 800-conjugated anti-rabbit secondary antibody (Tebu-Bio, Peterborough, UK). Antibody binding was visualized using an Odyssey® Sa Infrared Imaging System (LI-COR®). Protein quantification was performed using Odyssey® Image Studio™ software v5.0 (LI-COR®). Details of antibodies are given Tables 2 and 3.

Table 2. Details of primary antibodies used for experiments.

Antigen	Clone	Host	Supplier	Dilution	Molecular Weight (kDa)
Beta-actin	A5441	Mouse	Sigma Aldrich	1:10 000 (WB)	42
MT-1A	B01P	Mouse	Abnova	1:750 (WB)	6
MT-1M	17281-AP	Rabbit	ProteinTech	1 µg/mL (WB)	6

Table 3. Details of secondary antibodies used for experiments.

Antigen	Conjugate	Host	Supplier	Application
Anti-mouse IgG	Alexa 680	Goat	Life Technologies	WB
Anti-rabbit IgG	Alexa 800	Goat	Life Technologies	WB

5. Conclusions

MT-1 isoform expression has been characterized in normal human urothelium for the first time, and a unique expression profile described with the use of isoform-specific antibodies. Individual MT-1 genes demonstrated inducer-specific expression and two paralogs with cadmium-specific or -selective induction were identified as candidate biomarkers of cadmium exposure. With the potential for cadmium to interfere and substitute in the homeostatic regulation of zinc, new approaches are proposed for understanding cadmium-induced nongenotoxic carcinogenesis.

Supplementary Materials: Supplementary materials can be found at http://www.mdpi.com/1422-0067/20/6/1344/s1.

Author Contributions: Conceptualization, R.V.M., M.H., J.W.F.C., and J.S.; Methodology, R.V.M., M.H, A.S.M., and J.W.F.C.; Software, R.V.M. and A.S.M.; Validation, R.V.M. and J.S.; Formal Analysis, R.V.M. and A.S.M.; Investigation, R.V.M.; Resources, M.H., J.W.F.C., and J.S.; Data Curation, R.V.M. and J.S.; Writing—Original Draft Preparation, R.V.M.; Writing—Review and Editing, A.S.M, J.W.F.C., and J.S..; Visualization, R.V.M. and J.S.; Supervision, J.S.; Project Administration, R.V.M. and J.S.; Funding Acquisition, J.W.F.C and J.S.

Funding: This work was funded by Yorkshire Cancer Research (YCR) through a studentship award to R.V.M. Additional support was provided by York Against Cancer (YAC).

Conflicts of Interest: The authors declare no conflict of interest.

Abbreviations

HMOX1	Heme oxygenase-1
MT	Metallothionein
NHU	Normal human urothelial
SLC30A1	Solute carrier family A member 1
TEER	Trans-epithelial electrical resistance

References

1. Tchounwou, P.B.; Yedjou, C.G.; Patlolla, A.K.; Sutton, D.J. Heavy Metals Toxicity and the Environment. *EXS* **2012**, *101*, 133–164.

2. Feki-Tounsi, M.; Hamza-Chaffai, A. Cadmium as a possible cause of bladder cancer: A review of accumulated evidence. *Environ. Sci. Pollut. Res.* **2014**, *21*, 10561–10573. [CrossRef] [PubMed]

3. Waalkes, M.P. Cadmium carcinogenesis. *Mutat. Res.* **2003**, *533*, 107 120. [CrossRef] [PubMed]

4. Agency for Toxic Substances and Disease Registry Toxicological Profile for Cadmium. Available online: https://www.atsdr.cdc.gov/toxprofiles/tp.asp?id=48&tid=15 (accessed on 14 September 2016).

5. Coyle, P.; Philcox, J.C.; Carey, L.C.; Rofe, A.M. Metallothionein: The multipurpose protein. *Cell. Mol. Life Sci.* **2002**, *59*, 627–647. [CrossRef] [PubMed]

6. Sigel, A.; Sigel, H.; Sigel, R.K.O. *Metallothioneins and Related Chelators*; Metal Ions in Life Sciences; RSC Publishing: Cambridge, UK, 2009; Volume 5.

7. Klaassen, C.D.; Choudhuri, S.; McKim, J.M.; Lehman-McKeeman, L.D.; Kershaw, W.C. In vitro and in vivo studies on the degradation of metallothionein. *Environ. Health Perspect.* **1994**, *102*, 141–146. [PubMed]

8. Kellen, E.; Zeegers, M.P.; Hond, E.D.; Buntinx, F. Blood cadmium may be associated with bladder carcinogenesis: The Belgian case-control study on bladder cancer. *Cancer Detect. Prev.* **2007**, *31*, 77–82. [CrossRef] [PubMed]

9. Wolf, C.; Strenziok, R.; Kyriakopoulos, A. Elevated metallothionein-bound cadmium concentrations in urine from bladder carcinoma patients, investigated by size exclusion chromatography-inductively coupled plasma mass spectrometry. *Anal. Chim. Acta* **2009**, *631*, 218–222. [CrossRef]

10. Feki-Tounsi, M.; Olmedo, P.; Gil, F.; Khlifi, R.; Mhiri, M.-N.; Rebai, A.; Hamza-Chaffai, A. Cadmium in blood of Tunisian men and risk of bladder cancer: Interactions with arsenic exposure and smoking. *Environ. Sci. Pollut. Res. Int.* **2013**, *20*, 7204–7213. [CrossRef] [PubMed]

11. Chang, C.-H.; Liu, C.-S.; Liu, H.-J.; Huang, C.-P.; Huang, C.-Y.; Hsu, H.-T.; Liou, S.-H.; Chung, C.-J. Association between levels of urinary heavy metals and increased risk of urothelial carcinoma. *Int. J. Urol.* **2016**, *23*, 233–239. [CrossRef]

12. Achanzar, W.E.; Diwan, B.A.; Liu, J.; Quader, S.T.; Webber, M.M.; Waalkes, M.P. Cadmium-induced Malignant Transformation of Human Prostate Epithelial Cells. *Cancer Res.* **2001**, *61*, 455–458.

13. Takiguchi, M.; Achanzar, W.E.; Qu, W.; Li, G.; Waalkes, M.P. Effects of cadmium on DNA-(Cytosine-5) methyltransferase activity and DNA methylation status during cadmium-induced cellular transformation. *Exp. Cell Res.* **2003**, *286*, 355–365. [CrossRef]

14. Lei, Y.-X.; Wei, L.; Wang, M.; Wu, G.-R.; Li, M. Malignant transformation and abnormal expression of eukaryotic initiation factor in bronchial epithelial cells induced by cadmium chloride. *Biomed. Environ. Sci.* **2008**, *21*, 332–338. [CrossRef]

15. Sens, D.A.; Park, S.; Gurel, V.; Sens, M.A.; Garrett, S.H.; Somji, S. Inorganic Cadmium- and Arsenite-Induced Malignant Transformation of Human Bladder Urothelial Cells. *Toxicol. Sci.* **2004**, *79*, 56–63. [CrossRef] [PubMed]

16. Kreft, M.E.; Hudoklin, S.; Jezernik, K.; Romih, R. Formation and maintenance of blood–urine barrier in urothelium. *Protoplasma* **2010**, *246*, 3–14. [CrossRef] [PubMed]

17. Caldwell, J.; Gardner, I.; Swales, N. An Introduction to Drug Disposition: The Basic Principles of Absorption, Distribution, Metabolism, and Excretion. *Toxicol. Pathol.* **1995**, *23*, 102–114. [CrossRef] [PubMed]

18. Krause, M.; Rak-Raszewska, A.; Pietilä, I.; Quaggin, S.E.; Vainio, S. Signaling during Kidney Development. *Cells* **2015**, *4*, 112–132. [CrossRef]

19. Margoshes, M.; Vallee, B.L. A Cadmium Protein from Equine Kidney Cortex. *J. Am. Chem. Soc.* **1957**, *79*, 4813–4814. [CrossRef]

20. Kägi, J.H.; Schäffer, A. Biochemistry of metallothionein. *Biochemistry* **1988**, *27*, 8509–8515. [CrossRef]

21. Hunt, C.T.; Boulanger, Y.; Fesik, S.W.; Armitage, I.M. NMR analysis of the structure and metal sequestering properties of metallothioneins. *Environ. Health Perspect.* **1984**, *54*, 135–145. [CrossRef] [PubMed]

22. Capdevila, M.; Bofill, R.; Palacios, Ò.; Atrian, S. State-of-the-art of metallothioneins at the beginning of the 21st century. *Coord. Chem. Rev.* **2012**, *256*, 46–62. [CrossRef]

23. Dalton, T.; Fu, K.; Palmiter, R.D.; Andrews, G.K. Transgenic mice that overexpress metallothionein-I resist dietary zinc deficiency. *J. Nutr.* **1996**, *126*, 825–833. [CrossRef]

24. Kelly, E.J.; Quaife, C.J.; Froelick, G.J.; Palmiter, R.D. Metallothionein I and II protect against zinc deficiency and zinc toxicity in mice. *J. Nutr.* **1996**, *126*, 1782–1790.

25. Lee, D.K.; Geiser, J.; Dufner-Beattie, J.; Andrews, G.K. Pancreatic metallothionein-I may play a role in zinc homeostasis during maternal dietary zinc deficiency in mice. *J. Nutr.* **2003**, *133*, 45–50. [CrossRef]

26. Penkowa, M.; Cáceres, M.; Borup, R.; Nielsen, F.C.; Poulsen, C.B.; Quintana, A.; Molinero, A.; Carrasco, J.; Florit, S.; Giralt, M.; et al. Novel roles for metallothionein-I + II (MT-I + II) in defense responses, neurogenesis, and tissue restoration after traumatic brain injury: Insights from global gene expression profiling in wild-type and MT-I + II knockout mice. *J. Neurosci. Res.* **2006**, *84*, 1452–1474. [CrossRef] [PubMed]

27. Lazo, J.S.; Kondo, Y.; Dellapiazza, D.; Michalska, A.E.; Choo, K.H.; Pitt, B.R. Enhanced sensitivity to oxidative stress in cultured embryonic cells from transgenic mice deficient in metallothionein I and II genes. *J. Biol. Chem.* **1995**, *270*, 5506–5510. [CrossRef] [PubMed]

28. Karin, M.; Haslinger, A.; Holtgreve, H.; Richards, R.I.; Krauter, P.; Westphal, H.M.; Beato, M. Characterization of DNA sequences through which cadmium and glucocorticoid hormones induce human metallothionein-IIA gene. *Nature* **1984**, *308*, 513–519. [CrossRef]

29. Schulkens, I.A.; Castricum, K.C.M.; Weijers, E.M.; Koolwijk, P.; Griffioen, A.W.; Thijssen, V.L. Expression, regulation and function of human metallothioneins in endothelial cells. *J. Vasc. Res.* **2014**, *51*, 231–238. [CrossRef] [PubMed]

30. Yap, X.; Tan, H.-Y.; Huang, J.; Lai, Y.; Yip, G.W.-C.; Tan, P.-H.; Bay, B.-H. Over-expression of metallothionein predicts chemoresistance in breast cancer. *J. Pathol.* **2009**, *217*, 563–570. [CrossRef]

31. Liu, Z.-M.; van Hasselt, C.A.; Song, F.-Z.; Vlantis, A.C.; Cherian, M.G.; Koropatnick, J.; Chen, G.G. Expression of functional metallothionein isoforms in papillary thyroid cancer. *Mol. Cell. Endocrinol.* **2009**, *302*, 92–98. [CrossRef]

32. Ioachim, E.E.; Charchanti, A.V.; Stavropoulos, N.E.; Athanassiou, E.D.; Michael, M.C.; Agnantis, N.J. Localization of metallothionein in urothelial carcinoma of the human urinary bladder: An immunohistochemical study including correlation with HLA-DR antigen, p53, and proliferation indices. *Anticancer Res.* **2001**, *21*, 1757–1761. [PubMed]

33. Jin, R.; Chow, V.T.-K.; Tan, P.-H.; Dheen, S.T.; Duan, W.; Bay, B.-H. Metallothionein 2A expression is associated with cell proliferation in breast cancer. *Carcinogenesis* **2002**, *23*, 81–86. [CrossRef] [PubMed]

34. Varshney, U.; Jahroudi, N.; Foster, R.; Gedamu, L. Structure, organization, and regulation of human metallothionein IF gene: Differential and cell-type-specific expression in response to heavy metals and glucocorticoids. *Mol. Cell. Biol.* **1986**, *6*, 26–37. [CrossRef] [PubMed]

35. Boonprasert, K.; Ruengweerayut, R.; Aunpad, R.; Satarug, S.; Na-Bangchang, K. Expression of metallothionein isoforms in peripheral blood leukocytes from Thai population residing in cadmium-contaminated areas. *Environ. Toxicol. Pharmacol.* **2012**, *34*, 935–940. [CrossRef] [PubMed]

36. Mita, M.; Satoh, M.; Shimada, A.; Okajima, M.; Azuma, S.; Suzuki, J.S.; Sakabe, K.; Hara, S.; Himeno, S. Metallothionein is a crucial protective factor against Helicobacter pylori-induced gastric erosive lesions in a mouse model. *Am. J. Physiol. Gastrointest. Liver Physiol.* **2008**, *294*, G877–G884. [CrossRef]

37. Kägi, J.H.; Kojima, Y. Chemistry and biochemistry of metallothionein. *Exp. Suppl.* **1987**, *52*, 25–61.

38. Irvine, G.W.; Pinter, T.B.J.; Stillman, M.J. Defining the metal binding pathways of human metallothionein 1a: Balancing zinc availability and cadmium seclusion. *Metallomics* **2016**, *8*, 71–81. [CrossRef] [PubMed]

39. Kimura, T.; Kambe, T. The Functions of Metallothionein and ZIP and ZnT Transporters: An Overview and Perspective. *Int. J. Mol. Sci.* **2016**, *17*, 336. [CrossRef]

40. Miles, A.T.; Hawksworth, G.M.; Beattie, J.H.; Rodilla, V. Induction, Regulation, Degradation, and Biological Significance of Mammalian Metallothioneins. *Crit. Rev. Biochem. Mol. Biol.* **2000**, *35*, 35–70. [CrossRef]

41. Mehus, A.A.; Muhonen, W.W.; Garrett, S.H.; Somji, S.; Sens, D.A.; Shabb, J.B. Quantitation of Human Metallothionein Isoforms: A Family of Small, Highly Conserved, Cysteine-rich Proteins. *Mol. Cell. Proteom.* **2014**, *13*, 1020–1033. [CrossRef]

42. Conway, D.E.; Lee, S.; Eskin, S.G.; Shah, A.K.; Jo, H.; McIntire, L.V. Endothelial metallothionein expression and intracellular free zinc levels are regulated by shear stress. *Am. J. Physiol. Cell. Physiol.* **2010**, *299*, C1461–C1467. [CrossRef]

43. Jahroudi, N.; Foster, R.; Price-Haughey, J.; Beitel, G.; Gedamu, L. Cell-type specific and differential regulation of the human metallothionein genes. Correlation with DNA methylation and chromatin structure. *J. Biol. Chem.* **1990**, *265*, 6506–6511.

44. Miura, N.; Koizumi, S. Heavy metal responses of the human metallothionein isoform genes. *J. Pharm. Soc. Jpn.* **2007**, *127*, 665–673. [CrossRef]

45. Richards, R.I.; Heguy, A.; Karin, M. Structural and functional analysis of the human metallothionein-IA gene: Differential induction by metal ions and glucocorticoids. *Cell* **1984**, *37*, 263–272. [CrossRef]

46. Selvaraj, A.; Balamurugan, K.; Yepiskoposyan, H.; Zhou, H.; Egli, D.; Georgiev, O.; Thiele, D.J.; Schaffner, W. Metal-responsive transcription factor (MTF-1) handles both extremes, copper load and copper starvation, by activating different genes. *Genes Dev.* **2005**, *19*, 891–896. [CrossRef] [PubMed]

47. Sims, H.I.; Chirn, G.-W.; Marr, M.T. Single nucleotide in the MTF-1 binding site can determine metal-specific transcription activation. *PNAS* **2012**, *109*, 16516–16521. [CrossRef] [PubMed]

48. Sadhu, C.; Gedamu, L. Regulation of human metallothionein (MT) genes. Differential expression of MTI-F, MTI-G, and MTII-A genes in the hepatoblastoma cell line (HepG2). *J. Biol. Chem.* **1988**, *263*, 2679–2684.

49. Lehman-McKeeman, L.D.; Andrews, G.K.; Klaassen, C.D. Mechanisms of regulation of rat hepatic metallothionein-I and metallothionein-II levels following administration of zinc. *Toxicol. Appl. Pharmacol.* **1988**, *92*, 1–9. [CrossRef]

50. Klaassen, C.D.; Lehman-McKeeman, L.D. Regulation of the isoforms of metallothionein. *Biol. Trace Elem. Res.* **1989**, *21*, 119–129. [CrossRef]

51. Kim, J.-H.; Wang, S.-Y.; Kim, I.-C.; Ki, J.-S.; Raisuddin, S.; Lee, J.-S.; Han, K.-N. Cloning of a river pufferfish (Takifugu obscurus) metallothionein cDNA and study of its induction profile in cadmium-exposed fish. *Chemosphere* **2008**, *71*, 1251–1259. [CrossRef]

52. Jasani, B.; Schmid, K.W. Significance of metallothionein overexpression in human tumours. *Histopathology* **1997**, *31*, 131–136. [CrossRef]

53. Chaney, R.L. Cadmium and Zinc. In *Trace Elements in Soils*; Wiley: New York, NY, USA, 2010; pp. 409–440.

54. Malgieri, G.; Zaccaro, L.; Leone, M.; Bucci, E.; Esposito, S.; Baglivo, I.; Del Gatto, A.; Russo, L.; Scandurra, R.; Pedone, P.V.; et al. Zinc to cadmium replacement in the A. thaliana SUPERMAN Cys_2 His_2 zinc finger induces structural rearrangements of typical DNA base determinant positions. *Biopolymers* **2011**, *95*, 801–810. [PubMed]

55. Tang, L.; Qiu, R.; Tang, Y.; Wang, S. Cadmium–zinc exchange and their binary relationship in the structure of Zn-related proteins: A mini review. *Metallomics* **2014**, *6*, 1313–1323. [CrossRef] [PubMed]

56. Jeong, J.; Eide, D.J. The SLC39 family of zinc transporters. *Mol. Asp. Med.* **2013**, *34*, 612–619. [CrossRef] [PubMed]

57. Southgate, J.; Hutton, K.A.; Thomas, D.F.; Trejdosiewicz, L.K. Normal human urothelial cells in vitro: Proliferation and induction of stratification. *Lab. Investig.* **1994**, *71*, 583–594. [PubMed]

58. Cross, W.R.; Eardley, I.; Leese, H.J.; Southgate, J. A biomimetic tissue from cultured normal human urothelial cells: Analysis of physiological function. *Am. J. Physiol. Renal Physiol.* **2005**, *289*, F459–F468. [CrossRef]

59. Wang, Y.; Fang, J.; Leonard, S.S.; Rao, K.M.K. Cadmium inhibits the electron transfer chain and induces reactive oxygen species. *Free Radic. Biol. Med.* **2004**, *36*, 1434–1443. [CrossRef]

60. Heyno, E.; Klose, C.; Krieger-Liszkay, A. Origin of cadmium-induced reactive oxygen species production: Mitochondrial electron transfer versus plasma membrane NADPH oxidase. *New Phytol.* **2008**, *179*, 687–699. [CrossRef]

61. Durnam, D.M.; Palmiter, R.D. Induction of metallothionein-I mRNA in cultured cells by heavy metals and iodoacetate: Evidence for gratuitous inducers. *Mol. Cell. Biol.* **1984**, *4*, 484–491. [CrossRef]

62. Alam, J.; Smith, A. Heme-hemopexin-mediated induction of metallothionein gene expression. *J. Biol. Chem.* **1992**, *267*, 16379–16384.

63. Baird, S.K.; Kurz, T.; Brunk, U.T. Metallothionein protects against oxidative stress-induced lysosomal destabilization. *Biochem. J.* **2006**, *394*, 275–283. [CrossRef]

64. Palmiter, R.D. Regulation of metallothionein genes by heavy metals appears to be mediated by a zinc-sensitive inhibitor that interacts with a constitutively active transcription factor, MTF-1. *Proc. Natl. Acad. Sci. USA* **1994**, *91*, 1219–1223. [CrossRef] [PubMed]

65. Kheradmand, F.; Nourmohammadi, I.; Modarressi, M.H.; Firoozrai, M.; Ahmadi Faghih, M.A. Differential Gene-Expression of Metallothionein 1M and 1G in Response to Zinc in Sertoli TM4 Cells. *Iran Biomed. J.* **2010**, *14*, 9–15. [PubMed]

66. Chu, A.; Foster, M.; Ward, S.; Zaman, K.; Hancock, D.; Petocz, P.; Samman, S. Zinc-induced upregulation of metallothionein (MT)-2A is predicted by gene expression of zinc transporters in healthy adults. *Genes Nutr.* **2015**, *10*, 44. [CrossRef] [PubMed]

67. Chen, L.; Ma, L.; Bai, Q.; Zhu, X.; Zhang, J.; Wei, Q.; Li, D.; Gao, C.; Li, J.; Zhang, Z.; et al. Heavy metal-induced metallothionein expression is regulated by specific protein phosphatase 2A complexes. *J. Biol. Chem.* **2014**, *289*, 22413–22426. [CrossRef] [PubMed]

68. Heuchel, R.; Radtke, F.; Georgiev, O.; Stark, G.; Aguet, M.; Schaffner, W. The transcription factor MTF-1 is essential for basal and heavy metal-induced metallothionein gene expression. *EMBO J.* **1994**, *13*, 2870–2875. [CrossRef]

69. Zhou, X.D.; Sens, D.A.; Sens, M.A.; Namburi, V.B.R.K.; Singh, R.K.; Garrett, S.H.; Somji, S. Metallothionein-1 and -2 Expression in Cadmium- or Arsenic-Derived Human Malignant Urothelial Cells and Tumor Heterotransplants and as a Prognostic Indicator in Human Bladder Cancer. *Toxicol. Sci.* **2006**, *91*, 467–475. [CrossRef]

70. Irvine, G.W.; Stillman, M.J. Topographical analysis of As-induced folding of α-MT1a. *Biochem. Biophys. Res. Commun.* **2013**, *441*, 208–213. [CrossRef]

71. McMahon, R.J.; Cousins, R.J. Regulation of the zinc transporter ZnT-1 by dietary zinc. *Proc. Natl. Acad. Sci. USA* **1998**, *95*, 4841–4846. [CrossRef]

72. Holloway, A.F.; Stennard, F.A.; West, A.K. Human metallothionein gene MT1L mRNA is present in several human tissues but is unlikely to produce a metallothionein protein. *FEBS Lett.* **1997**, *404*, 41–44. [CrossRef]

73. Hahn, Y.; Lee, B. Human-specific nonsense mutations identified by genome sequence comparisons. *Hum. Genet.* **2006**, *119*, 169–178. [CrossRef]

74. Ryter, S.W.; Choi, A.M.K. Heme oxygenase-1: Redox regulation of a stress protein in lung and cell culture models. *Antioxid. Redox Signal.* **2005**, *7*, 80–91. [CrossRef]

75. Sarma, S.N.; Kim, Y.-J.; Song, M.; Ryu, J.-C. Induction of apoptosis in human leukemia cells through the production of reactive oxygen species and activation of HMOX1 and Noxa by benzene, toluene, and o-xylene. *Toxicology* **2011**, *280*, 109–117. [CrossRef]

76. Faurskov, B.; Bjerregaard, H.F. Effect of cadmium on active ion transport and cytotoxicity in cultured renal epithelial cells (A6). *Toxicol. In Vitro* **1997**, *11*, 717–722. [CrossRef]

77. Cao, X.; Lin, H.; Muskhelishvili, L.; Latendresse, J.; Richter, P.; Heflich, R.H. Tight junction disruption by cadmium in an in vitro human airway tissue model. *Respir. Res.* **2015**, *16*, 30. [CrossRef]

78. Thirumoorthy, N.; Manisenthil Kumar, K.-T.; Shyam Sundar, A.; Panayappan, L.; Chatterjee, M. Metallothionein: An overview. *World J. Gastroenterol.* **2007**, *13*, 993–996. [CrossRef]

79. Raudenska, M.; Gumulec, J.; Podlaha, O.; Sztalmachova, M.; Babula, P.; Eckschlager, T.; Adam, V.; Kizek, R.; Masarik, M. Metallothionein polymorphisms in pathological processes. *Metallomics* **2013**, *6*, 55–68. [CrossRef] [PubMed]

80. Palmiter, R.D.; Findley, S.D.; Whitmore, T.E.; Durnam, D.M. MT-III, a brain-specific member of the metallothionein gene family. *Proc. Natl. Acad. Sci. USA* **1992**, *89*, 6333–6337. [CrossRef] [PubMed]

81. Sens, M.A.; Somji, S.; Lamm, D.L.; Garrett, S.H.; Slovinsky, F.; Todd, J.H.; Sens, D.A. Metallothionein isoform 3 as a potential biomarker for human bladder cancer. *Environ. Health Perspect.* **2000**, *108*, 413–418. [CrossRef] [PubMed]

82. Zhou, X.D.; Sens, M.A.; Garrett, S.H.; Somji, S.; Park, S.; Gurel, V.; Sens, D.A. Enhanced expression of metallothionein isoform 3 protein in tumor heterotransplants derived from As^{+3}- and Cd^{+2}-transformed human urothelial cells. *Toxicol. Sci.* **2006**, *93*, 322–330. [CrossRef] [PubMed]

83. Somji, S.; Garrett, S.H.; Toni, C.; Zhou, X.D.; Zheng, Y.; Ajjimaporn, A.; Sens, M.A.; Sens, D.A. Differences in the epigenetic regulation of MT-3 gene expression between parental and Cd^{+2} or As^{+3} transformed human urothelial cells. *Cancer Cell Int.* **2011**, *11*, 2. [CrossRef]

84. Brazão-Silva, M.T.; Rodriguez, M.F.S.; Eisenberg, A.L.A.; Dias, F.L.; de Castro, L.M.; Nunes, F.D.; Faria, P.R.; Cardoso, S.V.; Loyola, A.M.; de Sousa, S.C.O.M. Metallothionein gene expression is altered in oral cancer and may predict metastasis and patient outcomes. *Histopathology* **2015**, *67*, 358–367. [CrossRef] [PubMed]

85. International Agency for Research on Cancer Beryllium, cadmium, mercury, and exposures in the glass manufacturing industry. In *IARC Monographs on the Evaluation of the Carcinogenic Risks to Humans*; IARC: Lyon, France, 1993; Volume 58.

86. Salnikow, K.; An, W.G.; Melillo, G.; Blagosklonny, M.V.; Costa, M. Nickel-induced transformation shifts the balance between HIF-1 and p53 transcription factors. *Carcinogenesis* **1999**, *20*, 1819–1823. [CrossRef]

87. Günther, V.; Lindert, U.; Schaffner, W. The taste of heavy metals: Gene regulation by MTF-1. *Biochim. Biophys. Acta (BBA) Mol. Cell Res.* **2012**, *1823*, 1416–1425. [CrossRef] [PubMed]

88. Kimura, T.; Itoh, N.; Andrews, G.K. Mechanisms of Heavy Metal Sensing by Metal Response Element-binding Transcription Factor-1. *J. Health Sci.* **2009**, *55*, 484–494. [CrossRef]

89. Otsuka, F. Molecular Mechanism of the Metallothionein Gene Expression Mediated by Metal-Responsive Transcription Factor 1. *J. Health Sci.* **2001**, *47*, 513–519. [CrossRef]

90. Langmade, S.J.; Ravindra, R.; Daniels, P.J.; Andrews, G.K. The transcription factor MTF-1 mediates metal regulation of the mouse ZnT1 gene. *J. Biol. Chem.* **2000**, *275*, 34803–34809. [CrossRef] [PubMed]

91. Guo, L.; Lichten, L.A.; Ryu, M.-S.; Liuzzi, J.P.; Wang, F.; Cousins, R.J. STAT5-glucocorticoid receptor interaction and MTF-1 regulate the expression of ZnT2 (Slc30a2) in pancreatic acinar cells. *Proc. Natl. Acad. Sci. USA* **2010**, *107*, 2818–2823. [CrossRef]

92. Bafaro, E.; Liu, Y.; Xu, Y.; Dempski, R.E. The emerging role of zinc transporters in cellular homeostasis and cancer. *Signal Transduct. Target. Ther.* **2017**, *2*, 17029. [CrossRef]

93. Urani, C.; Melchioretto, P.; Gribaldo, L. Regulation of metallothioneins and ZnT-1 transporter expression in human hepatoma cells HepG2 exposed to zinc and cadmium. *Toxicol. In Vitro* **2010**, *24*, 370–374. [CrossRef]

94. Urani, C.; Melchioretto, P.; Bruschi, M.; Fabbri, M.; Sacco, M.G.; Gribaldo, L. Impact of Cadmium on Intracellular Zinc Levels in HepG2 Cells: Quantitative Evaluations and Molecular Effects, Impact of Cadmium on Intracellular Zinc Levels in HepG2 Cells: Quantitative Evaluations and Molecular Effects. *BioMed Res. Int. BioMed Res. Int.* **2015**, *2015*, e949514.

95. Pedersen, M.Ø.; Larsen, A.; Stoltenberg, M.; Penkowa, M. The role of metallothionein in oncogenesis and cancer prognosis. *Prog. Histochem. Cytochem.* **2009**, *44*, 29–64. [CrossRef] [PubMed]

96. Hart, B.A.; Potts, R.J.; Watkin, R.D. Cadmium adaptation in the lung—A double-edged sword? *Toxicology* **2001**, *160*, 65–70. [CrossRef]

97. Eneman, J.D.; Potts, R.J.; Osier, M.; Shukla, G.S.; Lee, C.H.; Chiu, J.-F.; Hart, B.A. Suppressed oxidant-induced apoptosis in cadmium adapted alveolar epithelial cells and its potential involvement in cadmium carcinogenesis. *Toxicology* **2000**, *147*, 215–228. [CrossRef]

98. Potts, R.J.; Bespalov, I.A.; Wallace, S.S.; Melamede, R.J.; Hart, B.A. Inhibition of oxidative DNA repair in cadmium-adapted alveolar epithelial cells and the potential involvement of metallothionein. *Toxicology* **2001**, *161*, 25–38. [CrossRef]

99. Satoh, M.; Kloth, D.M.; Kadhim, S.A.; Chin, J.L.; Naganuma, A.; Imura, N.; Cherian, M.G. Modulation of Both Cisplatin Nephrotoxicity and Drug Resistance in Murine Bladder Tumor by Controlling Metallothionein Synthesis. *Cancer Res.* **1993**, *53*, 1829–1832.

100. Wülfing, C.; van Ahlen, H.; Eltze, E.; Piechota, H.; Hertle, L.; Schmid, K.-W. Metallothionein in bladder cancer: Correlation of overexpression with poor outcome after chemotherapy. *World J. Urol.* **2007**, *25*, 199–205. [CrossRef] [PubMed]

101. Yamasaki, Y.; Smith, C.; Weisz, D.; van Huizen, I.; Xuan, J.; Moussa, M.; Stitt, L.; Hideki, S.; Cherian, M.G.; Izawa, J.I. Metallothionein expression as prognostic factor for transitional cell carcinoma of bladder. *Urology* **2006**, *67*, 530–535. [CrossRef] [PubMed]

102. Southgate, J.; Masters, J.R.W.; Trejdosiewicz, L.K. Culture of Human Urothelium. In *Culture of Epithelial Cells*; John Wiley & Sons, Inc.: New York, NY, USA, 2002; pp. 381–399. ISBN 978-0-471-22120-3.

103. Rubenwolf, P.; Southgate, J. Permeability of differentiated human urothelium in vitro. *Methods Mol. Biol.* **2011**, *763*, 207–222.

104. Fishwick, C.; Higgins, J.; Percival-Alwyn, L.; Hustler, A.; Pearson, J.; Bastkowski, S.; Moxon, S.; Swarbreck, D.; Greenman, C.D.; Southgate, J. Heterarchy of transcription factors driving basal and luminal cell phenotypes in human urothelium. *Cell Death Differ.* **2017**, *24*, 809–818. [CrossRef] [PubMed]

105. Bray, N.L.; Pimentel, H.; Melsted, P.; Pachter, L. Near-optimal probabilistic RNA-seq quantification. *Nat. Biotechnol.* **2016**, *34*, 525–527. [CrossRef] [PubMed]

106. Soneson, C.; Love, M.I.; Robinson, M.D. Differential analyses for RNA-seq: Transcript-level estimates improve gene-level inferences. *F1000Research* **2015**, *4*, 1521. [CrossRef] [PubMed]

107. Pimentel, H.; Bray, N.L.; Puente, S.; Melsted, P.; Pachter, L. Differential analysis of RNA-seq incorporating quantification uncertainty. *Nat. Methods* **2017**, *14*, 687–690. [CrossRef] [PubMed]

108. Lobban, E.D.; Smith, B.A.; Hall, G.D.; Harnden, P.; Roberts, P.; Selby, P.J.; Trejdosiewicz, L.K.; Southgate, J. Uroplakin gene expression by normal and neoplastic human urothelium. *Am. J. Pathol.* **1998**, *153*, 1957–1967. [CrossRef]

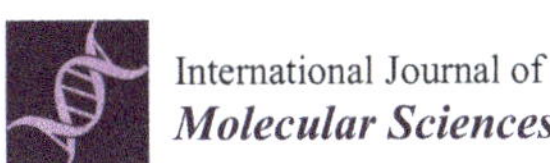
International Journal of
Molecular Sciences

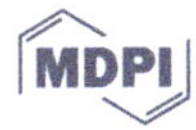

Review

Moving towards Personalized Medicine in Muscle-Invasive Bladder Cancer: Where Are We Now and Where Are We Going?

Juan Carlos Pardo [1,2,†], Vicenç Ruiz de Porras [2,3,†], Andrea Plaja [1,2], Cristina Carrato [4], Olatz Etxaniz [1,2], Oscar Buisan [5] and Albert Font [1,2,*]

[1] Department of Medical Oncology, Catalan Institute of Oncology, University Hospital Germans Trias i Pujol, Ctra. Can Ruti-Camí de les Escoles s/n, 08916 Badalona, Spain; jcpardor@iconcologia.net (J.C.P.); aplaja@iconcologia.net (A.P.); oetxaniz@iconcologia.net (O.E.)

[2] Catalan Institute of Oncology, Badalona Applied Research Group in Oncology (B·ARGO), Ctra. Can Ruti-Camí de les Escoles s/n, 08916 Badalona, Spain; vruiz@igtp.cat

[3] Germans Trias i Pujol Research Institute (IGTP), Ctra. Can Ruti-Camí de les Escoles s/n, 08916 Badalona, Spain

[4] Pathology Department, Hospital Germans Trias i Pujol, 08916 Badalona, Spain; criscarrato@gmail.com

[5] Urology Department, University Hospital Germans Trias i Pujol, 08916 Badalona, Spain; obuisan2903@gmail.com

* Correspondence: afont@iconcologia.net; Tel.: +34-93-497-8925; Fax: +34-93-497-8950

† These authors contribute equally to this work.

Received: 30 July 2020; Accepted: 28 August 2020; Published: 29 August 2020

Abstract: Neoadjuvant cisplatin-based chemotherapy followed by radical cystectomy is the recommended treatment, with the highest level of evidence, for patients with muscle-invasive bladder cancer (MIBC). However, only a minority of patients receive this treatment, mainly due to patient comorbidities, the relatively small survival benefit, and the lack of predictive biomarkers to select those patients most likely to benefit from this multimodal approach. In addition, adjuvant chemotherapy has been recommended for patients with high-risk MIBC, although randomized trials have not provided conclusive evidence on the impact of this approach. At present, however, this situation is changing, largely due to our improved knowledge of the molecular biology of bladder cancer, which has enabled us to identify new prognostic and predictive biomarkers that can be used to select the most appropriate treatment for each patient. Moreover, new active treatments, especially immunotherapy, have shown promising results in the neoadjuvant setting. In addition, the gene expression profile of bladder tumors can be used to classify them into different subtypes, which correlate with specific clinical-pathological characteristics and with treatment response or resistance. Therefore, the main objective for the near future is to introduce these translational breakthroughs into routine clinical practice in order to personalize treatment for each patient.

Keywords: muscle-invasive bladder cancer; chemotherapy; immunotherapy; personalized medicine; predictive biomarker

---

1. Neoadjuvant Therapy in Muscle-Invasive Bladder Cancer (MIBC): An Overview

The prognosis of bladder cancer (BC) has not improved significantly over the last 30 years, as few advances have been made in treatment options since the introduction of cisplatin-based chemotherapy in the mid-1980s. While it is true that platinum-based schemes have somewhat improved survival of patients with advanced disease, less than 50% of patients initially respond and most eventually develop resistance. In platinum-resistant patients, second-line chemotherapy provides poor survival expectations [1]. Despite these limitations, chemotherapy has been incorporated into the treatment of muscle-invasive bladder cancer (MIBC) in combination with local treatments, such as cystectomy or radiotherapy. However, the limited survival benefit and the absence of predictive biomarkers have led to some reluctance to incorporate these strategies into the routine management of the disease, especially with regard to the use of neoadjuvant chemotherapy (NAC) in MIBC. Although international clinical guidelines recommend NAC with cisplatin-based schemes with the highest level of evidence [2,3], less than 20% of patients with MIBC receive this treatment in clinical practice [4]. There are two main reasons for this: firstly, cisplatin-based chemotherapy is contraindicated in approximately 50% of patients due to renal failure or other comorbidities [5]; and secondly, there is a lack of clinical and pathological markers to identify patients who will benefit from NAC, while delaying local treatment in those who will not benefit can have a negative impact on prognosis [6].

Fortunately, this discouraging scenario has changed in recent years, mainly due to two advances. Firstly, the molecular characterization of BC has made it possible to identify potential prognostic and predictive biomarkers, as well as new therapeutic targets. Secondly, the recent introduction of new active therapies, especially immunotherapy, has expanded the therapeutic arsenal in BC beyond platinum-based chemotherapy.

Importantly, it is essential to identify biomarkers to select those patients likely to benefit from these novel treatment options, including immunotherapy—either alone or in combination with chemotherapy and/or biological therapies. This would also help to avoid the administration of ineffective treatments that may lead to unnecessary toxicities, delays in the administration of more effective therapies, and lowered cost-effectiveness. Studies with DNA and RNA sequencing have demonstrated the heterogeneity of bladder tumors at the molecular and genetic level and have identified specific profiles—based on differences in the type and frequency of mutations, in gene copy numbers, and in methylation patterns—that can help define patient prognosis and sensitivity to specific treatments [7]. However, despite these advances, only around 40% of bladder tumors present genomic alterations that are potentially treatable with targeted therapies. Moreover, in contrast to other cancers, such as melanoma, gastrointestinal stromal tumors, and breast and lung cancers, in which 20–60% of patients can be treated with therapies selected by the analysis of biomarkers [8], no biomarkers for BC have been approved for use in clinical practice. It is crucial, therefore, to transfer advances in molecular biology as quickly and efficiently as possible into clinical practice if we are to improve the survival of patients.

Here, we describe the potential applications of molecular biology in the diagnosis and treatment of BC, and especially of MIBC, based on the concept of precision medicine.

2. Predictive Biomarkers of Response to Cisplatin-Based Chemotherapy

Cisplatin-based chemotherapy remains the standard treatment for BC both for advanced disease and for the perioperative or conservative treatment of localized BC [2]. The antitumor mechanism of action of cisplatin is based on the formation of adducts that cause DNA damage, which prevents cell replication and induces cell death [9]. Cisplatin induces DNA damage either as single-strand breaks (SSBs), double-strand breaks (DSBs), or interstrand-crosslinks. However, cancer cells have several mechanisms to repair DNA damage. SSBs can be repaired by base excision repair, mismatch repair, or nucleotide excision repair (NER), while DSBs can be repaired by non-homologous end joining or homologous recombination (HR). The analysis of genes involved in the different pathways of DNA damage repair (DDR) may enable us to identify predictive biomarkers of response to cisplatin [10].

The NER pathway, which repairs SSBs, includes the ERCC excision repair 1 (ERCC1) and ERCC excision repair 2 (ERCC2) proteins. High levels of ERCC1 indicate a gain of NER pathway function, leading to greater repair of the DNA damage caused by cisplatin and thus decreased efficacy of the drug [11]. Bellmunt et al. demonstrated that in patients with metastatic BC treated with a cisplatin-based combination, those with high *ERCC1* expression had worse prognosis [12]. Several studies have analyzed the role of *ERCC2* mutations as predictive biomarkers in BC. *ERCC2* mutations are found in 12% of BCs, mostly in the helicase domain of the gene, and have been associated with a loss of NER pathway function in preclinical studies [13]. Interestingly, *ERCC2* mutations confer sensitivity to both cisplatin and carboplatin, but not to treatments with doxorubicin, ionizing radiation or poly (ADP-ribose) polymerase (PARP) inhibitors [13]. Whole exome sequencing of 50 MIBC tumor samples treated with cisplatin-based NAC demonstrated that *ERCC2* mutations were significantly associated with treatment response. Specifically, *ERCC2* mutations were detected in 36% of patients who responded to chemotherapy (<ypT1), while no mutations were detected in non-responders (>ypT2) [14]. These results were confirmed in a subsequent validation study [15]. In the joint analysis of the two series, *ERCC2* mutations were found in 38% (17/45) of responders and in only 6% (3/53) of non-responders [13]. Taken together, these data suggest that ERCC2 may well be a predictive biomarker of response to cisplatin-based chemotherapy. In this line, a recent study by the Memorial Sloan Kettering Cancer Center (MSKCC) compared the genomic profile of primary vs. secondary MIBC patients treated with NAC. They found that not only was the benefit of NAC limited to primary MIBC but also that *ERCC2* mutations were observed more frequently in primary MIBC (12% vs. 1.2%), which could explain the lack of benefit of NAC in secondary MIBC [13]. Other studies have also correlated mutations in the ATM serine/threonine kinase (*ATM*), RB transcriptional corepressor 1 (*RB1*) and FA complementation group C (*FANCC*) repair genes with efficacy of NAC in MIBC. In the study of Plimack et al., 13 of 15 cisplatin-responders (87%) presented mutations in some of these genes, while none of the non-responders harbored these mutations. In their validation study, 64% of responders presented some of these mutations as compared to only 15% of non-responders [16]. In a recent update of this study, a significant improvement in the five-year disease-specific survival was observed in carriers of at least one mutation compared to patients without mutations (90% vs. 49%, $p = 0.0015$) [17]. The presence of mutations in DDR pathways can identify patients likely to respond to NAC, who could be potential candidates for a bladder-sparing approach. The ongoing phase II RETAIN trial in patients treated with NAC aims to identify candidates for bladder preservation among patients who attain a complete response and have mutations in *ATM*, *RB1*, *FANCC*, or *ERCC2* (NCT02710734).

HR is used to repair DSBs. In a molecular profile analysis using the NGS600 testing platform, mutations in HR genes were detected in 17% of 17,566 tumors and in 23% of BCs, which had the third highest frequency of HR-DDR mutations (after endometrial and biliary tract carcinomas). The most frequently mutated genes in BC were AT-rich interaction domain 1A (*ARID1A*) (12.4%), *ATM* (4%), BRCA1 DNA repair associated (*BRCA1*) (3%), and BRCA2 DNA repair associated (*BRCA2*) (4.5%) [18]. More recently, 13% of patients with BC were found to harbor germline variants, 75% of which were located in DDR genes, mainly in *BRCA2*, mutS homolog 2 (*MSH2*), *BRCA1*, checkpoint kinase 2 (*CHEK2*), ERCC excision repair 3 (*ERCC3*), nibrin (*NBN*), and RAD50 double strand break repair protein (*RAD50*) [19]. In this line, a study by our group in 57 MIBC patients treated with NAC, increased *BRCA1* mRNA expression negatively correlated with pathological response and survival [20].

DDR is a complex process involving several different DNA repair pathways, making it necessary to analyze extensive panels of genes if we are to determine the predictive and prognostic value of the genes involved in each pathway. An MSKCC study analyzed a panel of 34 DDR genes in 100 patients with advanced BC treated with platinum-based chemotherapy and detected at least one alteration in one of the genes in 47 patients. Median overall survival was significantly higher in these patients than in those with no alterations (23.7 vs. 13.0 months, $p = 0.006$). Interestingly, the survival benefit was observed in both cisplatin- and carboplatin-treated patients [21]. A recent phase II trial in 49 patients treated with neoadjuvant dose-dense cisplatin plus gemcitabine analyzed a panel of 29 DDR genes and found that the presence of deleterious mutations, including *ERCC2* mutations, was associated with response to chemotherapy, with a positive predictive value of 89% and a two-year relapse-free survival of 100% [22].

In summary, current evidence indicates that the analysis of alterations in DNA repair pathways can provide prognostic and predictive information in BC patients. However, prospective studies including a larger number of patients are required to confirm these findings. In addition, given that cisplatin is contraindicated in approximately 50% of patients, it is important to analyze these biomarkers in patients treated with carboplatin as well. Finally, the study of these alterations will pave the way for the discovery of new prognostic and predictive biomarkers as well as the incorporation of new biological therapies, such as PARP inhibitors, which have been shown to be effective in ovarian and breast cancer patients harboring mutations in HR genes [23].

3. Therapeutic Implications of BC Molecular Subtypes

Several research groups have proposed various classifications of BC molecular subtypes based on the two reference subtypes, luminal and basal (Table 1). A group from Lund University analyzed a large number of non-MIBC and MIBC tumors and proposed five subtypes: urobasal A, urobasal B, genomically unstable, infiltrated, and squamous-like [24]. Urobasal A and B are characterized by the expression of biomarkers usually expressed in the normal urothelium, while the squamous-like subtype expresses keratin 5 (KRT5), keratin 6 (KRT6), and keratin 14 (KRT14), which are specific to squamous differentiation. The infiltrated subtype is characterized by stromal and immune cell infiltration. A group from the University of North Carolina (UNC) proposed another classification in which the basal subtype presents sarcomatoid characteristics and expresses high levels of both epidermal growth factor receptor (EGFR) and its ligands, while the luminal subtype expresses epithelial markers (E-cadherin (CDH1) and miR-200) and alterations in fibroblast growth factor receptor 3 (FGFR3) [25]. An MD Anderson (MDA) group added a third subtype, called p53-like, which is characterized by the presence of stromal markers and the activation of tumor protein p53 (TP53) [26]. The Cancer Genome Atlas (TCGA) proposed a classification based on four molecular subtypes called clusters (I–IV) [7]. Cluster I corresponds to the luminal phenotype and presents characteristics of papillary tumors, cluster II has the luminal phenotype but with a predominance of p53-like characteristics, and clusters III and IV correspond mainly to the basal subtype defined in the UNC and MD Anderson classifications [25,26]. A recent update of the TCGA study [27] defined five molecular subtypes: luminal papillary (35%), luminal infiltrated (19%), luminal (6%), basal-squamous (35%), and neuronal (5%). The TCGA luminal subtypes are characterized by a high expression of urothelial differentiation markers, such as forkhead box A1 (*FOXA1*), GATA binding protein 3 (*GATA3*), and peroxisome proliferator activated receptor gamma (*PPARG*). The luminal-papillary subtype has *FGFR3* mutations, amplifications, overexpression, and FGFR3-TACC3 fusions. The luminal-infiltrated subtype, which corresponds to cluster II in the original TCGA classification [7], is characterized by elevated expression of epithelial-mesenchymal transition (EMT) markers, such as twist family bHLH transcription factor 1 (*TWIST1*) and zinc finger E-box-binding homeobox 1 (*ZEB1*), and moderate expression of the immune markers Programmed death ligand 1 (*PDL1*), and cytotoxic T-lymphocyte associated protein 4 (*CTLA4*). The luminal subtype presents high expression of the keratin 20 (*KRT 20*). The basal-squamous subtype is defined by the expression of CD44 antigen (*CD44*), *KRT5*, *KRT6*, *KRT14*, is enriched in *TP53* mutations, and has the highest expression of the immune markers *PD-L1*, Programmed cell death 1 (*PD-1*) and *CTLA4*. Finally, the neuronal subtype has high expression of neuroendocrine and neuronal markers [27]. A Canadian study proposed four subtypes: basal, luminal, luminal-infiltrated, and claudin-low [28]. The claudin-low subtype corresponds to TCGA cluster IV [7] and has characteristics of the basal subtype, with the expression of EMT markers and immune infiltration. Recently, the Bladder Cancer Molecular Taxonomy Group (BCMTG) has proposed a consensus classification based on the analysis of 1750 transcriptomic profiles of the classifications published to date [29]: papillary luminal (24%), unspecified luminal (8%), unstable luminal (15%), stromal rich (15%), basal-SCC (35%), and neuroendocrine-like (3%). A web application of this model allows individual and anonymous classification of tumor samples according to this consensus (http://cit.ligue-cancer.net:3838/apps/consensusMIBC_web/).

Table 1. Summary of the main characteristics of molecular subtypes of bladder cancer according to different molecular classifications.

Molecular Classification	Patients (*n*)	Subtypes	Histological and Molecular Characteristics	Ref.
Lund University	308 BC	Urobasal A	High expression of *FGFR3*, *CCND1*, *TP63*, and *KRT5*	[24]
		Urobasal B		
		Genomically unstable (GU)	Frequent *TP53* mutations. *CCNE* and *ERBB2* expression and low cytokeratin expression	
		Squamous cell carcinoma-like (SCC)	High expression of basal keratins normally not expressed in the urothelium	
		Infiltrated	Stromal and immune cell infiltration	
UNC	262 High grade MIBC	Luminal	Expression of epithelial markers (E-cadherin/CDH1 and miR-200) and alterations in *FGFR3*	[25]
		Basal	Sarcomatoid features. High expression of EGFR and its ligands	
MDA	73 MIBC	Luminal	Features of active PPARγ and estrogen receptor transcription. *FGFR3* mutations	[26]
		Basal	p63 activation and squamous differentiation	
		p53-like	Presence of stromal markers and activation of p53 signature	
TCGA (2014)	131 High grade MIBC	Cluster I	Luminal phenotype; presence of papillary tumors features	[7]
		Cluster II	Tumors with luminal phenotype but with a predominance of p53-like subtype features	
		Cluster III	Correspond to basal subtype defined in the UNC and MD Anderson classifications	
		Cluster IV		
TCGA (2017)	412 T2-4, N0-3, M0-1 MIBC	Luminal papillary (35%)	*FOXA1*, *GATA3*, and *PPARG* expression. FGFR3 alterations	[27]
		Luminal infiltrate (19%)	*FOXA1*, *GATA3*, and *PPARG* expression. Expression of EMT (high) and immune (moderate) markers	
		Luminal (6%)	*FOXA1*, *GATA3*, and *PPARG* expression. High expression of *KRT 20*	
		Basal-SCC (35%)	High expression of immune response markers. *CD44*, *KRT5*, *KRT6* and *KRT14* expression. *TP53* mutations	
		Neuronal (5%)	High expression of neuroendocrine and neuronal markers	
BCMTG	1750 MIBC transcriptomic profiles	Luminal papillary (24%)	Papillary morphology. Expression of *FGFR3* and *PPARG*. Mutations in *FGFR3* and *KDM6A*	[29]
		Luminal non-specified (8%)	Micropapillary morphology. *PPARG* expression. Mutations in *ELF3*	
		Luminal unstable (15%)	Expression of *PPARG*, *E2F3*, and *ERBB2*. Genomic instability. Mutation in *TP53* and *ERCC2*	
		Stroma-rich (15%)	Stromal and immune cell (B cells) infiltration	
		Basal/squamous (35%)	*EGFR* expression. Mutations in *TP53* and *RB1*. Stromal and immune cell (CD8 T and NK cells) infiltration	
		Neuroendocrine-like (3%)	Neuroendocrine differentiation. Loss of TP53 and RB1. Mutations in *TP53* and *RB1*	

The molecular subtypes have been associated with specific clinical-pathological characteristics and differential sensitivity to treatments. Basal-SCC tumors, identified in the TCGA, UNC, and MD Anderson classifications [7,25,26], predominate in women and are associated with more aggressive tumors, more advanced disease stages, worse prognosis, and squamous cell features. In contrast, luminal tumors seem to be less aggressive but more resistant to NAC [27,28]. Recently, Lotan et al. showed that in early-stage MIBC treated with cystectomy, upstaging (≥pT3) is less likely in luminal than non-luminal tumors [30], suggesting that luminal tumors could be managed more conservatively with upfront cystectomy.

These molecular classifications can complement or help reconsider the standard histological classifications, since squamous differentiation might well be underreported. For example, only 42% of BCMTG [29] basal-SCC tumors had squamous cell features in the histological analysis. The histological, genomic, and transcriptional heterogeneity of BC has important clinical implications. Warrick et al. analyzed the intratumoral heterogeneity of different regions of primary MIBC tumors in relation to the Lund molecular subtypes [24] and histological variants. Nearly 40% of the tumors demonstrated molecular heterogeneity among the different histologies, especially the basal-squamous tumors, 78% of which co-occurred with either urothelial-like or genomically unstable tumors [31]. These results emphasize the need for an adequate tissue sampling that selects different areas of the tumor when establishing the molecular subtype.

Several studies have indicated that it is possible to classify BC into molecular subtypes using immunohistochemistry (IHC), which is less complex than transcriptomic analysis and could facilitate the use of molecular subtypes in clinical practice. Markers related to basal subtypes, such as KRT5/6, KRT14 and p63, and those associated with luminal phenotypes, such as GATA3, FOXA1, uroplakin and erb-b2 receptor tyrosine kinase 2 (HER2), have been proposed for an IHC-based classification. A meta-analysis found that by analyzing only GATA3 and KRT5/6 with IHC, it was possible to identify the basal and luminal subtypes with 91% reliability [32]. Recently, Makboul et al. stratified BC patients according to the Lund classification [24] using a simple IHC panel of five biomarkers (FGFR3, CK5, cyclin-B1, HER2, p53). More than 90% of tumors were classified without overlap and the different tumor subtypes significantly correlated with prognosis [33]. The different subtypes have also been correlated with response to chemotherapy. Basal tumors are associated with a better response to cisplatin-based chemotherapy, while tumors classified as p53-like or those in cluster II [7] have been associated with chemoresistance [26]. An MD Anderson study of 60 MIBC patients treated with neoadjuvant dose-dense methotrexate + vinblastine + doxorubicin + cisplatin (M-VAC) plus bevacizumab found that patients with basal tumors had more pathological complete responses (pCR) and longer survival than those with luminal or p53-like tumors. Five-year survival rates for patients with basal, luminal, and p53-like tumors were 91%, 73%, and 36%, respectively, probably due to the greater sensitivity to NAC in basal tumors, since achieving downstaging is a predictive factor for longer survival. Additionally, only patients with p53-like tumors presented bone metastases at disease progression. Interestingly, this study also found a greater frequency of the p53-like subtype in cystectomy samples than in transurethral resection (TUR) samples, especially in luminal tumors, suggesting that NAC can induce switching of tumor subtypes [34]. The Canadian study [28] analyzed the association between their four tumor subtypes (basal, luminal-infiltrated, luminal, claudin-low) and response to NAC. Patients with luminal tumors had the longest overall survival, while those with claudin-low tumors had the shortest, regardless of whether they received NAC or only cystectomy. In contrast, patients with basal tumors had longer survival but did not fare differently from luminal tumors if they were treated with NAC rather than only cystectomy. Recently, the same group has defined four subtypes by transcriptional analysis in residual tumor at cystectomy after NAC: CC1-basal, CC2-luminal, CC3-immune, and CC4-scar-like. The basal and luminal phenotypes observed in the residual disease were similar to the pretreatment subtypes. The CC3-immune tumors had the worst outcome and showed a high immune infiltration, suggesting a potential positive impact for immune checkpoint inhibitors (ICIs) as second-line treatment, whereas the CC4-scar-like tumors showed a low proliferation rate, expressed fibrosis, and had a good prognosis regardless of response to NAC [35]. These findings suggest that establishing molecular subtypes after NAC in residual tumor disease can be useful in selecting adjuvant treatment.

A recent study by our group, using IHC-based hierarchical clustering, classified MIBC patients treated with NAC in three clusters: BASQ-like (FOXA1/GATA3 low; KRT5/6/14 high), luminal-like (FOXA1/GATA3 high; KRT5/6/14 low), and mixed-cluster (FOXA1/GATA3 high; KRT5/6 high; KRT14 low). Patients with BASQ-like tumors were more likely to achieve a pathological response to NAC (OR 3.96; $p = 0.017$) [36].

Taken together, these findings indicate that the molecular classification of BC according to gene expression profiles can play an important role in selecting the most effective treatment for each patient. Thus, basal tumors would benefit most from chemotherapy, while luminal tumors would be associated with better prognosis but poor response to cisplatin-based chemotherapy, indicating that the best treatment option for these patients could be cystectomy. Molecular classification can thus provide additional information to the standard histological classification and better characterize BC for personalized treatment approaches.

In recent years, with the emergence of immunotherapy as a treatment option for BC, several studies have attempted to establish a correlation between tumor subtypes and immunotherapy efficacy. The revised TCGA classification [27] suggested that patients with luminal-infiltrated tumors and especially those with basal tumors can derive the greatest benefit from immunotherapy. Importantly, however, the TCGA patients had localized tumors and had not received any previous treatment, thus, these treatment strategies require validation in future studies. The IMvigor 210 study [37] demonstrated a greater benefit of treatment with atezolizumab, a PD-L1-blocking antibody, in advanced BC classified as TCGA cluster II [7], and in the CheckMate 275 study, basal tumors responded better to nivolumab, a PD-1-blocking antibody [38]. Surprisingly, tumors with high immune infiltration, classified as claudin-low, showed a poor response to immunotherapy [37,38]. This apparent paradox could be explained by the fact that there is a more effective suppression of T cells in cluster IV than in cluster II tumors [39]. Intriguingly, immunotherapy and chemotherapy seem to be effective in complementary patient populations. Patients with luminal-infiltrated tumors (cluster II) would benefit from immunotherapy, while in those with basal tumors (cluster IV), chemotherapy may be the treatment of choice. Although patients with neuronal-subtype tumors generally have a worse prognosis, a recent analysis of the IMvigor 210 trial showed that TCGA neuronal-subtype tumors [27] responded better to atezolizumab [40]. Moreover, this did not seem to be associated with other parameters related to immunotherapy response; for instance, the tumor mutational burden (TMB) and the load of tumor neo-antigens were lower in these tumors than in the other subtypes and none of the tumors were immunoinflammatory. In contrast, the neuronal subtype had low levels of transforming growth factor beta 1 (TGF-β1), which has been associated with improved response to immunotherapy [41]. In summary, while a molecular classification can help to select the best treatment option for each patient, it will be necessary to take into consideration other factors that may affect response to either chemotherapy or immunotherapy.

4. Predictive Biomarkers of Immunotherapy Response

The emergence of immunotherapy has highlighted the importance of biomarkers when deciding on the optimal treatment for each patient. In addition to molecular subtypes, many potential biomarkers have been correlated with the response to immunotherapy: PD-L1 expression, CD8$^+$ T-cell infiltration, DDR gene alterations, TMB, and immune and stromal gene expression signatures such as the interferon gamma (IFN-γ) signature [42]. To date, unfortunately, none of these markers has shown sufficiently consistent results to warrant incorporation into the routine management of BC.

PD-L1 expression is detected in 20–30% of bladder tumors and is associated with more advanced disease and worse prognosis [43]. Studies of advanced BC have shown conflicting results regarding the role of PD-L1 as a predictive biomarker of response to immunotherapy [44]. Importantly, since PD-L1 is a dynamic biomarker both in space and time, the analysis of a small tumor fragment in a biopsy may not be representative of the PD-L1 expression in the whole tumor. Moreover, prior treatment may influence PD-L1 expression. Therefore, IHC results of PD-L1 expression must be interpreted in the context of broader biomarker panels when selecting patients to receive immunotherapy.

Some biomarkers, such as the neutrophil/lymphocyte ratio, albumin levels, high C-reactive protein, and Interleukin-6 levels, can be easily incorporated into routine clinical practice, while others, such as gene expression signatures, are more complex [45]. In addition to the potential usefulness of the molecular subtypes in predicting response, the study of DDR pathways may be helpful, since defects in DDR have been associated with an increase in the TMB, and thus, with a greater immune response. An MSKCC study analyzed a panel of 34 DDR genes in patients with advanced BC treated with atezolizumab or nivolumab and found a significant benefit for immunotherapy in patients with deleterious mutations in the genes [46]. In addition, ICIs have recently been shown to be highly effective in tumors with defects in the MMR/microsatellite instability pathway [47]. In an effort to encompass these different biomarkers that may be related to immunotherapy response, an immunogram has recently been proposed that incorporates in seven main axes the different parameters related to immunotherapy response, which will help to predict the efficacy of ICIs in individual patients [48].

The possibility of incorporating immunotherapy in earlier stages of BC, where other treatments are currently available, makes it essential to identify biomarkers to select the most effective therapy for each patient. The solid rationale for exploring the efficacy of immunotherapy in early-stage disease has recently been elegantly reviewed [49]. Early stages have a greater integrity of the immune system and can induce greater T-cell expansion than advanced stages, where increased impairment of T-cell function is more evident and where cancer-associated inflammation has been linked to poor response to immunotherapy. Moreover, the neoadjuvant setting is optimal for exploring the role of potential predictive biomarkers to immunotherapy since tumor tissue can be obtained just before treatment initiation and the genomic profile can be compared before and after therapy.

Two recent phase II trials have explored the role of ICIs in the neoadjuvant setting. In the PURE-01 trial [50], 50 patients, most of whom were eligible for cisplatin therapy, were treated with three cycles of pembrolizumab, a PD-1-blocking antibody, followed by cystectomy. In the ABACUS trial [51], 95 patients who were ineligible for cisplatin-based NAC received two cycles of atezolizumab before cystectomy. A pCR was attained by 42% and 31% of patients in the PURE-01 and ABACUS trials, respectively. Both trials included detailed biomarker analyses to define potential predictive biomarkers of response to ICIs. In the PURE-01 study, a significant association between pCR and PD-L1 expression, TMB, and DDR and *RB1* gene alterations was observed. In the ABACUS trial, in contrast, these biomarkers did not correlate with pathological response; however, the quality of immune infiltration measured by CD8 and granzyme B (GZMB), a surrogate marker of activated CD8 cells, as well as an eight-gene cytotoxic T-cell transcriptional signature, significantly correlated with pCR. In addition, the inflamed and desert immune phenotypes, as described by Mariathasan et al. [41], correlated with response and resistance to atezolizumab, respectively. Interestingly, CD8 levels were higher in responding tumors, while high levels of fibroblast activation protein alpha (FAP), a surrogate marker of cancer-associated fibroblasts related to TGF-β, was associated with resistance to immunotherapy. PD-L1, CD8, GZMB, and FAP expression increased post-therapy. These results suggest a potential predictive role of response to ICIs for these markers although the contradictory findings of the two trials indicate a need for validation in a larger number of patients.

Both the PURE-01 and ABACUS trials showed promising results that suggest a level of efficacy for neoadjuvant immunotherapy comparable to that of NAC, making it a feasible treatment option for cisplatin-ineligible patients. This possibility raises the question of how to select cisplatin-eligible patients for NAC or immunotherapy or NAC-plus-immunotherapy, especially considering that many biomarkers, such as TMB and DDR alterations, are associated with the efficacy of both treatments [21,46]. A study exploring the association between the tumor microenvironment and outcome in MIBC patients found that higher T-cell inflamed and IFN-γ signature scores were associated with improved outcome in patients treated with bladder-sparing trimodality therapy (TMT) but with worse outcome in those treated with NAC-plus-RC, while high stromal infiltration was associated with poor prognosis in patients receiving NAC-plus-RC but not in those treated with TMT [52]. Along the same lines, immune signatures predicted response to neoadjuvant immunotherapy in patients included in the PURE-01 trial but not in patients treated with NAC [53]. An ongoing phase III trial (NCT03732677) exploring the combination of NAC and immunotherapy will shed further light on this issue.

A related question is how to integrate and sequence the different therapeutic options in the multimodality management of MIBC. Intriguingly, the cytotoxic effect of NAC can generate an immune effect through the activation of $CD8^+$ effector T cells and decreasing T_{regs} [54]. The concurrent administration of NAC and immunotherapy could thus hinder the T-cell response if T cells are killed by NAC. This phenomenon may partly explain the limited benefit obtained with NAC-plus-immunotherapy compared to NAC alone in advanced BC [55]. In contrast, a sequential administration of NAC followed by immunotherapy could be a more effective approach. In the TONIC trial in breast cancer, an upregulation of immune-related genes was detected after cisplatin-based chemotherapy, suggesting that NAC may induce a tumor microenvironment more conducive to immunotherapy response [56]. Finally, evidence suggests that neoadjuvant is more effective than adjuvant treatment, based on the greater tumor antigen exposition before tumor resection [49]. The recent results of the IMvigor 010 phase III trial showed that adjuvant atezolizumab did not demonstrate a significant benefit in high-risk MIBC patients treated with cystectomy [57].

5. Conclusions

In recent years, we have greatly broadened our understanding of the molecular biology of BC, which has allowed us to identify new prognostic and predictive biomarkers. We also have at our disposal novel therapeutic options, such as immunotherapy, which can improve patient outcome and quality of life. These new effective drugs show promising results but also highlight the question of how to select the optimal treatment for each patient. There is still no biomarker approved for clinical practice and it is crucial to incorporate into clinical practice all the advances in the field of molecular biology as efficiently and rapidly as possible. Only in this way, will we be able to achieve precision medicine and select the most effective treatment for each individual patient.

Author Contributions: Conceptualization, A.F., V.R.d.P., and J.C.P. Writing—Original draft preparation, A.F., V.R.d.P., and J.C.P. Writing—Review and editing, A.F., V.R.d.P., J.C.P., A.P., C.C., O.E. and O.B. All authors have read and agreed to the published version of the manuscript.

Funding: This research received no external funding.

Acknowledgments: We want to acknowledge Renée O'Brate for critical reading and language correction.

Conflicts of Interest: The authors declare no conflict of interest.

References

1. Bellmunt, J.; Fougeray, R.; Rosenberg, J.E.; von der Maase, H.; Schutz, F.A.; Salhi, Y.; Culine, S.; Choueiri, T.K. Long-term survival results of a randomized phase III trial of vinflunine plus best supportive care versus best supportive care alone in advanced urothelial carcinoma patients after failure of platinum-based chemotherapy. *Ann. Oncol.* **2013**, *24*, 1466–1472. [CrossRef]
2. Font, A.; Luque, R.; Villa, J.C.; Domenech, M.; Vazquez, S.; Gallardo, E.; Virizuela, J.A.; Beato, C.; Morales-Barrera, R.; Gelabert, A.; et al. The Challenge of Managing Bladder Cancer and Upper Tract Urothelial Carcinoma: A Review with Treatment Recommendations from the Spanish Oncology Genitourinary Group (SOGUG). *Target Oncol.* **2019**, *14*, 15–32. [CrossRef]
3. Alfred Witjes, J.; Lebret, T.; Comperat, E.M.; Cowan, N.C.; De Santis, M.; Bruins, H.M.; Hernandez, V.; Espinos, E.L.; Dunn, J.; Rouanne, M.; et al. Updated 2016 EAU Guidelines on Muscle-invasive and Metastatic Bladder Cancer. *Eur. Urol.* **2017**, *71*, 462–475. [CrossRef]

4. Reardon, Z.D.; Patel, S.G.; Zaid, H.B.; Stimson, C.J.; Resnick, M.J.; Keegan, K.A.; Barocas, D.A.; Chang, S.S.; Cookson, M.S. Trends in the use of perioperative chemotherapy for localized and locally advanced muscle-invasive bladder cancer: A sign of changing tides. *Eur. Urol.* **2015**, *67*, 165–170. [CrossRef] [PubMed]

5. Thompson, R.H.; Boorjian, S.A.; Kim, S.P.; Cheville, J.C.; Thapa, P.; Tarrel, R.; Dronca, R.; Costello, B.; Frank, I. Eligibility for neoadjuvant/adjuvant cisplatin-based chemotherapy among radical cystectomy patients. *BJU Int.* **2014**, *113*, E17–E21. [CrossRef] [PubMed]

6. Bhindi, B.; Frank, I.; Mason, R.J.; Tarrell, R.F.; Thapa, P.; Cheville, J.C.; Costello, B.A.; Pagliaro, L.C.; Karnes, R.J.; Thompson, R.H.; et al. Oncologic Outcomes for Patients with Residual Cancer at Cystectomy Following Neoadjuvant Chemotherapy: A Pathologic Stage-matched Analysis. *Eur. Urol.* **2017**, *72*, 660–664. [CrossRef] [PubMed]

7. Cancer Genome Atlas Research, N. Comprehensive molecular characterization of urothelial bladder carcinoma. *Nature* **2014**, *507*, 315–322. [CrossRef]

8. Hyman, D.M.; Taylor, B.S.; Baselga, J. Implementing Genome-Driven Oncology. *Cell* **2017**, *168*, 584–599. [CrossRef]

9. Siddik, Z.H. Cisplatin: Mode of cytotoxic action and molecular basis of resistance. *Oncogene* **2003**, *22*, 7265–7279. [CrossRef]

10. Curtin, N.J. DNA repair dysregulation from cancer driver to therapeutic target. *Nat. Rev. Cancer* **2012**, *12*, 801–817. [CrossRef]

11. Britten, R.A.; Liu, D.; Tessier, A.; Hutchison, M.J.; Murray, D. ERCC1 expression as a molecular marker of cisplatin resistance in human cervical tumor cells. *Int. J. Cancer* **2000**, *89*, 453–457. [CrossRef]

12. Bellmunt, J.; Paz-Ares, L.; Cuello, M.; Cecere, F.L.; Albiol, S.; Guillem, V.; Gallardo, E.; Carles, J.; Mendez, P.; de la Cruz, J.J.; et al. Spanish Oncology Genitourinary, G. Gene expression of ERCC1 as a novel prognostic marker in advanced bladder cancer patients receiving cisplatin-based chemotherapy. *Ann. Oncol.* **2007**, *18*, 522–528. [CrossRef] [PubMed]

13. Pietzak, E.J.; Zabor, E.C.; Bagrodia, A.; Armenia, J.; Hu, W.; Zehir, A.; Funt, S.; Audenet, F.; Barron, D.; Maamouri, N.; et al. Genomic Differences Between "Primary" and "Secondary" Muscle-invasive Bladder Cancer as a Basis for Disparate Outcomes to Cisplatin-based Neoadjuvant Chemotherapy. *Eur. Urol.* **2019**, *75*, 231–239. [CrossRef]

14. Van Allen, E.M.; Mouw, K.W.; Kim, P.; Iyer, G.; Wagle, N.; Al-Ahmadie, H.; Zhu, C.; Ostrovnaya, I.; Kryukov, G.V.; O'Connor, K.W.; et al. Somatic ERCC2 mutations correlate with cisplatin sensitivity in muscle-invasive urothelial carcinoma. *Cancer Discov.* **2014**, *4*, 1140–1153. [CrossRef] [PubMed]

15. Liu, D.; Plimack, E.R.; Hoffman-Censits, J.; Garraway, L.A.; Bellmunt, J.; Van Allen, E.; Rosenberg, J.E. Clinical Validation of Chemotherapy Response Biomarker ERCC2 in Muscle-Invasive Urothelial Bladder Carcinoma. *JAMA Oncol.* **2016**, *2*, 1094–1096. [CrossRef]

16. Plimack, E.R.; Dunbrack, R.L.; Brennan, T.A.; Andrake, M.D.; Zhou, Y.; Serebriiskii, I.G.; Slifker, M.; Alpaugh, K.; Dulaimi, E.; Palma, N.; et al. Defects in DNA Repair Genes Predict Response to Neoadjuvant Cisplatin-based Chemotherapy in Muscle-invasive Bladder Cancer. *Eur. Urol.* **2015**, *68*, 959–967. [CrossRef]

17. Miron, B.; Hoffman-Censits, J.H.; Anari, F.; O'Neill, J.; Geynisman, D.M.; Zibelman, M.R.; Kutikov, A.; Viterbo, R.; Greenberg, R.E.; Chen, D.; et al. Defects in DNA Repair Genes Confer Improved Long-term Survival after Cisplatin-based Neoadjuvant Chemotherapy for Muscle-invasive Bladder Cancer. *Eur. Urol. Oncol.* **2020**. [CrossRef]

18. Heeke, A.L.; Pishvaian, M.J.; Lynce, F.; Xiu, J.; Brody, J.R.; Chen, W.J.; Baker, T.M.; Marshall, J.L.; Isaacs, C. Prevalence of Homologous Recombination-Related Gene Mutations Across Multiple Cancer Types. *JCO Precis. Oncol.* **2018**, *2018*. [CrossRef]

19. Carlo, M.I.; Ravichandran, V.; Srinavasan, P.; Bandlamudi, C.; Kemel, Y.; Ceyhan-Birsoy, O.; Mukherjee, S.; Mandelker, D.; Chaim, J.; Knezevic, A.; et al. Cancer Susceptibility Mutations in Patients with Urothelial Malignancies. *J. Clin. Oncol.* **2020**, *38*, 406–414. [CrossRef]

20. Font, A.; Taron, M.; Gago, J.L.; Costa, C.; Sanchez, J.J.; Carrato, C.; Mora, M.; Celiz, P.; Perez, L.; Rodriguez, D.; et al. BRCA1 mRNA expression and outcome to neoadjuvant cisplatin-based chemotherapy in bladder cancer. *Ann. Oncol.* **2011**, *22*, 139–144. [CrossRef]

21. Teo, M.Y.; Bambury, R.M.; Zabor, E.C.; Jordan, E.; Al-Ahmadie, H.; Boyd, M.E.; Bouvier, N.; Mullane, S.A.; Cha, E.K.; Roper, N.; et al. DNA Damage Response and Repair Gene Alterations Are Associated with Improved Survival in Patients with Platinum-Treated Advanced Urothelial Carcinoma. *Clin. Cancer Res.* **2017**, *23*, 3610–3618. [CrossRef] [PubMed]

22. Iyer, G.; Balar, A.V.; Milowsky, M.I.; Bochner, B.H.; Dalbagni, G.; Donat, S.M.; Herr, H.W.; Huang, W.C.; Taneja, S.S.; Woods, M.; et al. Multicenter Prospective Phase II Trial of Neoadjuvant Dose-Dense Gemcitabine Plus Cisplatin in Patients with Muscle-Invasive Bladder Cancer. *J. Clin. Oncol.* **2018**, *36*, 1949–1956. [CrossRef] [PubMed]

23. Romeo, M.; Pardo, J.C.; Martinez-Cardus, A.; Martinez-Balibrea, E.; Quiroga, V.; Martinez-Roman, S.; Sole, F.; Margeli, M.; Mesia, R. Translational Research Opportunities Regarding Homologous Recombination in Ovarian Cancer. *Int. J. Mol. Sci.* **2018**, *19*, 3249. [CrossRef] [PubMed]

24. Sjodahl, G.; Lauss, M.; Lovgren, K.; Chebil, G.; Gudjonsson, S.; Veerla, S.; Patschan, O.; Aine, M.; Ferno, M.; Ringner, M.; et al. A molecular taxonomy for urothelial carcinoma. *Clin. Cancer Res.* **2012**, *18*, 3377–3386. [CrossRef] [PubMed]

25. Damrauer, J.S.; Hoadley, K.A.; Chism, D.D.; Fan, C.; Tiganelli, C.J.; Wobker, S.E.; Yeh, J.J.; Milowsky, M.I.; Iyer, G.; Parker, J.S.; et al. Intrinsic subtypes of high-grade bladder cancer reflect the hallmarks of breast cancer biology. *Proc. Natl. Acad. Sci. USA* **2014**, *111*, 3110–3115. [CrossRef]

26. Choi, W.; Porten, S.; Kim, S.; Willis, D.; Plimack, E.R.; Hoffman-Censits, J.; Roth, B.; Cheng, T.; Tran, M.; Lee, I.L.; et al. Identification of distinct basal and luminal subtypes of muscle-invasive bladder cancer with different sensitivities to frontline chemotherapy. *Cancer Cell* **2014**, *25*, 152–165. [CrossRef] [PubMed]

27. Robertson, A.G.; Kim, J.; Al-Ahmadie, H.; Bellmunt, J.; Guo, G.; Cherniack, A.D.; Hinoue, T.; Laird, P.W.; Hoadley, K.A.; Akbani, R.; et al. Comprehensive Molecular Characterization of Muscle-Invasive Bladder Cancer. *Cell* **2018**, *174*, 1033. [CrossRef]

28. Seiler, R.; Ashab, H.A.D.; Erho, N.; van Rhijn, B.W.G.; Winters, B.; Douglas, J.; Van Kessel, K.E.; Fransen van de Putte, E.E.; Sommerlad, M.; Wang, N.Q.; et al. Impact of Molecular Subtypes in Muscle-invasive Bladder Cancer on Predicting Response and Survival after Neoadjuvant Chemotherapy. *Eur. Urol.* **2017**, *72*, 544–554. [CrossRef]

29. Kamoun, A.; de Reynies, A.; Allory, Y.; Sjodahl, G.; Robertson, A.G.; Seiler, R.; Hoadley, K.A.; Groeneveld, C.S.; Al-Ahmadie, H.; Choi, W.; et al. Bladder Cancer Molecular Taxonomy, G. A Consensus Molecular Classification of Muscle-invasive Bladder Cancer. *Eur. Urol.* **2020**, *77*, 420–433. [CrossRef]

30. Lotan, Y.; Boorjian, S.A.; Zhang, J.; Bivalacqua, T.J.; Porten, S.P.; Wheeler, T.; Lerner, S.P.; Hutchinson, R.; Francis, F.; Davicioni, E.; et al. Molecular Subtyping of Clinically Localized Urothelial Carcinoma Reveals Lower Rates of Pathological Upstaging at Radical Cystectomy Among Luminal Tumors. *Eur. Urol.* **2019**, *76*, 200–206. [CrossRef]

31. Warrick, J.I.; Sjodahl, G.; Kaag, M.; Raman, J.D.; Merrill, S.; Shuman, L.; Chen, G.; Walter, V.; DeGraff, D.J. Intratumoral Heterogeneity of Bladder Cancer by Molecular Subtypes and Histologic Variants. *Eur. Urol.* **2019**, *75*, 18–22. [CrossRef] [PubMed]

32. Dadhania, V.; Zhang, M.; Zhang, L.; Bondaruk, J.; Majewski, T.; Siefker-Radtke, A.; Guo, C.C.; Dinney, C.; Cogdell, D.E.; Zhang, S.; et al. Meta-Analysis of the Luminal and Basal Subtypes of Bladder Cancer and the Identification of Signature Immunohistochemical Markers for Clinical Use. *EBioMedicine* **2016**, *12*, 105–117. [CrossRef] [PubMed]

33. Makboul, R.; Hassan, H.M.; Refaiy, A.; Abdelkawi, I.F.; Shahat, A.A.; Hameed, D.A.; Morsy, A.; Salah, T.; Ahmed Mohammed, R.A. A Simple Immunohistochemical Panel Could Predict and Correlate to Clinicopathologic and Molecular Subgroups of Urinary Bladder Urothelial Carcinoma. *Clin. Genitourin Cancer* **2019**, *17*, e712–e719. [CrossRef] [PubMed]

34. McConkey, D.J.; Choi, W.; Shen, Y.; Lee, I.L.; Porten, S.; Matin, S.F.; Kamat, A.M.; Corn, P.; Millikan, R.E.; Dinney, C.; et al. A Prognostic Gene Expression Signature in the Molecular Classification of Chemotherapy-naive Urothelial Cancer is Predictive of Clinical Outcomes from Neoadjuvant Chemotherapy: A Phase 2 Trial of Dose-dense Methotrexate, Vinblastine, Doxorubicin, and Cisplatin with Bevacizumab in Urothelial Cancer. *Eur. Urol.* **2016**, *69*, 855–862.

35. Seiler, R.; Gibb, E.A.; Wang, N.Q.; Oo, H.Z.; Lam, H.M.; van Kessel, K.E.; Voskuilen, C.S.; Winters, B.; Erho, N.; Takhar, M.M.; et al. Divergent Biological Response to Neoadjuvant Chemotherapy in Muscle-invasive Bladder Cancer. *Clin. Cancer Res.* **2019**, *25*, 5082–5093. [CrossRef]

36. Font, A.; Domenech, M.; Benitez, R.; Rava, M.; Marques, M.; Ramirez, J.L.; Pineda, S.; Dominguez-Rodriguez, S.; Gago, J.L.; Badal, J.; et al. Immunohistochemistry-Based Taxonomical Classification of Bladder Cancer Predicts Response to Neoadjuvant Chemotherapy. *Cancers* **2020**, *12*, 1784.

37. Rosenberg, J.E.; Hoffman-Censits, J.; Powles, T.; van der Heijden, M.S.; Balar, A.V.; Necchi, A.; Dawson, N.; O'Donnell, P.H.; Balmanoukian, A.; Loriot, Y.; et al. Atezolizumab in patients with locally advanced and metastatic urothelial carcinoma who have progressed following treatment with platinum-based chemotherapy: A single-arm, multicentre, phase 2 trial. *Lancet* **2016**, *387*, 1909–1920. [CrossRef]

38. Sharma, P.; Retz, M.; Siefker-Radtke, A.; Baron, A.; Necchi, A.; Bedke, J.; Plimack, E.R.; Vaena, D.; Grimm, M.O.; Bracarda, S.; et al. Nivolumab in metastatic urothelial carcinoma after platinum therapy (CheckMate 275): A multicentre, single-arm, phase 2 trial. *Lancet Oncol.* **2017**, *18*, 312–322. [CrossRef]

39. Kardos, J.; Chai, S.; Mose, L.E.; Selitsky, S.R.; Krishnan, B.; Saito, R.; Iglesia, M.D.; Milowsky, M.I.; Parker, J.S.; Kim, W.Y.; et al. Claudin-low bladder tumors are immune infiltrated and actively immune suppressed. *JCI Insight* **2016**, *1*, e85902. [CrossRef]

40. Kim, J.; Kwiatkowski, D.; McConkey, D.J.; Meeks, J.J.; Freeman, S.S.; Bellmunt, J.; Getz, G.; Lerner, S.P. The Cancer Genome Atlas Expression Subtypes Stratify Response to Checkpoint Inhibition in Advanced Urothelial Cancer and Identify a Subset of Patients with High Survival Probability. *Eur. Urol.* **2019**, *75*, 961–964. [CrossRef]

41. Mariathasan, S.; Turley, S.J.; Nickles, D.; Castiglioni, A.; Yuen, K.; Wang, Y.; Kadel, E.E., III; Koeppen, H.; Astarita, J.L.; Cubas, R.; et al. TGFbeta attenuates tumour response to PD-L1 blockade by contributing to exclusion of T cells. *Nature* **2018**, *554*, 544–548. [CrossRef] [PubMed]

42. Hussain, S.A.; Birtle, A.; Crabb, S.; Huddart, R.; Small, D.; Summerhayes, M.; Jones, R.; Protheroe, A. From Clinical Trials to Real-life Clinical Practice: The Role of Immunotherapy with PD-1/PD-L1 Inhibitors in Advanced Urothelial Carcinoma. *Eur. Urol. Oncol.* **2018**, *1*, 486–500. [CrossRef] [PubMed]

43. Boorjian, S.A.; Sheinin, Y.; Crispen, P.L.; Farmer, S.A.; Lohse, C.M.; Kuntz, S.M.; Leibovich, B.C.; Kwon, E.D.; Frank, I. T-cell coregulatory molecule expression in urothelial cell carcinoma: Clinicopathologic correlations and association with survival. *Clin. Cancer Res.* **2008**, *14*, 4800–4808. [CrossRef] [PubMed]

44. Aggen, D.H.; Drake, C.G. Biomarkers for immunotherapy in bladder cancer: A moving target. *J. Immunother. Cancer* **2017**, *5*, 94. [CrossRef]

45. Ayers, M.; Lunceford, J.; Nebozhyn, M.; Murphy, E.; Loboda, A.; Kaufman, D.R.; Albright, A.; Cheng, J.D.; Kang, S.P.; Shankaran, V.; et al. IFN-gamma-related mRNA profile predicts clinical response to PD-1 blockade. *J. Clin. Investig.* **2017**, *127*, 2930–2940. [CrossRef]

46. Teo, M.Y.; Seier, K.; Ostrovnaya, I.; Regazzi, A.M.; Kania, B.E.; Moran, M.M.; Cipolla, C.K.; Bluth, M.J.; Chaim, J.; Al-Ahmadie, H.; et al. Alterations in DNA Damage Response and Repair Genes as Potential Marker of Clinical Benefit From PD-1/PD-L1 Blockade in Advanced Urothelial Cancers. *J. Clin. Oncol.* **2018**, *36*, 1685–1694. [CrossRef]

47. Le, D.T.; Uram, J.N.; Wang, H.; Bartlett, B.R.; Kemberling, H.; Eyring, A.D.; Skora, A.D.; Luber, B.S.; Azad, N.S.; Laheru, D.; et al. PD-1 Blockade in Tumors with Mismatch-Repair Deficiency. *N. Engl. J. Med.* **2015**, *372*, 2509–2520. [CrossRef]

48. van Dijk, N.; Funt, S.A.; Blank, C.U.; Powles, T.; Rosenberg, J.E.; van der Heijden, M.S. The Cancer Immunogram as a Framework for Personalized Immunotherapy in Urothelial Cancer. *Eur. Urol.* **2019**, *75*, 435–444. [CrossRef]

49. Versluis, J.M.; Long, G.V.; Blank, C.U. Learning from clinical trials of neoadjuvant checkpoint blockade. *Nat. Med.* **2020**, *26*, 475–484. [CrossRef]

50. Necchi, A.; Anichini, A.; Raggi, D.; Briganti, A.; Massa, S.; Luciano, R.; Colecchia, M.; Giannatempo, P.; Mortarini, R.; Bianchi, M.; et al. Pembrolizumab as Neoadjuvant Therapy Before Radical Cystectomy in Patients With Muscle-Invasive Urothelial Bladder Carcinoma (PURE-01): An Open-Label, Single-Arm, Phase II Study. *J. Clin. Oncol.* **2018**, *36*, 3353–3360. [CrossRef]

51. Powles, T.; Kockx, M.; Rodriguez-Vida, A.; Duran, I.; Crabb, S.J.; Van Der Heijden, M.S.; Szabados, B.; Pous, A.F.; Gravis, G.; Herranz, U.A.; et al. Clinical efficacy and biomarker analysis of neoadjuvant atezolizumab in operable urothelial carcinoma in the ABACUS trial. *Nat. Med.* **2019**, *25*, 1706–1714. [CrossRef] [PubMed]

52. Efstathiou, J.A.; Mouw, K.W.; Gibb, E.A.; Liu, Y.; Wu, C.L.; Drumm, M.R.; da Costa, J.B.; du Plessis, M.; Wang, N.Q.; Davicioni, E.; et al. Impact of Immune and Stromal Infiltration on Outcomes Following Bladder-Sparing Trimodality Therapy for Muscle-Invasive Bladder Cancer. *Eur. Urol.* **2019**, *76*, 59–68. [CrossRef] [PubMed]
53. Necchi, A.; Raggi, D.; Gallina, A.; Ross, J.S.; Fare, E.; Giannatempo, P.; Marandino, L.; Colecchia, M.; Luciano, R.; Bianchi, M.; et al. Impact of Molecular Subtyping and Immune Infiltration on Pathological Response and Outcome Following Neoadjuvant Pembrolizumab in Muscle-invasive Bladder Cancer. *Eur. Urol.* **2020**, *77*, 701–710. [CrossRef]
54. Krantz, D.; Hartana, C.A.; Winerdal, M.E.; Johansson, M.; Alamdari, F.; Jakubczyk, T.; Huge, Y.; Aljabery, F.; Palmqvist, K.; Zirakzadeh, A.A.; et al. Neoadjuvant Chemotherapy Reinforces Antitumour T cell Response in Urothelial Urinary Bladder Cancer. *Eur. Urol.* **2018**, *74*, 688–692. [CrossRef] [PubMed]
55. Galsky, M.D.; Arija, J.A.A.; Bamias, A.; Davis, I.D.; De Santis, M.; Kikuchi, E.; Garcia-Del-Muro, X.; De Giorgi, U.; Mencinger, M.; Izumi, K.; et al. Atezolizumab with or without chemotherapy in metastatic urothelial cancer (IMvigor130): A multicentre, randomised, placebo-controlled phase 3 trial. *Lancet* **2020**, *395*, 1547–1557. [CrossRef]
56. Voorwerk, L.; Slagter, M.; Horlings, H.M.; Sikorska, K.; van de Vijver, K.K.; de Maaker, M.; Nederlof, I.; Kluin, R.J.C.; Warren, S.; Ong, S.; et al. Immune induction strategies in metastatic triple-negative breast cancer to enhance the sensitivity to PD-1 blockade: The TONIC trial. *Nat. Med.* **2019**, *25*, 920–928. [CrossRef]
57. Hussain, M.H.A.; Powles, T.; Albers, P.; Castellano, D.; Daneshmand, S.; Gschwend, J.; Nishiyama, H.; Oudard, S.; Tayama, D.; Davarpanah, N.N.; et al. IMvigor010: Primary analysis from a phase III randomized study of adjuvant atezolizumab (atezo) versus observation (obs) in high-risk muscle-invasive urothelial carcinoma (MIUC). *J. Clin. Oncol.* **2020**, *38*, 5000. [CrossRef]

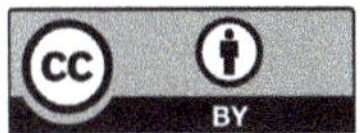

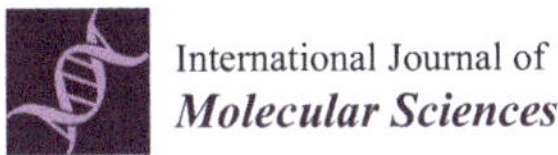

International Journal of
Molecular Sciences

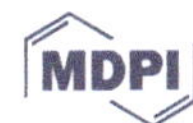

Review

Activating Telomerase *TERT* Promoter Mutations and Their Application for the Detection of Bladder Cancer

Maria Zvereva [1,2,*], Eduard Pisarev [3], Ismail Hosen [4], Olga Kisil [5], Simon Matskeplishvili [6], Elena Kubareva [7], David Kamalov [6], Alexander Tivtikyan [6], Arnaud Manel [8], Emmanuel Vian [9], Armais Kamalov [6], Thorsten Ecke [10] and Florence Le Calvez-Kelm [2]

1. Chair of Chemistry of Natural Compounds, Department of Chemistry, Lomonosov Moscow State University, 119991 Moscow, Russia
2. International Agency for Research on Cancer (IARC), 69372 Lyon, France; lecalvezf@iarc.fr
3. Faculty of Bioengineering and Bioinformatics, Lomonosov Moscow State University, 119234 Moscow, Russia; profard95@gmail.com
4. Department of Biochemistry and Molecular Biology, Faculty of Biological Sciences, University of Dhaka, Dhaka 1000, Bangladesh; ismail.hosen@du.ac.bd
5. Gause Institute of New Antibiotics, 119021 Moscow, Russia; olvv@mail.ru
6. Medical Research and Education Center, Lomonosov Moscow State University, 119992 Moscow, Russia; simonmats@yahoo.com (S.M.); davidffm@mail.ru (D.K.); aleksandertivtikyan@yandex.ru (A.T.); kamalov@mc.msu.ru (A.K.)
7. Belozersky Institute of Physico-Chemical Biology, Moscow State University, 119992 Moscow, Russia; kubareva@belozersky.msu.ru
8. Le Creusot Hospital, 71200 Le Creusot, France; manelarnaud69@gmail.com
9. Department of Urology, Protestant Clinic of Lyon, 69300 Lyon, France; emmanuel.vian@gmail.com
10. Department of Urology, HELIOS Hospital Bad Saarow, D-15526 Bad Saarow, Germany; thorsten.ecke@helios-gesundheit.de
* Correspondence: mzvereva@chem.msu.ru; Tel.: +7-49-5939-4533

Received: 31 July 2020; Accepted: 18 August 2020; Published: 21 August 2020

Abstract: This review summarizes state-of-the-art knowledge in early-generation and novel urine biomarkers targeting the telomerase pathway for the detection and follow-up of bladder cancer (BC). The limitations of the assays detecting telomerase reactivation are discussed and the potential of transcription-activating mutations in the promoter of the *TERT* gene detected in the urine as promising simple non-invasive BC biomarkers is highlighted. Studies have shown good sensitivity and specificity of the urinary *TERT* promoter mutations in case-control studies and, more recently, in a pilot prospective cohort study, where the marker was detected up to 10 years prior to clinical diagnosis. However, large prospective cohort studies and intervention studies are required to fully validate their robustness and assess their clinical utility. Furthermore, it may be interesting to evaluate whether the clinical performance of urinary *TERT* promoter mutations could increase when combined with other simple urinary biomarkers. Finally, different approaches for assessment of *TERT* promoter mutations in urine samples are presented together with technical challenges, thus highlighting the need of careful technological validation and standardization of laboratory methods prior to translation into clinical practice.

Keywords: bladder cancer; biomarkers; non-invasive detection; telomerase; somatic mutations; *TERT* promoter region

---

1. Introduction

More than 300 thousand new cases of bladder cancer (BC) are diagnosed in the world annually [1]. Currently, the gold standard of BC diagnosis and monitoring is cystoscopy, which is an invasive, painful, and relatively expensive procedure [2]. In the last few years, urine components have attracted the intense focus of investigators aiming to discover novel biomarkers for detection of BC, as urine is in direct contact with potentially malignant urothelium, is easy to obtain, and its testing should potentially be much more cost-effective.

Molecular markers for such analyses can be of different nature (nucleic acids, proteins, small-molecular-weight compounds), but should be directly linked to the cell processes that are altered during neoplastic transformation (for example, avoidance of programmed cell death through disruption of the telomerase pathway). The characterization of molecular genetic alteration changes, associated with the malignant cell transformation, in differentiation or metastatic potential has provided insights into the interplay of these oncogenic processes and the activation of telomerase and its components [3]. This activation is directly related to the disruption of the cell division control system and, therefore, leads to uncontrolled cell growth. It has been widely demonstrated that telomerase activity is enhanced in 85–90% of tumor cell types [4]. There are multiple underlying mechanisms of telomerase activation [5], but genetic alterations in the promoter region of telomerase reverse transcriptase (*TERT*), leading to both increased gene expression and activity of the enzyme, are considered the most frequent. Therefore, they are considered highly promising putative biomarkers of cancer [6]. The process of reactivating the telomerase enzyme includes alterations in the gene promoter of the catalytic subunit of telomerase caused by methylation [7] and somatic mutations [8], both leading to its overexpression.

In this review, we trace the history of the early-generation of urine BC biomarkers identified in the telomerase pathway, discuss the limitations of the detection of related assays, and highlight the potential of transcription-activating mutations in the promoter of the *TERT* gene detected in the urine as promising simple non-invasive biomarkers for the detection of BC and surveillance for its relapse. Mutations in the *TERT* promoter have been shown to occur in many histological tumor types, making these alterations the most frequent somatic abnormalities detected in cancer so far. In BC particularly, they are detected in 60–85% of cases in all stages and grades of the disease. These mutations have been detected in the intracellular and extracellular DNA fragments from urine samples collected both at the time of primary clinical diagnosis of BC and during post-surgical follow-up. Therefore, they represent promising biomarkers to detect and monitor BC [9]. Recent publications reveal an important short-term clinical perspective of the use of *TERT* promoter mutations as BC urinary biomarkers [10,11]. However, additional validations in large prospective cohort studies and interventional studies are necessary to fully assess their clinical performance and utility. Moreover, it is necessary to evaluate whether the sensitivity of the urinary *TERT* promoter mutations in detecting BC is increased when combined with other urinary biomarkers. Finally, careful technological validation and standardization of laboratory methods for assessing *TERT* promoter mutations in urine samples are critical for their clinical implementation.

2. Telomerase Reactivation in Bladder Cancer and Early-Generation of Telomerase Urinary-Based Biomarkers

Telomerase reactivation in BC has been first described in the mid-1990s [12]. Telomerase is an RNA-protein machinery that synthesizes repeating telomeric DNA. Telomeres are special structures at the ends of chromosomes where DNA interacts with specific proteins, shaping the "cap" to protect chromosome ends from degradation and to maintain their integrity [13]. Human telomerase contains a protein component (reverse transcriptase or hTERT) and a matrix RNA constituent (telomerase RNA, hTR), which, together with other proteins, form the active holoenzyme whose function is to extend telomeric DNA with new repeats and, therefore, revert the progressive loss of sequences at the ends of chromosomes associated with incomplete DNA replication [14]. In differentiated human cells, telomeres are typically shortened with every cell division up to a programmed critical length that leads to cell aging and apoptosis. During tumorigenesis, the mechanism leading to critical telomere shortening is counteracted by telomerase activation, thus preventing cell death.

Enhanced through genetic or epigenetic changes, telomerase activity is, therefore, a telltale sign of malignancy [15]. Bladder cancer cells have shorter telomeres than adjacent normal urothelium [12]. Telomerase activity was shown to be high in BC tumor samples but not in the normal epithelium of patients with BC. Therefore, in many early studies, the measurement of telomerase activity as a biomarker of cancer diagnosis was considered. A relatively simple and accurate test called the Telomere Repeat Amplification Protocol (TRAP) was established to determine telomerase activity in cells and tissue samples [16]. The method relies on the amplification and measurement of the total number of telomeric repeats newly synthesized by the telomerase on a telomere-like oligonucleotide. Due to its direct contact to the urothelium, urine provides the most easily accessible reservoir of potential biomarkers to study urological diseases, so the possibility to use the TRAP assay to detect increased levels of telomerase secreted into the urine by bladder cancer cells has been tested. A case-control study involving 134 primary BC cases and 84 controls demonstrated promising performance of the urine TRAP assay with a sensitivity of 90% and specificity of 88% (when telomerase activity is 50 arbitrary enzymatic units (AEU)) in detecting the presence of bladder tumors in men [17]. While other studies reported a high sensitivity (70–90%) compared to the current standard urine cytology, specificity proved to be lower, ranging from 66% to 88% [17–20]. The suboptimal of specificity has been attributed to the inherent telomerase activity in inflammatory or non-urothelial cells present in urine samples [21], which results in a significant variability in telomerase activity in urine of healthy individuals but also in cancer patients. This was observed by the same authors who reported an average value of telomerase activity of 27 AEU (total range of 0–88) in urine of healthy individuals and 112 AEU (total range of 30–382) in bladder cancer patients [17]. Another limitation of this method, which possibly reflects the lack of reproducibility between studies, includes the sensitivity of urine samples to inactivating agents that rapidly reduce the activity of the enzyme, giving rise to the need for strict protocols of handling samples at special conditions between sample collection and processing in order to maintain stability of the RNA-protein complex. Therefore, the lack of standardization of the TRAP assay and difficulties due to the technical requirements limit its use as a clinical biomarker for bladder cancer detection [22]. A recent alternative method to determine telomerase activity in human urine samples using the hybridization chain reaction and dynamic light scattering has been developed for the detection of bladder cancer [23]. Preliminary findings indicate a high specificity in cellular models and in few healthy individuals and patients with malignancies other than bladder cancer [24–26], but this needs to be confirmed in large case-control studies.

Another existing method to analyze telomerase reactivation is the quantitative measurement of the expression level of telomerase subunits TERT and telomerase RNA (TR) using real-time reverse transcription polymerase chain reaction (qRT-PCR). High expressions of these mRNAs have been observed consistently across many different malignancies, suggesting a promising avenue for early cancer detection in body fluids, especially in urine samples of patients with BC [27]. The quantitative analysis of TR and TERT in urine samples had an overall sensitivity of 77.0% and 55.2%, respectively, and a specificity of 72.1% and 85.0%, and determining both TERT mRNA and TR levels turned out to be more sensitive but less specific than urine cytology [28]. More recently, a protocol of combined modified TRAP and qRT-PCR methods to interrogate urine sediments gave encouraging results for the non-invasive detection of BC [29]. However, obstacles remain before urine telomerase activity-based assays can be translated into clinical practice [30]: (1) A high false-positive rate due to the telomerase activity of blood cells or non-urothelial cells in urine, which, despite attempts to sort out positive non-tumor cells, is yet to be solved; (2) an inconsistent correlation between TERT mRNA and telomerase activity in some tissues [31]; (3) a low number of telomerase-positive cells in urine in early stages of BC, and (4) a possible high rate of telomerase or RNA degradation in the urine and serious technical constraints to maintain their stability. Based on the above considerations, it was of clinical interest to search for novel non-telomerase activity-based urinary biomarkers for the detection and surveillance of BC. Nowadays, several urine-based bladder cancer biomarkers have received FDA-approval: (1) The immunoassays based on the detection of the Nuclear matrix protein 22

(NMP22® BC and its improved variant, the NMP22® BladderChek®, Alere, Waltham, MA, USA) [32] and the detection of the complement factor H-related protein (BTA stat® and BTA TRAK®); (2) the immunofluorescence assays based on the detection of the carcinoembryonic antigen and 2 mucins (ImmunoCyt™/uCyt), and (3) the multitarget fluorescence in situ hybridization (FISH) assay based on the detection of aneuploidy of several chromosomal regions (UroVysion) [33]. Other interesting commercially available biomarkers are emerging: The UBC® rapid (IDL, Bromma, Sweden) test to measure soluble fragments of cytokeratins 8 and 18 in urine [34] and the CxBladder test to identify the presence of five mRNAs (MDK, HOXA13, CDC2, IGFBP5, and CXCR2) in the urine [35]. Only few studies compared the performance of telomerase-based assays with FDA-approved tests for BC detection [32,36,37]. The UroVysion assay (FISH) had higher specificity than the TRAP assays and other urine markers; meanwhile, Bravaccini and colleagues showed that the combination of urine cytology and FISH to the TRAP assay had some potential in discriminating patients with bladder cancer from individuals with other urinary symptoms [36]. Another study conducted in a group of workers employed in the production of tires and, therefore, exposed to various potential bladder carcinogens, and in a control group of unexposed subjects showed that the two-step design using the TRAP assay with standard urine cytology and comet assay as the primary screening tool, and then FISH (UroVysion) in TRAP-positive cases increased the accuracy for the detection of BC as compared to the conventional urine cytology [38].

However, based on performance and cost considerations, none of the commercially available urine biomarkers to date are recommended as reliable diagnostic targets both by the European Association of Urology (link to NMIBC guideline https://uroweb.org/guideline/non-muscle-invasive-bladder-cancer/#5; link to MIBC guideline https://uroweb.org/guideline/bladder-cancer-muscle-invasive-and-metastatic/#6) and American Urological Association (link to NMIBC guideline https://www.auanet.org/guidelines/bladder-cancer-non-muscle-invasive-guideline#x2517) for routine BC clinical management or for screening in high-risk populations [39–42]. The absence of urine biomarkers that can be clinically exploited and the fact that the re-activation of telomerase is a crucial mechanism of urothelial carcinogenesis (observed in 99% of urothelial carcinomas) rekindled the interest in further research on other markers indirectly influencing telomerase activation, for example, through recurrent genetic changes that have been identified in the regulatory elements of the *TERT* gene.

3. Urinary *TERT* Promoter Mutations: The Holy Grail of a Biomarker for Bladder Cancer Detection and Surveillance?

3.1. TERT Promoter Mutations and Biological Significance in Bladder Carcinogenesis

Since their discovery in 2013 in melanoma samples, mutations in the promoter region of the *TERT* gene have been found to be frequent in several tumor types [43]. Their functional impact has been well-characterized in vitro and associated with the creation of new binding sites to numerous cellular transcription factors, resulting in an increase in *TERT* expression and telomerase reactivation. [44,45]. The introduction of mutations in the *TERT* promoter sequence caused a two- to four-fold increase in promoter activity in reporter cell lines [44]. Thus, detection of such mutations can be seen as an indirect measure of telomerase reactivation and neoplastic transformation of cells.

Two hotspot mutations of the *TERT* promoter have been detected with high frequency in bladder cancer but not in neighboring normal tissues [43,46,47]. These mutations occur at two positions upstream of the transcription starting site, at −124 bp (nucleotide polymorphism G > A, g.1295228 (chr5, 1, 295, 228 assembly GRCh37) or g.1295113 (chr5, 1, 295, 113 assembly GRCh38)) and −146 bp (nucleotide polymorphism G > A, g.1295250 (chr5, 1, 295, 250, assembly GRCh37) or g.1295135 (chr5, 1, 295, 135 assembly GRCh38)) in a GC-rich genome region, which specifies its alternative organization (Figure 1). Reported to be mutually exclusive, somatic mutations in *TERT* promoter occur in 60–80% cases of all stages and grades of BC [40,48–53]. Specifically, Kinde et al. were the first to show that *TERT* promoter mutations occur frequently in low-grade, high-grade papillary tumors and carcinoma in situ lesions [54]. Allory et al. reported a *TERT* promoter mutation frequency of 87% in cell lines and of 83% in bladder tumors, regardless of stages or the risk associated with disease. Mutation frequency was virtually the same for low-risk non-muscle-invading bladder cancer (NMIBC) (73%), high-risk NMIBC (74%), and muscle-invading bladder cancer (MIBC) (53%). These mutations occurred more frequently than any other genomic changes in both NMIBC risk categories. *TERT* promoter mutations were not shown to be associated with age, sex, or smoking [48]. In addition to urothelial carcinomas, these mutations have also been reported in other rare histological variants of primary BC, such as squamous cell carcinoma (SCC) [55], small cell carcinoma [56], adenocarcinoma of non-enteric type [57], and plasmacytoid urothelial carcinoma [58].

Furthermore, it has been shown that the two single nucleotide substitutions C228T and C250T together account for 99% of *TERT* promoter mutations in BC. Of the two-thirds of bladder tumors carrying a *TERT* promoter mutation, Rachakonda P.S. and colleagues observed that the C228T mutation (G > A) was the most frequent change in BC followed by the C250T mutation, identified in 53.5% and 11.6% of all tumors, respectively [53]. Two additional rare nucleotide mutations were C228A (number of tumors, *n* = 3) and 57A > C (T > G) −57 (nucleotide polymorphism A > C, g.1295161 (chr5, 1, 295, 161 assembly GRCh37) or g.1295046 (chr5, 1, 295, 046 assembly GRCh38), (*n* = 1)). Mutations in all positions −57, −124, and −146 were mutually exclusive and resulted in the creation of a new common binding site de novo for transcription factors Ets/TCF. Similar results were obtained by Allory and colleagues [48]. The most frequent mutation was C228T (*n* = 65) followed by C250T (*n* = 10), and two additional rare mutations were C242T/C243T (*n* = 2) and C228A (*n* = 1). All mutations were mutually exclusive.

With regard to their potential as prognostic markers, one study investigated the relation between the disease-specific survival of patients with urothelial cancer and (1) the presence of C228T and C250T mutations in the *TERT* promoter; and (2) the level of TERT mRNA expression in two independent cohorts of previously untreated patients (*n* = 35 and *n* = 87). A significant decline in survival was strongly correlated with increased TERT mRNA level, but not with the presence of mutation in the *TERT* promoter [59]. Interestingly, the authors also demonstrated that the presence of a *TERT* mutation was associated with an increase in TERT mRNA expression level, leading to the enhancement in telomerase activity and telomere elongation. It has been hypothesized that this unexpected effect is due to the alternative functions of the telomerase catalytic subunit [60], and the existence of alternative mechanisms, other than mutations in the *TERT* promoter, such as epigenetic changes, also contribute to telomerase activation.

3.2. Analytical Methods for Detecting Mutations in the TERT Promoter: Comparison of Analytical Performance and Bias

There is a wide range of established analytical approaches for detecting mutations in the *TERT* promoter. However, the detection of these mutations is complicated by the composition and the structure of the *TERT* promoter genomic region, which is characterized by the highly GC-rich sequence and alternative structures of double stranded DNA in the form of G-quadruplexes, as illustrated in Figure 1 [61]. Another challenge is the detection of low-abundance tumor-derived mutations in body fluids. The DNA fragments carrying the tumor-specific alterations can represent a very small fraction of the total DNA. In blood samples, for example, the circulating tumor DNA fraction has been reported to be as low as 0.5% [62]. The analytical sensitivity of the assays is, therefore, critical in such settings. Despite such constraints, many quantitative PCR-based diagnostics described below have been successfully applied to human biological fluids, e.g., whole blood [63], urine (see Table 1), and urine samples of patients with hematuria (Table S4).

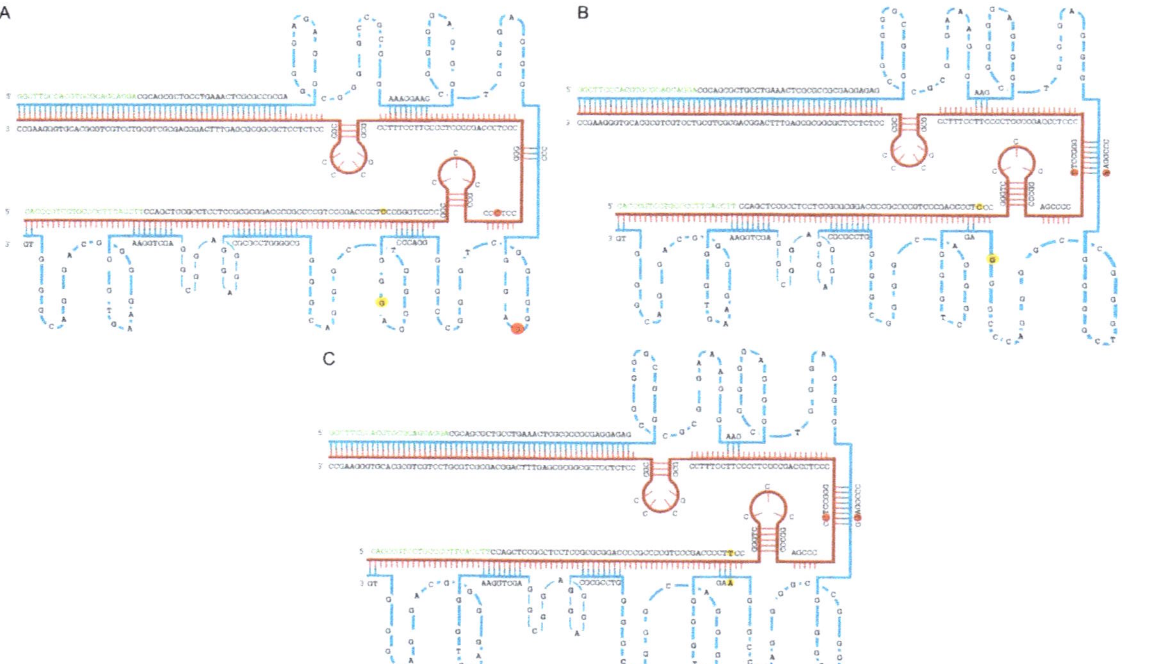

Figure 1. Predicted intramolecular distribution of putative Quadruplex forming G-Rich Sequences (QGRS) in the *TERT* promoter sequence. (**A**) the structure of wild type (WT) DNA; (**B**) only with mutation C228T; (**C**) only with mutation C250T. The two nucleotides at −124 and −146 positions from the ATG start site are highlighted with red and yellow circles respectively. These two hotspots affected by mutations predominantly including C228T and C250T are of the interest for both fundamental research and clinical diagnostics. G-strand and C-strand are marked in blue and claret lines respectively. Regions corresponding to the primers applied to amplify this fragment are marked in green. Despite the close resemblance between all three types of structures they differ substantially. The structures were obtained using online programs "QGRS Mapper" [64] (output data are provided in Tables S1–S3). In this manner both G- and C-strands were analyzed, however only G-strand contains G-quadruplexes. Procedure and software used to calculate and create the structures are described in the Supplementary Materials in more detail.

Currently, the used method for detecting known genetic changes in clinical research is real-time PCR (quantitative PCR and its modifications). Yet, they often lack the sensitivity to detect underrepresented genetic alterations, so-called low mutant allelic fraction (MAF), which are often found diluted with wild-type DNA fragments originating from non-malignant cells or non-mutated cells. Furthermore, the heterogeneous composition of DNA fragments found in 'liquid biopsy' samples may also complicate the analysis. Studies that used real-time PCR to detect *TERT* promoter mutations in tumor and urine samples are shown in Table 1. Successful application of a qPCR-based method known as castPCR was described by Wang and co-workers [61]. In comparison to Sanger-sequencing, castPCR demonstrated dramatically higher sensitivity and specificity in a wide range of tumors of the urinary system (Table 1). The most recent progress with regard to the detection of *TERT* promoter mutations by qPCR has been achieved by Batista and colleagues who demonstrated that their sensitive, urine-based assay called Uromonitor® (Uromonitor Maia, Portugal) based on competitive allele-specific discrimination PCR was capable of detecting trace amounts of *TERT* promoter mutations in urine samples [65].

Next-generation sequencing (NGS) can simultaneously analyze millions of DNA copies. The identification of low-allelic somatic mutations requires ultra-deep sequencing so that the few sequencing reads with the mutant allele can be generated within the pool of wild-type reads. To achieve such high sequencing coverage of the screened genomic region(s), sequencing must be targeted. Traditional NGS-based targeted sequencing is able to detect mutant DNA forms at or higher than 2% allelic fraction against the background of the wild type DNA [66], but recent developments of NGS systems, such as Safe-SeqS [54,67], Tam-Seq [68,69], and CAPP-seq [70], improved threshold limits, the latter reaching an analytical sensitivity of 0.0025% MAF. Avogbe et al. recently developed UroMuTERT, a simple, non-invasive, and sensitive NGS-based assay for the detection of low-level *TERT* promoter mutations. Combined with a specific algorithm developed by the same group, called Needlestack [71], UroMuTERT achieved detection thresholds of 0.8% and 0.5% mutant allelic fraction MAFs for C228T and C250T mutations, respectively [10].

In addition to the next-generation sequencing methods, another platform that can detect low-abundance mutant DNA molecules against a background of the thousand-fold excess of wild-type molecules is droplet-digital PCR (ddPCR). It combines the short hands-on-time and easy laboratory workflows and does not require complex bioinformatic analysis (Table 1), making it highly suitable for implementation into clinical practice.

Figure 1 shows a possible organization of the *TERT* promoter region. This model was generated in the online server "QGRS Mapper" and the particular fragment shown on the picture was described [61] to determine mutations C228T and C250T in upper tract urothelial carcinomas (UTUC) using PCR in conjunction with subsequent Sanger sequencing. All the analytical approaches described above include an amplification step of genomic regions containing −124 and −146 sites from the ATG starting codon, whose length may vary according to primer design. The occurrence of C228T and C250T mutations can distort the double-stranded structure of this region, and the amplification efficiency may also be subject to the ability of primers to anneal and extend template DNA in such complex regions with secondary structures. This could explain the wide ranges of reported sensitivities and specificities.

To develop diagnostic approaches based on the identification of mutations in the promoter region of the *TERT* gene, it will be critical to compare the performance of screening methods and provide harmonized and standardized laboratory procedures.

Table 1. Accuracy and methodological characteristics of tests for detecting the *TERT* promoter mutations in the urine for various neoplasias of the urinary system.

Article	Tumor Type	Method	Number of Patients	Size of Control Group	Sensitivity %	Specificity %	Length of PCR Product	Primers (Sequences Are Presented from 5′ End to End) and Probes
[56]	Small cell carcinoma (SCC)	PCR+ Sanger sequencing	11	3	100	100	163	CAGCGCTGCCTGAAACTC; GTCCTGCCCCTTCACCTT
[61]	Ureter carcinoma (UC)	PCR+ Sanger sequencing	20	0	94	10	193	CACCCGTCCTGCCCCTTCACCTT; GGCTTCCCACGTGCGCAGCAGGA-
	Renal pelvic carcinoma (RPC)		16	0	93.8	25	193	
	UTUC (RPC + UC) C228T	PCR+ Sanger sequencing	10	37	60	97	193	dnp
		castPCR	10	37	90	92	dnp *	
	BC (C228T)	PCR+ Sanger sequencing	36	33	47	100	193	CACCCGTCCTGCCCCTTCACCTT; GGCTTCCCACGTGCGCAGCAGGA
		castPCR	36	33	86	97	dnp	dnp
	UTUC + BC	PCR+ Sanger sequencing	46	70	50	98	193	CACCCGTCCTGCCCCTTCACCTT; GGCTTCCCACGTGCGCAGCAGGA
		castPCR	46	70	89	96	dnp	dnp
[10]	Urothelial cancer (UC) primary	UroMuTERT (NGS)	45	94	86.7	94.7	147	CTTCCAGCTCCGCCTCCTCCGCGCGG; AGCGCTGCCTGAAACTCGCGCC
	Urothelial cancer (UC) recurrence		48	94	87.5	94.7	147	
	UC (Diaguro)		93	94	87.1	94.7	147	
[72]	Urothelial bladder carcinoma	ddPCR	99	376	81.8	83.5	52 60	C228T: CGGAAAGGAAGGGGAGGG;GTCCCCGGCCCAGC Mut: [6FAM]-CCC+C+T+T+CCGG-[BHQ_1] WT: [HEX]-CCCC+T+C+CGGG-[BHQ_1] C250T: TGGGAGGGCCCGGAG;GACCCCGCCCCGT Mut: [6FAM]CCC+C+T+T+CCGG[BHQ_1] WT: [HEX]CCCC+T+C+CCGG[BHQ_1]
[55]	Squamous cell carcinoma Benign transurethral bladder biopsy samples	Safe-SeqS	15 0 [i]	94 [ii] 8	80	dnp	125 dnp	1st couple: CACACAGGAAACAGCTAT GACCATGGGCCGCGGAAAGGAAG; CGACGTAAAACGACGGCCAGTNNNNNNN NNNNNNNNCGTCCTGCCCCTTCACC ** 2nd couple: CACACAGGAAACAGCTATGAC CATGGCGGAAAGGAAAGGGAG; CGACGTAAAACGACGGCCAGTNNNNNN NNNNNNNNCCGTCCCGACCCCTC
[73]	NMIBC primary	SNaPshot assay	230	0	69	52	dnp	dnp

Table 1. *Cont.*

Article	Tumor Type	Method	Number of Patients	Size of Control Group	Sensitivity %	Specificity %	Length of PCR Product	Primers (Sequences Are Presented from 5′ End to End) and Probes
[48]	BC (primary)	SNaPshot assay	118	0	62	–	155	AGCGCTGCCTGAAACTCG; CCCTTCACCTTCCAGCTC
	BC (recurrence)		113	0	42	–	155	Probes: for C228T/A T_{23}GGCTGGGAGGGCCCGGA
	BC (recurrence-free samples)		0	218	–	73	155	for C250T T_{39}CTGGGCCGGGGACCCGG
[74]	Renal pelvic carcinoma (RPC)		5	0	60	dnp	193	CACCCGTCCTGCCCCTTCACCTT; GGCTTCCCACGTGCGCAGCAGGA
	UTUC		14	0	29	dnp	193	
	Chromophobe renal cell carcinoma (CRCC)		8	0	13	dnp	193	
	Ureter carcinoma (UC)		9	0	11	dnp	193	
	Clear cell renal cell carcinoma (CCRCC)		96	0	9.3	dnp	193	
	Renal cell carcinoma [iii] (RCC)		109	0	9.2	dnp	193	
[75]	BC early detection	PCR + Illumina sequencing	570	188	57	99.4	126	GGCCGCGGAAAGGAAG; CGTCCTGCCCCTTCACC
	UTUC		56	188	29	99.4		
	BC surveillance		322	188	57	99.4		
[11]	BC	UroMuTERT and ddPCR	30	101	46.7	100	65	C228T: CCCTCCCGGGTCC; CCGCGGAAAGGAAGG; probes: Mut: CCCGGAaGGGGCTG (FAM_lowaBlack); WT: CGGAgGGGGCTGG (HEX_IowaBlack). C250T CTTCACCTTCCAGCTCC; GAGGGCCCGGAGG; probes: Mut: CCCGGaAGGGGTCG (FAM_lowBlack); WT: ACCCGGgAGGGGT (HEX_IowaBlack).
[47]	UTUC	ddPCR	56	50	46.4	96	113	dnp
[76]	BC (supernatant)	NGS	92	0	46	100		NGS-primers: ACCTTCCAGCTCCGCCTCCTCCGCGCGGAC; AGAGGGCGGGGCCGCGGAAAGGAAGGGGAG
	BC (sediment)		92	0	48	100		
	Non-cancer hematuria		0	33				
[57]	Primary bladder adenocarcinoma	Safe-SeqS	14	94 [iv]	28.6	dnp	125	1st couple: CACACAGGAAACAGCTATGAC CATGGGCCGCGGAAAGGAAG; CGACGTAAAACGACGGCCAGTNNNNNNN NNNNNNNCGTCCTGCCCCTTCACC 2nd couple: CACACAGGAAACAGCTATGAC CATGGCGGAAAGGAAAGGGAG; CGACGTAAAACGACGGCCAGTNNNNNN NNNNNNNNCCGTCCCGACCCCTC
	Benign transurethral bladder biopsy samples		0	8			dnp	
[53]	Urothelial cell carcinoma	PCR+ Sanger sequencing	327	0	dnp	65.4	343	AGCACCTCGCGGTAGTGG; GGATTCGCGGGCACAGAC

* "dnp"–data not provided; ** "N" is a degenerate base (it can be A, T, G, or C with equal likelihood); [i]. Table fields with "Number of patients 0" correspond to control group or additional control group; [ii]. Peripheral blood; [iii]. In this study, 6 subtypes of RCC tumor were investigated. In the table data only about 2 subtypes (ccRCC and chRCC) are presented. 4 remaining RCC tumors did not harbor *TERT* promoter mutations; [iv]. Peripheral blood.

3.3. Predictive Significance of Determining TERT Promoter Mutations in Urine

The high frequency and the localization of mutations in a small region of the *TERT* promoter provided an extraordinary opportunity for a simple non-invasive assay for early detection or monitoring the recurrence or progression of disease in the patients whose tumors carry one of those variants. This is especially pertinent for the conception of an early detection test as *TERT* promoter mutations have been reported to be early events in the BC tumorigenesis process [54]. Normal urothelium cells and extracellular DNA (also called cell-free DNA or cfDNA) are constantly released into the urine. Malignant transformation of bladder tissue will lead to exfoliated tumor cells and circulating tumor DNA (also called ctDNA) to mix with normal cells and cfDNA in the urine.

TERT promoter mutations (C228T and C250T) have been previously detected in DNA from urinary exfoliated cells (cellDNA) collected prior to diagnosis and during post-surgical follow-up, with sensitivities and specificities varying from 52% to 82% and from 83% to 99%, respectively, in patients with incident or early BC and from 42% to 74% and 73% to 93%, respectively, in patients with recurrent BC [48,54,72,73,75,77]. Two studies reported a sensitivity of 80% using pre-surgery urine cellDNA but no information was provided on the primary or recurrence status [46,50]. The first indication these mutations detected in urine samples during follow-up was associated with recurrence and, therefore, could potentially serve as markers to monitor the disease status that was provided by the study conducted by Kinde et al. [54]. While limited in size, the authors showed that among patients whose tumors harbored *TERT* promoter mutations ($n = 11$), the same mutations were present in urine collected for follow-up in seven of eight patients with relapse but in none of the six patients without recurrence [54]. In line with these findings, Descotes and colleagues showed that, in particular, the presence of *TERT* mutant DNA forms in post-surgical urine samples was associated with recurrence in 100 patients initially diagnosed with NMIBC [46].

The association held true in a limited subset of patients with negative cystoscopy ($n = 6$), suggesting that *TERT* promoter mutations in urine could be a promising avenue for early detection of recurrence in patients under surveillance for BC. The same research group also showed that the detection of urinary mutations could be used as a dynamic monitoring of recurrence. This was illustrated in one patient for whom the absence of the initially detected C250T mutation was noted in post-diagnostic serial urine samples for 7 years before being detectable at the time of recurrence confirmed by cystoscopy. However, Allory et al. reported a relatively low specificity for the prediction of recurrence as mutations were detected in 27% of recurrence-free patients under surveillance for BC [48]. The high false-positive rate may reflect a timeline that is suboptimal for follow-up, which, if prolonged, may contribute to increase specificity, as patients with clinically undetectable tumors at the time of a *TERT* promoter mutation positive test may present with clinically detectable tumors later on. More well-powered longitudinal studies with sufficient follow-up durations and serial post-surgery urine samples are required to fully assess the true performance of these biomarkers for the prediction of BC recurrence.

There is growing evidence supporting the utility of urinary *TERT* promoter mutations to detect primary BC. Allory and colleagues first reported a sensitivity of 62% for the detection of primary BC with a specificity of 90% in individuals with hematuria but no bladder tumor [48] (Table 1 and Table S4). Combining urinary *TERT* promoter mutations with other DNA-based markers was also evaluated [72,75]. In a prospective blinded study, urine samples from 475 patients with gross hematuria collected at the time of standard urological examination (flexible cystoscopy and computed tomography urography) were tested for DNA mutation (*TERT* and *FGFR3*) and methylation biomarkers (*SALL3, ONECUT2, CCNA1, BCL2, EOMES,* and *VIM*) to determine whether a urine-based DNA test could replace flexible cystoscopy in the initial assessment of the most common BC symptom, i.e., gross hematuria. Of the 99 (20.8%) patients presenting urothelial bladder tumors, the DNA test had a sensitivity of 97.0% and a specificity of 76.9%. Detection of mutations in the *TERT* promoter showed the highest sensitivity (81.8%), but at the same time, the lowest specificity (83.5%) for individuals with hematuria [72] (Table 1 and Table S4). The *FGFR3* gene is the most frequently mutated gene in NMIBC with a total frequency of 70%. While they are much less frequent than *TERT* promoter mutations, they could still represent a putative interesting combined biomarker for the detection of BC. The added value of their combination with *TERT* promoter mutations for the comprehensive non-invasive detection of BC has to still be demonstrated in independent study. A combined DNA-based biomarker approach was also recently evaluated in a screening study conducted by Springer et al. where they assessed the performance of a multigene panel assay that includes the screening of *TERT* promoter mutations and regions of interest in ten other somatically mutated genes (UROSEEK) for detecting BC 0–18 months prior to clinical diagnosis in high-risk symptomatic patients. The authors reported a sensitivity of 83% and a specificity of 93% for their panel, while *TERT* promoter mutations were detected in 57% of the cases. Specifically, the sensitivity and specificity of the *TERT* promoter mutation in urine samples of individuals with hematuria were 55% and 90%, respectively (Table S4) [75]. In a recent case-control study, Avogbe et al. used their developed single-plex ultrasensitive UroMuTERT assay to test the urinary DNA samples (both cfDNA or cellDNA) of 93 primary and recurrent cases with urothelial cancer and 94 controls, and compare its performance to that of urine cytology for the detection of urothelial cancer [10]. C228T or C250T mutations were detected in urinary cfDNA or cellDNA with 87.1% sensitivity and 94.7% specificity. The UroMuTERT sensitivity was consistent across primary and recurrent cases, and tumor stages and grades, and highest for urinary cfDNA and cellDNA combined. It also significantly outperformed the sensitivity of urine cytology, especially for detection of low-grade early-stage urothelial cancer [10]. In addition, the UroMuTERT single-gene assay demonstrated comparable performance to that of the UroSEEK multiple markers assay (including C228T and C250T) for the detection of primary or early urothelial cancer (sensitivity of 86.7% versus 83%; specificity of 94.7% versus 93%). Therefore, more studies are required to understand whether the observed differences in the detection rate of urinary *TERT* promoter mutations may originate from pre-analytical procedures or from the use of multiple urinary DNA sources versus one or from differences in prevalence of *TERT* promoter mutations in BC across populations. This has important implications as a simple single-gene assay with harmonized and standardized procedures for urine collection and processing might be able to achieve the same clinical performance for the detection of BC as complex multi-gene assays, which are more expensive and clinically less easily implemented.

While most studies conducted so far have focused on the evaluation of urinary cellDNA, there is, in addition to what Avogbe and colleagues reported [10], accumulating evidence that urinary cfDNA could be a reliable alternative source of urinary DNA for non-invasive genomic profiling of BC. While being based on recurrent clinically actionable genomic aberrations rather than on the assessment on *TERT* promoter mutations, a study reported that the use of urinary cfDNA led to higher analytical sensitivity (90%), as well as the use of urinary cellDNA (61%) for the detection of UC tumor-associated alterations [78]. These findings are in line with an initial study from 2007 reporting the superiority of urinary cfDNA over cellDNA for the detection of genetic alterations of patients with urothelial cancer [78,79]. Applied to the detection of the *TERT* promoter mutations, two recent studies highlighted the potential of the marker in urinary cfDNA for the detection of BC [80,81]. Specifically, of 77 patients whose tumor cells carried the 228 G > A/T mutation, the same mutation was detected by ddPCR in urinary cfDNA of 71 individuals (92%) and the mutation was absent in cfDNA of 26 of 27 healthy patients (specificity of 96%). Patients with false-negative results had an early-stage tumor, and increased mutant allelic fraction was found to correlate with increased stages of the disease. Concordant mutational status between tumor tissues and liquid biopsy was obtained in 92% of cases [80]. However, in studies comparing the analytical sensitivity of both forms of urinary DNAs, the results are sparse. Stasik and colleagues demonstrated a better sensitivity in using cellDNA (83%) than in using cfDNA (77%), but, overall, the *TERT* mutation allelic frequencies (MAF) were highly correlated, suggesting little added value in using cfDNA as an alternative source of urinary DNA [2]. This observation is in agreement with the results from Ward et al. who demonstrated an equal ability to detect somatic tumor mutations in cfDNA and cellDNA [82]. Avogbe and co-workers also reported an overall high concordance between cfDNA and cellDNA results but still observed the highest sensitivity for the combined source of DNA (87.1%) as opposed to cfDNA only (81.8%) and cellDNA (83.5%), highlighting the potential utility of combining multiple sources of DNA for the assessment of the marker in rare cases presenting with discordant results between cfDNA and cellDNA [10]. Interestingly, Stastik et al. observed a potential advantage of using urinary cfDNA in leukocyte-rich urines where the mutant allelic fractions of *TERT* promoter mutations were higher in cfDNA than in cellDNA [2].

In order to validate promising biomarkers, expert groups recommend a nested case-control study design within prospective cohorts in which samples collected at enrolment within the targeted population will be tested for the biomarker(s) in asymptomatic individuals who will develop cancer later and those who will not [83,84]. This sort of study was recently conducted by Hosen et al. who investigated the potential of urinary *TERT* promoter mutations as early detection biomarkers for bladder cancer in asymptomatic individuals in a case-control study nested within a longitudinal population-based prospective cohort of 50,045 Iranian individuals (the Golestan Cohort Study). *TERT* promoter mutations were assessed in baseline urine samples (1.9–4.5 mL) from 38 individuals who subsequently developed primary BC and 152 matched controls using the UroMuTERT and droplet digital PCR assays. Sequencing results were obtained for 30 cases and 101 controls. *TERT* promoter mutations were detected in 14 pre-clinical cases (sensitivity 46.67%) and none of the controls (specificity 100.00%). Most notably, the mutations were detectable up to 10 years prior to clinical diagnosis, indicating that detecting pre-clinical BC using cost-effective urinary *TERT* biomarkers may provide a valuable opportunity for BC screening and management [11].

Avogbe and colleagues [10] developed a predictive assay UroMuTERT, based on NGS (single-plex assay) of the hTERT promoter and the certain algorithm for detecting mutations of low-allelic fractions. Mutations in the *TERT* promoter in the urine DNA (cfDNA or cellDNA) showed superior sensitivity and specificity compared to all the methods described above, significantly surpassing the urine cytology especially for detecting early-stage NMIBC, which allowed the authors to propose modifications to the classic diagnostic protocol. The high recurrence rates of bladder cancer require frequent follow-ups involving expensive and invasive cystoscopic examination, thus further increasing the already high initial expenses for the management of bladder cancer [85,86]. The average costs of cystoscopy are around $206, and the cost of non-invasive urine cytology is around $56 [87]. By contrast, the cost of the NGS-based and ddPCR assays for detecting urinary *TERT* promoter mutations in bladder cancer developed by our group [10,11] is about 24€ per sample, and, therefore, has the potential to be easily implemented for cost-effective bladder cancer management strategies.

4. Conclusions

In summary, urinary *TERT* promoter mutations have demonstrated significant potential to be used as reliable, inexpensive, and non-invasive biomarkers for early detection and monitoring of BC. Moreover, urine ddPCR-based assays have been shown to be capable of detecting very low levels of these mutations, cost-effective, and simple to use, and would therefore represent an attractive method for clinical practice. The fact that *TERT* promoter mutations have been identified in urine years prior to the primary clinical diagnosis of BC and in some relapse-free patients under surveillance reflects the early occurrence of the mutations in the primary carcinogenic and in the relapse processes, providing a window of opportunity for early molecular detection and intervention. It may also explain the lack of specificity in some studies with the insufficient duration of follow-up. Therefore, large studies with a long-duration follow-up should further assess the robustness of these biomarkers for both detection and surveillance of BC. In particular, it should be evaluated whether a clinical diagnosis can be made through cystoscopy or urography in asymptomatic individuals or patients under surveillance presenting with a positive urinary *TERT* promoter mutations assay, or they would benefit from regular *TERT* mutation screening until the tumor becomes detectable.

Studies have shown that screening the high-risk population for bladder cancer with robust urinary markers, while not recommended by urological societies at present, could be cost-effective. Should their clinical relevance be demonstrated in individuals at high-risk of developing the disease (i.e., subjects with symptoms, mainly hematuria and/or lower urinary tract symptoms, or subjects with occupational exposure to certain chemicals), this may increase awareness of bladder cancer risk and facilitate the implementation of screening strategies in defined high-risk groups who would benefit from close surveillance with a non-invasive test. Furthermore, early detection of primary or recurrent BC using urinary *TERT* promoter mutations as a primary tool should lead to timely therapeutic intervention and better survival. It should also reduce both the numbers of unnecessary cystoscopy procedures in patients with a *TERT* promoter mutation negative test and the cost of clinical management of suspected BCs. In addition, as it is unlikely that *TERT* promoter mutations in BC could be detected in urine in all BC cases, it would be important to evaluate whether the clinical performance of this promising and already successfully applied biomarker could further increase when combined with existing urinary biomarkers, which alone lacks the sensitivity and specificity for clinical utility.

Finally, the origin of the occurrence of the *TERT* promoter mutations and their correlation to the BC phenotype still have to be elucidated. Future research on the etiologies of mutations occurrence in certain parts of the genome leading to enhanced activity of the *TERT* promoter will result in a new practical understanding of the biology of BC and possibly the development of preventive approaches. With regard to potential therapeutic applications, it is worth noting that the region of the *TERT* promoter that frequently carries *TERT* promoter mutations in BC, which are absent in normal bladder cells, can presumably become the target of anti-cancer therapy, including novel TERT-based immunotherapies, which could be tailored to patients whose tumors harbor these mutations [88,89].

Supplementary Materials: The following are available online at http://www.mdpi.com/1422-0067/21/17/6034/s1, Table S1: G-quadruplexes of WT G-strand, Table S2: G-quadruplexes of G-strand with C228T, Table S3: G-quadruplexes of G-strand with C250T, Table S4: Applicability of different test systems to mutation analysis in patients with hematuria.

Funding: This research was supported by the Russian Foundation for Basic Research (grant no. 18-29-08040), the French Cancer League and the International Agency for Research on Cancer.

Conflicts of Interest: Where authors are identified as personnel of the International Agency for Research on Cancer/World Health Organization, the authors alone are responsible for the views expressed in this article and they do not necessarily represent the decisions, policy or views of the International Agency for Research on Cancer/World Health Organization.

Abbreviations

BC	Bladder cancer
NMIBC	Non-muscle-invasive bladder cancer
MIBC	Muscle-invasive bladder cancer
HTERT	Human telomerase reverse transcriptase
NGS	Next-generation sequencing
ddPCR	Droplet digital polymerase chain reaction

References

1. Antoni, S.; Ferlay, J.; Soerjomataram, I.; Znaor, A.; Jemal, A.; Bray, F. Bladder Cancer Incidence and Mortality: A Global Overview and Recent Trends. *Eur. Urol.* **2017**, *71*, 96–108. [CrossRef] [PubMed]
2. Stasik, S.; Salomo, K.; Heberling, U.; Froehner, M.; Sommer, U.; Baretton, G.B.; Ehninger, G.; Wirth, M.P.; Thiede, C.; Fuessel, S. Evaluation of TERT promoter mutations in urinary cell-free DNA and sediment DNA for detection of bladder cancer. *Clin. Biochem.* **2019**, *64*, 60–63. [CrossRef] [PubMed]
3. Hannen, R.; Bartsch, J.W. Essential roles of telomerase reverse transcriptase hTERT in cancer stemness and metastasis. *FEBS Lett.* **2018**, *592*, 2023–2031. [CrossRef] [PubMed]
4. Jafri, M.A.; Ansari, S.A.; Alqahtani, M.H.; Shay, J.W. Roles of telomeres and telomerase in cancer, and advances in telomerase-targeted therapies. *Genome Med.* **2016**, *8*, 69. [CrossRef] [PubMed]
5. Yuan, X.; Larsson, C.; Xu, D. Mechanisms underlying the activation of TERT transcription and telomerase activity in human cancer: Old actors and new players. *Oncogene* **2019**, *38*, 6172–6183. [CrossRef] [PubMed]

6. Leao, R.; Apolonio, J.D.; Lee, D.; Figueiredo, A.; Tabori, U.; Castelo-Branco, P. Mechanisms of human telomerase reverse transcriptase (hTERT) regulation: Clinical impacts in cancer. *J. Biomed. Sci.* **2018**, *25*, 22. [CrossRef] [PubMed]

7. Lee, D.D.; Leao, R.; Komosa, M.; Gallo, M.; Zhang, C.H.; Lipman, T.; Remke, M.; Heidari, A.; Nunes, N.M.; Apolonio, J.D.; et al. DNA hypermethylation within TERT promoter upregulates TERT expression in cancer. *J. Clin. Investig.* **2019**, *129*, 223–229. [CrossRef]

8. Chiba, K.; Lorbeer, F.K.; Shain, A.H.; McSwiggen, D.T.; Schruf, E.; Oh, A.; Ryu, J.; Darzacq, X.; Bastian, B.C.; Hockemeyer, D. Mutations in the promoter of the telomerase gene TERT contribute to tumorigenesis by a two-step mechanism. *Science* **2017**, *357*, 1416–1420. [CrossRef]

9. Gunes, C.; Wezel, F.; Southgate, J.; Bolenz, C. Implications of TERT promoter mutations and telomerase activity in urothelial carcinogenesis. *Nat. Rev. Urol.* **2018**, *15*, 386–393. [CrossRef]

10. Avogbe, P.H.; Manel, A.; Vian, E.; Durand, G.; Forey, N.; Voegele, C.; Zvereva, M.; Hosen, M.I.; Meziani, S.; De Tilly, B.; et al. Urinary TERT promoter mutations as non-invasive biomarkers for the comprehensive detection of urothelial cancer. *EBioMedicine* **2019**, *44*, 431–438. [CrossRef]

11. Hosen, M.I.; Sheikh, M.; Zvereva, M.; Scelo, G.; Forey, N.; Durand, G.; Voegele, C.; Poustchi, H.; Khoshnia, M.; Roshandel, G.; et al. Urinary TERT promoter mutations are detectable up to 10 years prior to clinical diagnosis of bladder cancer: Evidence from the Golestan Cohort Study. *EBioMedicine* **2020**, *53*, 17. [CrossRef] [PubMed]

12. Kamata, S.; Kageyama, Y.; Yonese, J.; Oshima, H. Significant telomere reduction in human superficial transitional cell carcinoma. *Br. J. Urol.* **1996**, *78*, 704–708. [CrossRef] [PubMed]

13. Turner, K.J.; Vasu, V.; Griffin, D.K. Telomere Biology and Human Phenotype. *Cells* **2019**, *8*, 73. [CrossRef]

14. Zvereva, M.I.; Shcherbakova, D.M.; Dontsova, O.A. Telomerase: Structure, functions, and activity regulation. *Biochemistry* **2010**, *75*, 1563–1583. [CrossRef]

15. Schmidt, J.C.; Cech, T.R. Human telomerase: Biogenesis, trafficking, recruitment, and activation. *Genes Dev.* **2015**, *29*, 1095–1105. [CrossRef] [PubMed]

16. Kim, N.W.; Piatyszek, M.A.; Prowse, K.R.; Harley, C.B.; West, M.D.; Ho, P.L.; Coviello, G.M.; Wright, W.E.; Weinrich, S.L.; Shay, J.W. Specific association of human telomerase activity with immortal cells and cancer. *Science* **1994**, *266*, 2011–2015. [CrossRef]

17. Sanchini, M.A.; Gunelli, R.; Nanni, O.; Bravaccini, S.; Fabbri, C.; Sermasi, A.; Bercovich, E.; Ravaioli, A.; Amadori, D.; Calistri, D. Relevance of urine telomerase in the diagnosis of bladder cancer. *JAMA* **2005**, *294*, 2052–2056. [CrossRef]

18. Landman, J.; Chang, Y.; Kavaler, E.; Droller, M.J.; Liu, B.C. Sensitivity and specificity of NMP-22, telomerase, and BTA in the detection of human bladder cancer. *Urology* **1998**, *52*, 398–402. [CrossRef]

19. Kinoshita, H.; Ogawa, O.; Kakehi, Y.; Mishina, M.; Mitsumori, K.; Itoh, N.; Yamada, H.; Terachi, T.; Yoshida, O. Detection of telomerase activity in exfoliated cells in urine from patients with bladder cancer. *J. Natl. Cancer Inst.* **1997**, *89*, 724–730. [CrossRef]

20. Yoshida, K.; Sugino, T.; Tahara, H.; Woodman, A.; Bolodeoku, J.; Nargund, V.; Fellows, G.; Goodison, S.; Tahara, E.; Tarin, D. Telomerase activity in bladder carcinoma and its implication for noninvasive diagnosis by detection of exfoliated cancer cells in urine. *Cancer* **1997**, *79*, 362–369. [CrossRef]

21. Sanchini, M.A.; Bravaccini, S.; Medri, L.; Gunelli, R.; Nanni, O.; Monti, F.; Baccarani, P.C.; Ravaioli, A.; Bercovich, E.; Amadori, D.; et al. Urine telomerase: An important marker in the diagnosis of bladder cancer. *Neoplasia* **2004**, *6*, 234–239. [CrossRef] [PubMed]

22. Sullivan, P.S.; Chan, J.B.; Levin, M.R.; Rao, J. Urine cytology and adjunct markers for detection and surveillance of bladder cancer. *Am. J. Transl. Res.* **2010**, *2*, 412–440. [PubMed]

23. Li, T.; Zou, L.; Zhang, J.; Li, G.; Ling, L. Non-invasive diagnosis of bladder cancer by detecting telomerase activity in human urine using hybridization chain reaction and dynamic light scattering. *Anal. Chim. Acta* **2019**, *13*, 90–97. [CrossRef] [PubMed]

24. Ludlow, A.T.; Robin, J.D.; Sayed, M.; Litterst, C.M.; Shelton, D.N.; Shay, J.W.; Wright, W.E. Quantitative telomerase enzyme activity determination using droplet digital PCR with single cell resolution. *Nucleic Acids Res.* **2014**, *42*, e104. [CrossRef] [PubMed]

25. Vukašinović, A.R.; Kotur-Stevuljević, J.M.; Mlakar, V.; Sopić, M.D.; Cvetković, Z.P.; Petković, M.R.; Spasojević-Kalimanovska, V.V.; Bogavac-Stanojević, N.B.; Ostanek, B. Telomerase stability and evaluation of real-time telomeric repeat amplification protocol. *Scand. J. Clin. Lab. Investig.* **2019**, *79*, 188–193. [CrossRef]

26. Su, D.; Huang, X.; Dong, C.; Ren, J. Quantitative Determination of Telomerase Activity by Combining Fluorescence Correlation Spectroscopy with Telomerase Repeat Amplification Protocol. *Anal. Chem.* **2018**, *90*, 1006–1013. [CrossRef]

27. Müller, M. Telomerase: Its clinical relevance in the diagnosis of bladder cancer. *Oncogene* **2002**, *21*, 650–655. [CrossRef]

28. Weikert, S.; Krause, H.; Wolff, I.; Christoph, F.; Schrader, M.; Emrich, T.; Miller, K.; Müller, M. Quantitative evaluation of telomerase subunits in urine as biomarkers for noninvasive detection of bladder cancer. *Int. J. Cancer* **2005**, *117*, 274–280. [CrossRef]

29. Glukhov, A.I.; Grigorieva, Y.E.; Gordeev, S.A.; Vinarov, A.Z.; Potoldykova, N.V. Development of noninvasive bladder cancer diagnosis on basis of telomerase and it's subunits hTERT and hTR detection. *Biomed. Khim.* **2015**, *61*, 150–160. [CrossRef]

30. Tilki, D.; Burger, M.; Dalbagni, G.; Grossman, H.B.; Hakenberg, O.W.; Palou, J.; Reich, O.; Roupret, M.; Shariat, S.F.; Zlotta, A.R. Urine markers for detection and surveillance of non-muscle-invasive bladder cancer. *Eur. Urol.* **2011**, *60*, 484–492. [CrossRef]

31. Liu, K.; Hodes, R.J.; Weng, N. Cutting edge: Telomerase activation in human T lymphocytes does not require increase in telomerase reverse transcriptase (hTERT) protein but is associated with hTERT phosphorylation and nuclear translocation. *J. Immunol.* **2001**, *166*, 4826–4830. [CrossRef] [PubMed]

32. March-Villalba, J.A.; Panach-Navarrete, J.; Herrero-Cervera, M.J.; Aliño-Pellicer, S.; Martínez-Jabaloyas, J.M. hTERT mRNA expression in urine as a useful diagnostic tool in bladder cancer. Comparison with cytology and NMP22 BladderCheck Test®. *Actas Urológicas Españolas (Engl. Ed.)* **2018**, *42*, 524–530. [CrossRef]

33. Clinton, T.; Lotan, Y. Review of the Clinical Approaches to the Use of Urine-based Tumor Markers in Bladder Cancer. *Rambam Maimonides Med. J.* **2017**, *8*, e0040. [CrossRef] [PubMed]

34. Ecke, T.H.; Weiß, S.; Stephan, C.; Hallmann, S.; Arndt, C.; Barski, D.; Otto, T.; Gerullis, H. UBC(®) Rapid Test-A Urinary Point-of-Care (POC) Assay for Diagnosis of Bladder Cancer with a focus on Non-Muscle Invasive High-Grade Tumors: Results of a Multicenter-Study. *Int. J. Mol. Sci.* **2018**, *19*, 3841. [CrossRef] [PubMed]

35. O'Sullivan, P.; Sharples, K.; Dalphin, M.; Davidson, P.; Gilling, P.; Cambridge, L.; Harvey, J.; Toro, T.; Giles, N.; Luxmanan, C.; et al. A multigene urine test for the detection and stratification of bladder cancer in patients presenting with hematuria. *J. Urol.* **2012**, *188*, 741–747. [CrossRef] [PubMed]

36. Bravaccini, S.; Casadio, V.; Gunelli, R.; Bucchi, L.; Zoli, W.; Amadori, D.; Silvestrini, R.; Calistri, D. Combining cytology, TRAP assay, and FISH analysis for the detection of bladder cancer in symptomatic patients. *Ann. Oncol.* **2011**, *22*, 2294–2298. [CrossRef]

37. Halling, K.C.; King, W.; Sokolova, I.A.; Karnes, R.J.; Meyer, R.G.; Powell, E.L.; Sebo, T.J.; Cheville, J.C.; Clayton, A.C.; Krajnik, K.L.; et al. A comparison of BTA stat, hemoglobin dipstick, telomerase and Vysis UroVysion assays for the detection of urothelial carcinoma in urine. *J. Urol.* **2002**, *167*, 2001–2006. [CrossRef]

38. Cavallo, D.; Casadio, V.; Bravaccini, S.; Iavicoli, S.; Pira, E.; Romano, C.; Fresegna, A.M.; Maiello, R.; Ciervo, A.; Buresti, G.; et al. Assessment of DNA damage and telomerase activity in exfoliated urinary cells as sensitive and noninvasive biomarkers for early diagnosis of bladder cancer in ex-workers of a rubber tyres industry. *Biomed. Res. Int.* **2014**, *2014*, 370907. [CrossRef]

39. Schmitz-Dräger, B.J.; Droller, M.; Lokeshwar, V.B.; Lotan, Y.; Hudson, M.A.; van Rhijn, B.W.; Marberger, M.J.; Fradet, Y.; Hemstreet, G.P.; Malmstrom, P.U.; et al. Molecular markers for bladder cancer screening, early diagnosis, and surveillance: The WHO/ICUD consensus. *Urol. Int.* **2015**, *94*, 1–24. [CrossRef]

40. Larré, S.; Catto, J.W.; Cookson, M.S.; Messing, E.M.; Shariat, S.F.; Soloway, M.S.; Svatek, R.S.; Lotan, Y.; Zlotta, A.R.; Grossman, H.B. Screening for bladder cancer: Rationale, limitations, whom to target, and perspectives. *Eur. Urol.* **2013**, *63*, 1049–1058. [CrossRef]

41. Xylinas, E.; Kluth, L.A.; Rieken, M.; Karakiewicz, P.I.; Lotan, Y.; Shariat, S.F. Urine markers for detection and surveillance of bladder cancer. *Urol. Oncol.* **2014**, *32*, 222–229. [CrossRef] [PubMed]

42. Shegay, P.V.; Zhavoronkov, A.A.; Gaifullin, N.M.; Vorob'ev, N.V.; Alekseev, B.Y.; Popov, S.V.; Garazha, A.V.; Buzdin, A.A.; Kaprin, A.D. Potentialities of MicroRNA Diagnosis in Patients with Bladder Cancer. *Bull. Exp. Biol. Med.* **2017**, *164*, 106–108. [CrossRef] [PubMed]

43. Killela, P.J.; Reitman, Z.J.; Jiao, Y.; Bettegowda, C.; Agrawal, N.; Diaz, L.A., Jr.; Friedman, A.H.; Friedman, H.; Gallia, G.L.; Giovanella, B.C.; et al. TERT promoter mutations occur frequently in gliomas and a subset of tumors derived from cells with low rates of self-renewal. *Proc. Natl. Acad. Sci. USA* **2013**, *110*, 6021–6026. [CrossRef] [PubMed]

44. Horn, S.; Figl, A.; Rachakonda, P.S.; Fischer, C.; Sucker, A.; Gast, A.; Kadel, S.; Moll, I.; Nagore, E.; Hemminki, K.; et al. TERT promoter mutations in familial and sporadic melanoma. *Science* **2013**, *339*, 959–961. [CrossRef]
45. Huang, F.W.; Hodis, E.; Xu, M.J.; Kryukov, G.V.; Chin, L.; Garraway, L.A. Highly recurrent TERT promoter mutations in human melanoma. *Science* **2013**, *339*, 957–959. [CrossRef]
46. Descotes, F.; Kara, N.; Decaussin-Petrucci, M.; Piaton, E.; Geiguer, F.; Rodriguez-Lafrasse, C.; Terrier, J.E.; Lopez, J.; Ruffion, A. Non-invasive prediction of recurrence in bladder cancer by detecting somatic TERT promoter mutations in urine. *Br. J. Cancer* **2017**, *117*, 583–587. [CrossRef]
47. Hayashi, Y.; Fujita, K.; Matsuzaki, K.; Matsushita, M.; Kawamura, N.; Koh, Y.; Nakano, K.; Wang, C.; Ishizuya, Y.; Yamamoto, Y.; et al. Diagnostic potential of TERT promoter and FGFR3 mutations in urinary cell-free DNA in upper tract urothelial carcinoma. *Cancer Sci.* **2019**, *110*, 1771–1779. [CrossRef]
48. Allory, Y.; Beukers, W.; Sagrera, A.; Flandez, M.; Marques, M.; Marquez, M.; van der Keur, K.A.; Dyrskjot, L.; Lurkin, I.; Vermeij, M.; et al. Telomerase reverse transcriptase promoter mutations in bladder cancer: High frequency across stages, detection in urine, and lack of association with outcome. *Eur. Urol.* **2014**, *65*, 360–366. [CrossRef]
49. Eich, M.-L.; Rodriguez Pena, M.D.C.; Springer, S.U.; Taheri, D.; Tregnago, A.C.; Salles, D.C.; Bezerra, S.M.; Cunha, I.W.; Fujita, K.; Ertoy, D.; et al. Incidence and distribution of UroSEEK gene panel in a multi-institutional cohort of bladder urothelial carcinoma. *Mod. Pathol.* **2019**, *32*, 1544–1550. [CrossRef]
50. Hurst, C.; Platt, F.; Knowles, M. Abstract 2240: TERT promoter mutations are highly prevalent in bladder cancer and represent a potential new urinary biomarker. *Cancer Res.* **2014**, *74*, 2240.
51. Kurtis, B.; Zhuge, J.; Ojaimi, C.; Ye, F.; Cai, D.; Zhang, D.; Fallon, J.T.; Zhong, M. Recurrent TERT promoter mutations in urothelial carcinoma and potential clinical applications. *Ann. Diagn. Pathol.* **2016**, *21*, 7–11. [CrossRef] [PubMed]
52. Pietzak, E.J.; Bagrodia, A.; Cha, E.K.; Drill, E.N.; Iyer, G.; Isharwal, S.; Ostrovnaya, I.; Baez, P.; Li, Q.; Berger, M.F.; et al. Next-generation Sequencing of Nonmuscle Invasive Bladder Cancer Reveals Potential Biomarkers and Rational Therapeutic Targets. *Eur. Urol.* **2017**, *72*, 952–959. [CrossRef] [PubMed]
53. Rachakonda, P.S.; Hosen, I.; de Verdier, P.J.; Fallah, M.; Heidenreich, B.; Ryk, C.; Wiklund, N.P.; Steineck, G.; Schadendorf, D.; Hemminki, K.; et al. TERT promoter mutations in bladder cancer affect patient survival and disease recurrence through modification by a common polymorphism. *Proc. Natl. Acad. Sci. USA* **2013**, *110*, 17426–17431. [CrossRef] [PubMed]
54. Kinde, I.; Munari, E.; Faraj, S.F.; Hruban, R.H.; Schoenberg, M.; Bivalacqua, T.; Allaf, M.; Springer, S.; Wang, Y.; Diaz, L.A., Jr.; et al. TERT promoter mutations occur early in urothelial neoplasia and are biomarkers of early disease and disease recurrence in urine. *Cancer Res.* **2013**, *73*, 7162–7167. [CrossRef]
55. Cowan, M.; Springer, S.; Nguyen, D.; Taheri, D.; Guner, G.; Rodriguez, M.A.; Wang, Y.; Kinde, I.; VandenBussche, C.J.; Olson, M.T.; et al. High prevalence of TERT promoter mutations in primary squamous cell carcinoma of the urinary bladder. *Mod. Pathol.* **2016**, *29*, 511–515. [CrossRef]
56. Zheng, X.; Zhuge, J.; Bezerra, S.M.; Faraj, S.F.; Munari, E.; Fallon, J.T., 3rd; Yang, X.J.; Argani, P.; Netto, G.J.; Zhong, M. High frequency of TERT promoter mutation in small cell carcinoma of bladder, but not in small cell carcinoma of other origins. *J. Hematol. Oncol.* **2014**, *7*, 014–0047. [CrossRef]
57. Cowan, M.L.; Springer, S.; Nguyen, D.; Taheri, D.; Guner, G.; Mendoza Rodriguez, M.A.; Wang, Y.; Kinde, I.; Del Carmen Rodriguez Pena, M.; VandenBussche, C.J.; et al. Detection of TERT promoter mutations in primary adenocarcinoma of the urinary bladder. *Hum. Pathol.* **2016**, *53*, 8–13. [CrossRef]
58. Palsgrove, D.N.; Taheri, D.; Springer, S.U.; Cowan, M.; Guner, G.; Mendoza Rodriguez, M.A.; Rodriguez Pena, M.D.C.; Wang, Y.; Kinde, I.; Ricardo, B.F.P.; et al. Targeted sequencing of plasmacytoid urothelial carcinoma reveals frequent TERT promoter mutations. *Hum. Pathol.* **2019**, *85*, 1–9. [CrossRef]
59. Borah, S.; Xi, L.; Zaug, A.J.; Powell, N.M.; Dancik, G.M.; Cohen, S.B.; Costello, J.C.; Theodorescu, D.; Cech, T.R. Cancer. TERT promoter mutations and telomerase reactivation in urothelial cancer. *Science* **2015**, *347*, 1006–1010. [CrossRef]
60. Ségal-Bendirdjian, E.; Geli, V. Non-canonical Roles of Telomerase: Unraveling the Imbroglio. *Front. Cell Dev. Biol.* **2019**, *7*, 332. [CrossRef]
61. Wang, K.; Liu, T.; Ge, N.; Liu, L.; Yuan, X.; Liu, J.; Kong, F.; Wang, C.; Ren, H.; Yan, K.; et al. TERT promoter mutations are associated with distant metastases in upper tract urothelial carcinomas and serve as urinary biomarkers detected by a sensitive castPCR. *Oncotarget* **2014**, *5*, 12428–12439. [CrossRef] [PubMed]

62. Bettegowda, C.; Sausen, M.; Leary, R.J.; Kinde, I.; Wang, Y.; Agrawal, N.; Bartlett, B.R.; Wang, H.; Luber, B.; Alani, R.M.; et al. Detection of Circulating Tumor DNA in Early- and Late-Stage Human Malignancies. *Sci. Transl. Med.* **2014**, *6*, 224ra24. [CrossRef] [PubMed]

63. Srisuwan, W.; Tatu, T. A Simple Whole-Blood Polymerase Chain Reaction without DNA Extraction for Thalassemia Diagnosis. *Hemoglobin* **2018**, *42*, 178–183. [CrossRef]

64. Kikin, O.; D'Antonio, L.; Bagga, P.S. QGRS Mapper: A web-based server for predicting G-quadruplexes in nucleotide sequences. *Nucl. Acids Res.* **2006**, *34*, W676–W682. [CrossRef]

65. Batista, R.; Vinagre, J.; Prazeres, H.; Sampaio, C.; Peralta, P.; Conceição, P.; Sismeiro, A.; Leão, R.; Gomes, A.; Furriel, F.; et al. Validation of a Novel, Sensitive, and Specific Urine-Based Test for Recurrence Surveillance of Patients With Non-Muscle-Invasive Bladder Cancer in a Comprehensive Multicenter Study. *Front. Genet.* **2019**, *10*, 1237. [CrossRef] [PubMed]

66. Siravegna, G.; Marsoni, S.; Siena, S.; Bardelli, A. Integrating liquid biopsies into the management of cancer. *Nat. Rev. Clin. Oncol.* **2017**, *14*, 531–548. [CrossRef] [PubMed]

67. Kinde, I.; Wu, J.; Papadopoulos, N.; Kinzler, K.W.; Vogelstein, B. Detection and quantification of rare mutations with massively parallel sequencing. *Proc. Natl. Acad. Sci. USA* **2011**, *108*, 9530–9535. [CrossRef]

68. Forshew, T.; Murtaza, M.; Parkinson, C.; Gale, D.; Tsui, D.W.Y.; Kaper, F.; Dawson, S.-J.; Piskorz, A.M.; Jimenez-Linan, M.; Bentley, D.; et al. Noninvasive Identification and Monitoring of Cancer Mutations by Targeted Deep Sequencing of Plasma DNA. *Sci. Transl. Med.* **2012**, *4*, 136ra68. [CrossRef]

69. Gale, D.; Lawson, A.R.J.; Howarth, K.; Madi, M.; Durham, B.; Smalley, S.; Calaway, J.; Blais, S.; Jones, G.; Clark, J.; et al. Development of a highly sensitive liquid biopsy platform to detect clinically-relevant cancer mutations at low allele fractions in cell-free DNA. *PLoS ONE* **2018**, *13*, e0194630. [CrossRef]

70. Newman, A.M.; Bratman, S.V.; To, J.; Wynne, J.F.; Eclov, N.C.; Modlin, L.A.; Liu, C.L.; Neal, J.W.; Wakelee, H.A.; Merritt, R.E.; et al. An ultrasensitive method for quantitating circulating tumor DNA with broad patient coverage. *Nat. Med.* **2014**, *20*, 548–554. [CrossRef]

71. Delhomme, T.M.; Avogbe, P.H.; Gabriel, A.A.G.; Alcala, N.; Leblay, N.; Voegele, C.; Vallée, M.; Chopard, P.; Chabrier, A.; Abedi-Ardekani, B.; et al. Needlestack: An ultra-sensitive variant caller for multi-sample next generation sequencing data. *NAR Genom. Bioinform.* **2020**, *2*, 20. [CrossRef] [PubMed]

72. Dahmcke, C.M.; Steven, K.E.; Larsen, L.K.; Poulsen, A.L.; Abdul-Al, A.; Dahl, C.; Guldberg, P. A Prospective Blinded Evaluation of Urine-DNA Testing for Detection of Urothelial Bladder Carcinoma in Patients with Gross Hematuria. *Eur. Urol.* **2016**, *70*, 916–919. [CrossRef] [PubMed]

73. Critelli, R.; Fasanelli, F.; Oderda, M.; Polidoro, S.; Assumma, M.B.; Viberti, C.; Preto, M.; Gontero, P.; Cucchiarale, G.; Lurkin, I.; et al. Detection of multiple mutations in urinary exfoliated cells from male bladder cancer patients at diagnosis and during follow-up. *Oncotarget* **2016**, *7*, 67435–67448. [CrossRef] [PubMed]

74. Wang, K.; Liu, T.; Liu, L.; Liu, J.; Liu, C.; Wang, C.; Ge, N.; Ren, H.; Yan, K.; Hu, S.; et al. TERT promoter mutations in renal cell carcinomas and upper tract urothelial carcinomas. *Oncotarget* **2014**, *5*, 1829–1836. [CrossRef]

75. Springer, S.U.; Chen, C.-H.; Rodriguez Pena, M.D.C.; Li, L.; Douville, C.; Wang, Y.; Cohen, J.D.; Taheri, D.; Silliman, N.; Schaefer, J.; et al. Non-invasive detection of urothelial cancer through the analysis of driver gene mutations and aneuploidy. *eLife* **2018**, *7*, e32143. [CrossRef]

76. Ou, Z.; Li, K.; Yang, T.; Dai, Y.; Chandra, M.; Ning, J.; Wang, Y.; Xu, R.; Gao, T.; Xie, Y.; et al. Detection of bladder cancer using urinary cell-free DNA and cellular DNA. *Clin. Transl. Med.* **2020**, *9*, 4. [CrossRef]

77. Ward, D.G.; Baxter, L.; Gordon, N.S.; Ott, S.; Savage, R.S.; Beggs, A.D.; James, J.D.; Lickiss, J.; Green, S.; Wallis, Y.; et al. Multiplex PCR and Next Generation Sequencing for the Non-Invasive Detection of Bladder Cancer. *PLoS ONE* **2016**, *11*, e0149756. [CrossRef]

78. Togneri, F.S.; Ward, D.G.; Foster, J.M.; Devall, A.J.; Wojtowicz, P.; Alyas, S.; Vasques, F.R.; Oumie, A.; James, N.D.; Cheng, K.K.; et al. Genomic complexity of urothelial bladder cancer revealed in urinary cfDNA. *Eur. J. Hum. Genet.* **2016**, *24*, 1167–1174. [CrossRef]

79. Szarvas, T.; Kovalszky, I.; Bedi, K.; Szendroi, A.; Majoros, A.; Riesz, P.; Fule, T.; Laszlo, V.; Kiss, A.; Romics, I. Deletion analysis of tumor and urinary DNA to detect bladder cancer: Urine supernatant versus urine sediment. *Oncol. Rep.* **2007**, *18*, 405–409. [CrossRef]

80. Russo, I.J.; Ju, Y.; Gordon, N.S.; Zeegers, M.P.; Cheng, K.K.; James, N.D.; Bryan, R.T.; Ward, D.G. Toward Personalised Liquid Biopsies for Urothelial Carcinoma: Characterisation of ddPCR and Urinary cfDNA for the Detection of the TERT 228 G > A/T Mutation. *Bladder Cancer* **2018**, *4*, 41–48. [CrossRef]

81. Hayashi, Y.; Fujita, K.; Matsuzaki, K.; Eich, M.L.; Tomiyama, E.; Matsushita, M.; Koh, Y.; Nakano, K.; Wang, C.; Ishizuya, Y.; et al. Clinical Significance of Hotspot Mutation Analysis of Urinary Cell-Free DNA in Urothelial Bladder Cancer. *Front. Oncol.* **2020**, *10*, 755. [CrossRef] [PubMed]

82. Ward, D.G.; Gordon, N.S.; Boucher, R.H.; Pirrie, S.J.; Baxter, L.; Ott, S.; Silcock, L.; Whalley, C.M.; Stockton, J.D.; Beggs, A.D.; et al. Targeted deep sequencing of urothelial bladder cancers and associated urinary DNA: A 23-gene panel with utility for non-invasive diagnosis and risk stratification. *BJU Int.* **2019**, *124*, 532–544. [CrossRef] [PubMed]

83. Pepe, M.S.; Etzioni, R.; Feng, Z.; Potter, J.D.; Thompson, M.L.; Thornquist, M.; Winget, M.; Yasui, Y. Phases of biomarker development for early detection of cancer. *J. Natl. Cancer Inst.* **2001**, *93*, 1054–1061. [CrossRef] [PubMed]

84. Pesch, B.; Brüning, T.; Johnen, G.; Casjens, S.; Bonberg, N.; Taeger, D.; Müller, A.; Weber, D.G.; Behrens, T. Biomarker research with prospective study designs for the early detection of cancer. *Biochim. Biophys. Acta* **2014**, *5*, 874–883. [CrossRef] [PubMed]

85. Svatek, R.S.; Hollenbeck, B.K.; Holmäng, S.; Lee, R.; Kim, S.P.; Stenzl, A.; Lotan, Y. The economics of bladder cancer: Costs and considerations of caring for this disease. *Eur. Urol.* **2014**, *66*, 253–262. [CrossRef] [PubMed]

86. Leal, J.; Luengo-Fernandez, R.; Sullivan, R.; Witjes, J.A. Economic Burden of Bladder Cancer Across the European Union. *Eur. Urol.* **2016**, *69*, 438–447. [CrossRef] [PubMed]

87. Lotan, Y.; Svatek, R.S.; Sagalowsky, A.I. Should we screen for bladder cancer in a high-risk population?: A cost per life-year saved analysis. *Cancer* **2006**, *107*, 982–990. [CrossRef]

88. Zanetti, M. A second chance for telomerase reverse transcriptase in anticancer immunotherapy. *Nat. Rev. Clin. Oncol.* **2017**, *14*, 115–128. [CrossRef]

89. Carrozza, F.; Santoni, M.; Piva, F.; Cheng, L.; Lopez-Beltran, A.; Scarpelli, M.; Montironi, R.; Battelli, N.; Tamberi, S. Emerging immunotherapeutic strategies targeting telomerases in genitourinary tumors. *Crit. Rev. Oncol. Hematol.* **2018**, *131*, 1–6. [CrossRef]

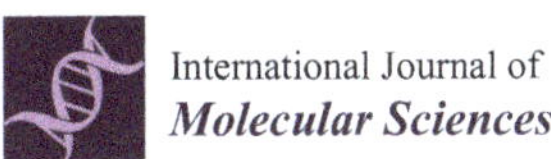
International Journal of
Molecular Sciences

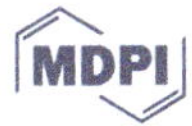

Review

Diagnostic and Prognostic Potential of Biomarkers CYFRA 21.1, ERCC1, p53, FGFR3 and TATI in Bladder Cancers

Milena Matuszczak and Maciej Salagierski *

Department of Urology, Collegium Medicum, University of Zielona Góra, 65-046 Zielona Góra, Poland; matuszczakmilena@gmail.com
* Correspondence: m.salagierski@cm.uz.zgora.pl

Received: 16 April 2020; Accepted: 5 May 2020; Published: 9 May 2020

Abstract: The high occurrence of bladder cancer and its tendency to recur in combination with a lifelong surveillance make the treatment of superficial bladder cancer one of the most expensive and time-consuming. Moreover, carcinoma in situ often leads to muscle invasion with an unfavorable prognosis. Currently, invasive methods including cystoscopy and cytology remain a gold standard. The aim of this study was to explore urine-based biomarkers to find the one with the best specificity and sensitivity, which would allow optimizing the treatment plan. In this review, we sum up the current knowledge about Cytokeratin fragments (CYFRA 21.1), Excision Repair Cross-Complementation 1 (ERCC1), Tumour Protein p53 (Tp53), Fibroblast Growth Factor Receptor 3 (FGFR3), Tumor-Associated Trypsin Inhibitor (TATI) and their potential applications in clinical practice.

Keywords: biomarkers; bladder cancer; tumor markers; prognosis

1. Introduction: Bladder Cancer Issues and Biomarkers

Bladder cancer is the most common urinary site of malignancy and the second most common reason of cancer deaths from the genitourinary tract after prostate cancer in the United States, with 81,400 new cases and 17,980 deaths in the year 2020 [1]. Globally there are about 430,000 new cases diagnosed each year [2].

Favorably, non-invasive lesions constitute approximately 75–80% of newly diagnosed urothelial bladder cancers (UBC). More than 50% of UBCs are caused by smoking. Other important factors include occupational exposure to aromatic amines and polycyclic hydrocarbons. Less evident is the impact of diet and environmental pollution. Increasing data indicate that genetic predisposition plays a role in UBC pathogenesis [2–4].

There are two major groups of patients with distinct prognosis and molecular features.

Carcinoma in situ (CIS) and tumors staged as Ta, T1 are grouped as non-muscle-invasive bladder cancers (NMIBC) [5]. NMIBC patients generally have a significant risk of recurrence and potential clinical course for progression [6] but their life expectancy is long and the cancer rarely progresses to muscle invasion. For NMIBC, the major problem is that after the initial transurethral resection of the bladder (TURB), they characteristically recur in 50–70% of cases, with only approximately 10–20% of cases progressing to muscle-invasive bladder cancer (MIBC) [7].

Muscle-invasive tumors very often metastasize and are usually diagnosed de novo, the prognosis is unfavorable and for decades there has been made no major innovation in therapy. Papillary non-invasive cancers (pTa) grow up from carcinoma in situ (CIS) of the urothelium (frequently TP53-mutated, a high-grade lesion) and often metastasize and evolve into muscle invasion [8]. Robertson et al. demonstrated that MIBC shows high overall mutation rates but fortunately most of them seem to be passenger variation without any functional meaning, or repeated genetic alterations including the *TP53, FGFR3, PIK3CA* and *RB1* genes' mutations [4,9].

Muscle-invasive bladder cancer (MIBC) is a high risk but potentially curable disease. Unfortunately, still nearly half of patients die from MIBC despite getting the appropriate treatment [10,11]. The major problem in the management of superficial bladder cancer is its tendency to recur. Lifelong surveillance with a relatively long-life expectancy (5-year survival rate > 90%) makes it the most expensive and time-consuming malignancy to treat.

In recent years, a great effort has been put in the search for new potential biomarkers such as protein 53 (p53), ERCC1, CYFRA 21.1, FGFR3 and TATI in the prognosis and prediction of bladder cancer. The *FGFR3* mutations could be a marker of low-grade and early stage tumors, while the changes in p53 appear better in detecting high-grade or advanced cancers.

2. Diagnostic and Prognostic Potential of Bladder Cancer Biomarkers

2.1. Cytokeratin Fragment 21.1 (CYFRA 21.1)

Cytokeratin fragments (CYFRA 21.1) is an ELISA-based assay that detects the concentration of a soluble fragment of cytokeratin 19 by using two monoclonal antibodies [12]. The studies have shown that the differentiation between liquid biopsies of healthy (non-cancer) individuals and BC patients may be done using this biomarker.

Authors [13] concluded that both serum and urine CYFRA 21.1 present decisive indexes for bladder cancer diagnosis. They made a systematic analysis which indicated the pooled sensitivities and specificities for the serum and urine CYFRA 21.1 were of 42%, 82%, 94% and 80%, respectively. The areas under the receiver operating characteristic curves (AUC) for the serum and urine CYFRA 21.1 were in sequence 0.88 and 0.87 (Table 1).

In an extensive meta-analysis of three case–control studies Kuang [14] confirmed that urinary or serum samples containing CYFRA21.1 can be used as diagnostic biomarkers and for the distinction between local and metastatic bladder cancer. In this meta-analysis, all healthy individuals had a lower CYFRA21.1 level than patients with bladder cancer. The locally invasive disease showed also lower CYFRA 21.1 levels than the subgroup with metastatic bladder cancer. Notwithstanding, between patients with bladder cancer stage I and stage II, and among the group of patients with local stage II and III were no significant differences in the CYFRA21.1 level. Therefore, CYFRA 21.1 cannot be useful in differentiating grades I–III of local bladder cancer but may be used as a diagnostic biomarker and to detect metastases.

Nisman [15] evaluated that for detecting transitional cell tumors that were grade 1 with CYFRA 21.1 measured in urine samples gave a three-times higher sensitivity compared with the sensitivity of cytology.

CYFRA 21.1 has a high sensitivity for identifying high-grade and CIS tumors and a greater accuracy for the detection of primary tumors than for the recurrence, but it cannot be used for an early detection of BC. The specificity of this test is between 73% and 86% and the sensitivity is between 70% and 90% [12,15,16].

Andreadis and colleagues [17] analyzed a group of 142 patients with invasive bladder cell carcinoma, including 56 patients with stage T1-4 N0 M0 and 86 with involved lymph nodes or distant metastases. The control group contained 33 healthy volunteers. Seven per cent of patients with the locally advanced disease and 66% of patients with the metastatic disease had an elevated level of this biomarker. CYFRA 21.1 may also be a useful tool in indicating the response to chemotherapy.

Importantly, Nisman and colleagues [15] showed that CYFRA 21.1 detected 100% of CIS, 92.8% of invasive bladder tumors (T2 or higher classification) and 91.9% of grade 3 tumors. The CYFRA 21.1 assay identified almost all tumors (with the exception of only one) that had a positive cytology. Moreover, the assay detected 65% of recurrent tumors and 71% of primary tumors that were omitted by cytopathology.

Unfortunately, CYFRA 21.1 is a false positive in the group of patients with urinary tract infections, stones, history of pelvic radiotherapy, urethral catheterization or BCG intravesical instillation within the three previous months. Even years following intravesical immunotherapy with the BCG level of urinary CYFRA 21.1 may be elevated.

Importantly, the abnormal serum level of CYFRA 21.1 [18] corresponds with a worse response.

In conclusion, Washino [19] observed that serum CYFRA 21.1 might be a marker of high-grade and advanced urothelial carcinoma. On the contrary, CEA and CA19-9 were not demonstrated as potential tumor markers.

The centrifugation step in the methodology is the very important one to improve the precision of this assay by removing cells' debris that contains a large amount of CYFRA 21.1, i.e., after this process, a significant decrease in the number of true positive and false positive results can be observed [20].

CYFRA 21.1 is considered as one of the best urinary markers for bladder cancer. Jeong and colleagues noticed that CYFRA 21.1 and NMP22 are the most effective at predicting bladder cancer [21]. However, there is a disadvantage being that the concentrations of both markers are strongly influenced by benign urological diseases, intravesical instillations and also a disappointing performance in low-stage bladder cancer.

Table 1. Predictive capacity of bladder cancer biomarkers.

Protein Name	Gene Symbol	Purpose	Diagnostic Value	Prognostic Value	FDA Approved	Method	Samples Used (No. Patients)	Predicitive Capacity	Reference
CYFRA 21.1	*KRT19*	Diagnostic and surveillance	Both serum and urine CYFRA 21.1 levels provide an effective index for the diagnosis of BC.	High risk of malignancy- significantly higher serum level of CYFRA 21.1 according to tumour stage ($p < 0.01$) and grade ($p < 0.05$). Patients with increased CYFRA 21.1 level had significantly worse disease-specific survival ($p < 0.0001$, log rank test) [19]. Moreover, patients with metastases had a higher CYFRA 21.1 level than those with locally invasive BC [14].	No	Meta-analysis performed using STATA 12.0 on the base of studies had published before 2 November 2014 in EMBASE, Web of Science and Medline databases. Quality of the studies was assessed by revised QUADAS tools, all of selected studies were English language publications and evaluate diagnostic accuracy of CYFRA 21.1 in patients with BC. Systematic review included 13 studies and 1,262 BC and 1,233 non-bladder cancer patients. 8 studies measured urine and 5 serum level of CYFRA 21.1. In serum detection of CYFRA 21.1 471 BC and 296 non- bladder cancer patients were analyzed. Urine CYFRA 21.1 studies included 538 BC and 678 non-bladder cancer patients.	Urine (n = 538 BC/678 control) Serum (n = 471 BC/296 control)	Sensitivity = 82% Specificity = 80% AUC = 0.87 Sensitivity = 42% Specificity = 94% AUC = 0.88	[12–14,19]
DNA EXCISION REPAIR PROTEIN ERCC-1	*ERCC1*	Diagnostic and surveillance	71.3% (308/432) of cases was ERCC1 positive. Ta = 3.2% T1 = 11.7% T2 = 21.4% T3 = 45.1% T4 = 18.5% CIS = 8.1% LG = 20.8% HG = 79.2%	ERCC positive tumour had significantly better disease-free survival (HR 0.7, $p = 0.028$) than ERCC1 negative tumours. ERCC1 positive tumours has significantly reduced risk of recurrences (HR 0.71, $p = 0.021$). The 5-year DFS and CSS were better for ERCC1 positive than negative, and were respectively 62% vs 49% and 70% vs 59%. However, there was no important outcomes of adjuvant cisplatin-based chemotherapy by ERCC1 status.	No	Study cohort had 432 patients and 308 of tumours expressed ERCC1. Staining was conducted using Abcam® mouse monoclonal antibody and expression of ERCC1was evaluated by 2 pathologists. Chi-square test was made to assessed differences between ERCC1 expression. All analyses were performed with STATA®, version 13.1. Primary tumour samples collected at RC, cells were lysed and total RNA was extracted with Qiagen® kit. ERCC1 mRNA expression was measured by RNA sequencing and confirmed by qPCR using TaqMan® gene expression assays.	UCB cell lines in vitro (n = 432)	No data	[22]
TUMOR SUPPRESSOR P53	*TP53* gene	Diagnostic (as a complementary tool) and surveillance	54% (56/103) of cases had TP53 mutations. Ta = 40% T1 = 52% T2 = 80% CIS = 55% LG = 34% HG = 62%	High risk of malignancy-significant difference of TP53 mutations according to tumour stage ($p = 0.005$) and to cellular grade ($p < 0.001$).	No	Sample collection of urine and tumours from 103 patients. Extraction of mRNA was made by Micro mRNA Purification Kit. Then Verso Kit® were used to reverse transcription, amplification was performed by PCR PrimeStar®. FASAY assay was used to detect *TP53* mutations in tumour tissues and urinary cells. Statistical test was performed using SPSS software®, version 17.	Primary bladder tumours and associated urine (n = 103)	Sensitivity = 34% Specificity = 87% PPV = 0.76 NPV = 0.53	[23]

Table 1. *Cont.*

Protein Name	Gene Symbol	Purpose	Diagnostic Value	Prognostic Value	FDA Approved	Method	Samples Used (No. Patients)	Predicitive Capacity	Reference
FIBROBLAST GROWTH FACTOR RECEPTOR 3	FGFR3 gene	Diagnostic (as a complementary tool) and surveillance	36% (37/103) of cases had FGFR3 mutations. Ta = 55% T1 = 29% T2 = 19% CIS = 10% LG = 62% HG = 26%	Low risk of malignancy-negative association of FGFR3 mutations based on tumour stage ($p = 0.002$) and cellular grade ($p < 0.001$) [23]. Low level of FGFR3 expression is an independent predictor of cancer progression and is associated with HG tumours [24].	No *	Sample collection of urine and tumours from 103 patients. Extraction of genomic DNA was performed by QIAamp Viral RNA® Mini kit. Multiplex PCR Kit were used to amplification. Snapshot ® kit was used to detect FGFR3 eight most frequent mutations hotspots in tumour tissues and urinary cells (two independent analysis were carried out). Statistical test was performed using SPSS software®, version 17.	Primary bladder tumours and associated urine ($n = 103$)	Sensitivity = 43% Specificity = 98% PPV = 0.94 NPV =0.76	[23]
								Sensitivity = 97.6% Specificity = 84.8% AUC = 0.96 NPV = 0.996 (1)	[25]
TUMOR-ASSOCIATED TRYPSIN INHIBITOR	SPINK1 gene	Diagnostic and surveillance	49.1% (54/110) of cases had TATI expression. Stage <T2 = 66.7% Stage ≥T2 = 44.9% LG = 76.2% HG = 44.9%	Low risk of malignancy- negative association of TATI expression was positively correlated based on tumour stage ($p = 0.048$) and poor differentiation ($p = 0.013$). Significant differences were observed between TATI-positive and negative specimens in PFS and OS (Log-rank test, $p = 0.003, 0.003$). In a group of patients with BC undergoing RC TATI expression was independent protective factor. Moreover, TATI expression could enhance prognostic value of p53.	No	Study cohort had 110 patients and 54 of tumours, undergone RC, expressed TATI. Staining was conducted using Abcam® anti-TATI monoclonal antibody and expression of TATI was evaluated by 2 pathologists. Proportion of immune-positive cells and their staining intensity was scored in two scales and used to evaluation of TATI expression. All analyses were performed with SPSS software, version 21.	Tissue microarrays from UCB ($n = 110$)	No data	[26]
						Study cohort consisted of 160 patients, divided into 3 groups. Group 1 had 80 primary HG UBC. Group 2 of 40 healthy volunteers and group 3 of 40 benign UBC. TATI was measured using a radioimmunoassay according to the manufacturer's instructions (Orion Diagnostica). Analyses were performer with STATA®, statistical software, version 6.0	Urine ($n = 160$)	Sensitivity = 85.7% Specificity = 77.5%	[27]

(1) Using a logistic regression analysis with a model consisting of the 3 markers' methylation values, FGFR3 status, age and known smoker status at the diagnosis time. * It is available THERASCREEN® FGFR RGQ RT-PCR KIT. Abbreviations: HR—Hazarc Ratio, n—number of patients participating in study, p—calculated probability, CIS—carcinoma in situ, HG—high grade, LG—low grade, FASAY—Functional Analysis of Separated Allele in Yeast, ELISA—enzyme-linked immunosorbent assay, IHC—immunohistochemistry, RC—radical cystectomy, BC—bladder cancer, CCS—cancer specific survival, DFS—disease-free survival, UCB—urothelial carcinoma of bladder, qPCR—quantitative polymerase chain reaction, PPV—positive predictive value, NPV—negative predictive value.

2.2. Excision Repair Cross-Complementation 1 (ERCC1)

The nucleotide excision repair (NER) pathway is important for the protection of genomic stability and for the removal of platinum-induced DNA adducts and cisplatin resistance [28,29]. The key molecules in this pathway belong to the excision repair cross-complementing group 1 (ERCC1) [30].

The ERCC1 role is detecting, repairing and rate-limiting the interstrand cross-links in DNA [31]. Therefore, this enzyme may be representative for the crucial DNA damage repair ability of the cell [32,33]. In a group of patients treated with a surgical resection, ERCC1 as the DNA repair protein may also be engaged in weakening the malignancy of tumors by reducing the amount of mutations. Moreover, genetic testing of ERCC1 expression levels could personalize the chemotherapy by selecting the patients who would benefit from platinum-based chemotherapy. A variety of tumors, including bladder tumors, show that the ERCC1 level is strongly associated with cisplatin resistance [34].

One of the first reports in the literature presenting the impact of ERCC1 expression on the survival of oncologically treated patients was the study of George R. Simon. In 2005, Simon's analysis included 51 patients who were operated on for non-small cell lung cancer and determined their ERCC1 expression. The median survival in the ERCC1 positive expression group was found to be significantly longer—94.9 months compared with 35.5 months in the negative ERCC1 group. The conclusions were that the ERCC1 expression might be an independent prognostic factor for survival in lung cancer [32].

In 2006, Olaussen's work on a large group of patients was published, which included the results of a study of 761 patients after radical lung cancer surgery. The goal was to identify a group of patients who might take an advantage from adjuvant treatment. The study showed that the benefit of adjuvant chemotherapy concerned the patients with a negative ERCC1 expression. An interesting finding was that in the group that did not receive chemotherapy but was only treated surgically, patients with a positive ERCC1 expression had a longer survival compared with those with a negative ERCC1 expression [31].

In advanced non-small cell lung cancer, the ERCC1 expression has a significant prognostic value and its high level is associated with a longer survival in patients who do not receive chemotherapy after a complete resection [31,32]. Piljić et al. indicated that the ERCC1 expression in all stages of lung carcinoma has a great value in monitoring patients receiving chemotherapy based on platinum [35]. Li et al. indicated that in a group of patients with advanced non-small cell lung cancer, ERCC1-negative had better progression-free survival (PFS) ($p = 0.016$) and overall survival (OS) ($p = 0.030$) in comparison with positive patients [36].

The value of ERCC1 has also been confirmed in other cancers. ERCC1 is one of the most frequent in 84% or even more of colon cancers, and reductions of a DNA repair gene has been observed [37,38]. In 40% of the crypts within 10 cm on each side of colonic adenocarcinomas, ERCC1 was found to be deficient [37]. The literature data presented above show a significant relationship between the ERCC1 expression and survival in different types of cancer.

In 2012, Sun [39] analyzed 93 patients with BC who underwent radical cystectomy and they demonstrated that ERCC1 can be used as a prognostic and predictive biomarker in this group. An ERCC1-positive expression was found in 58% of patients, and the study group was divided into those who received additional adjuvant chemotherapy and those without chemotherapy. It was found that patients after radical cystectomy without adjuvant chemotherapy with a high ERCC1 expression have a significantly longer five-year survival than those with a low expression, 84% to 49%, respectively. It has also been reported that ERCC1-negative patients potentially may benefit from adjuvant chemotherapy.

Klatte and colleagues [22] presented the work assessing ERCC1 as a prognostic and predictive biomarker of bladder cancer after cystectomy. In a group of 432 patients, a positive expression was found in 71% of patients. Patients with an ERCC1-positive expression had a significantly better five-year disease-free survival (DFS) than those with an ERCC1-negative expression, 62% to 49%, and cancer-specific survival (CSS), 70% to 59%, respectively. In the ERCC1-positive group, the risk of bladder cancer (BC) recurrence and death due to BC was 30% lower. Patients undergoing radical cystectomy with an ERCC1-positive expression had better survival values than those with a negative expression. Therefore, ERCC1 may be an independent prognostic marker for bladder cancer.

Similar conclusions were made in Hemdan's report. They evaluated a group of 244 patients who underwent radical cystectomy or neoadjuvant chemotherapy and radical cystectomy. Negative ERCC1 correlated with a worse overall survival in the group with only surgical treatment. It was noted that neoadjuvant chemotherapy would benefit mainly patients with an ERCC1-negative expression, while for those who were ERCC1-positive, the influence was minimal [40].

Another meta-analysis was published by Urun [41], performed on 1425 patients from 13 studies, and patients with an ERCC1-positive expression constituted 24–76% of the examined populations. The role of ERCC1 as a prognostic factor of survival was assessed in patients with advanced bladder cancer treated with platinum-based chemotherapy. The conclusions were that a positive ERCC1 expression is not significantly related to overall survival, but has a significant impact on worse progression-free survival, and may be an indicator of worse survival in patients with advanced bladder cancer, but large prospective studies are needed to consider ERCC1 as a prognostic marker in patients with advanced bladder cancer.

Sakano [42] suggested that, in the group of patients with bladder cancer undergoing a combined trimodality approach, the disease-specific survival might be predicted by the expression of ERCC1 and XRCC1. A positive expression of these molecules was connected with better disease-specific survival rates but further research is needed to confirm these results.

Analyzing the previous studies, gives controversial information about predicting the prognostic role of ERCC1 in the treatment of advanced bladder cancer. In 2018, Eldehna [34] conducted a descriptive study on 80 patients with muscle-invasive bladder cancer (stages T2–T4a) who received platinum-based chemotherapy. The results of their research showed a significant relationship between a platinum-based treatment response and the ERCC1 expression in bladder cancer tissue samples ($p = 0.013$). It was an indicative association between a negative immuno-expression and more favorable outcome but no difference between the ERCC1 expression and mean overall survival or progression-free survival in different immune-expression levels in patients was apparent. Therefore, ERCC1 may be a potential predictive but not prognostic marker and for this reason, genetic testing could personalize chemotherapy by selecting the patients who would benefit from a platinum-based treatment in bladder cancer.

In summary, ERCC1-positive tumors were associated with better prognosis in cases without chemotherapies. However, in cases with chemotherapies, ERCC1-negative tumors were associated with a better outcome.

The most possible explanation for the above scenario seems related to the function of this enzyme, which appears crucial in the DNA damage repair ability of the cell. The above DNA repair, related to the ERCC1 activity, is, however, non-beneficial for patients treated with chemotherapy, potentially leading to an "antichemotherapeutic" activity.

2.3. Tumour Protein p53 (TP53)

The common oncosuppressor gene mutated in all human cancers and the most frequently mutated gene in MIBC is the tumor protein p53 (*TP53*) [43]. Genomic integrity and stability are maintained by *TP53* via triggering a cell-cycle arrest, apoptosis, autophagy and DNA repair. Mutant p53 proteins silence the autophagy related gene (ATG) which affects the autophagic flow, and therefore suppresses regulation to the autophagic vesicles formation and their fusion with lysosomes [44]. Additionally, p53 preferentially binds to the AMPKα subunit and inhibits the AMPK activation. Mutp53s become oncogenic via the activation of AMPK [45].

Bladder carcinogenesis is closely associated with tumor suppressor dysfunction and the inactivation of *TP53* [46]. Therefore, p53 has been studied as a marker of urothelial cell carcinoma recurrence and progression.

Cheap and simple methods to detect the abnormal function of p53 is immunohistochemistry staining (IHC). The short half-life of wild-type p53 prevents its intra-nuclear accumulation [47].

Increased p53 accumulation in the cell nucleus is a result of *TP53* mutations.

Immunohistochemical patterns of *TP53* mutations are strongly associated with the progression of urothelial cell carcinoma. Plenty of data illustrate that from non-missense mutations (i.e., nonsense, insertion and deletion) to wild-type *TP53*, the expression of p53's IHC increases. That promotes the grow up of an invasive phenotype of bladder cancer [48]. The high expression of p53 has been associated with features of tumor aggressiveness and correlated with poor oncological outcomes [43,49]. Therefore, this protein level was higher in more advanced bladder cancer [50,51]. Plenty of studies have indicated that p53 can be useful to assess the level of progress and to prognose urothelial cell carcinoma [49,51].

However, Ciccasese and colleagues [52] published a study with a contradictory opinion. In their opinion, the single p53 marker is not good enough as a prognostic marker of MIBC.

Moreover, the most aggressive T1 high-grade cancers appear to be also associated with the expression of this protein. The progression from T1 NMIBC to T1HG can be predicted by a p53 overexpression [53].

Authors [51] collected data from 70 patients and showed that 16% of patients with low-grade and 91% of patients with high-grade lesions were p53-positive. There was 33% positivity in Tis, 55% in T1, 72% in T2 and 100% in T3a and T3b. These results indicated a strong intensification of p53 staining—94.6% of high-grade and 5.4% of low-grade tumors. Moreover, the p53 accumulation in the nucleus, in a group treated with radical cystectomy and in other MIBCs, has a prognostic value [54].

Another study showed that an aggressive tumor phenotype is strongly associated with the overexpression of p53 [43]. MIBC and CIS correlated with a high level of *TP53* deletion and mutation [55]. According to the TCGA cohort data [4], 89% of MIBCs have an inactivated TP53 cell-cycle pathway, with *TP53* mutations in 48%. Bladder epithelial cells become malignant by the TP53/RB1 pathway or the FGFR3/RAS pathway [55].

2.4. Fibroblast Growth Factor Receptor 3 (FGFR3)

Fibroblast growth factor receptor 3 (FGFR3) alternations are associated with urothelial cell carcinoma pathogenesis [56,57]. FGFR3 is activated by the mutation or overexpression in many bladder tumors at any stage, but is predominantly active in low-grade NMIBCs [58,59]. Higher levels of FGFR3 expression were observed in low-grade, non-invasive tumors and recurrent non-invasive tumors than in invasive and non-invasive high-grade carcinoma [57].

This marker is associated with a lower chance of progression to a muscle-invasive disease and it is like a hallmark of the low-grade pathway. FGFR3 alternations occur mainly in non-invasive tumors [59,60], specifically in the luminal-papillary subtype (35%), which has the best overall survival and is characterized by a papillary morphology [59,61]. Moreover, many studies indicated that *FGFR3* mutation and the risk of progression are an inverse interaction. Therefore, patients with MIBC and the *FGFR3* mutation have better survival rates [62]. Another study suggests that also the progression in pT1 tumors is in negative correlation with the *FGFR3* mutation [63]. Many studies confirm that *FGFR3* mutations correlate with an overall benign effect [59,63,64]. Moreover, in the risk stratification, surveillance and diagnosis of low- or high-risk NMIBC patients, *FGFR3* mutations combined with the promoter hyper-methylation of *HS3ST2*, *SEPTIN9* and *SLIT2* have shown 97.6% sensitivity and 84.8% specificity (Table 1) [25]. The presence of the *FGFR3* mutation in urine is observed not only in low-grade tumors but it also seems to be associated with future recurrence [65,66].

FGFR3 is involved in tumorigenesis in ~40% of invasive bladder cancer and in the majority (~80%) of low-grade non-invasive (stage Ta) bladder cancers [59]. Tomlinson et al. observed an FGFR3 overexpression in nearly 40% of MIBC, whereas mutations occurred in 21% of MIBC [67]. Sung [56] observed that an FGFR3 overexpression results in the worst overall survival and disease-free survival in a group of patients with adjuvant chemotherapy. In a group without this treatment, no prognostic significance was observed.

High levels of FGFR3- and PIK3CA-mutated DNA in urine can be useful in predicting later metastasis and progression in NMIBC [68]. Choi et al. indicated that *FGFR3* mutations are characteristic for the luminal type of MIBC [69]. In conclusion, FGFR3 may be an important therapeutic target in both non-invasive and invasive BC [58,59].

In the results of their research, Beukers [60] confirmed that mutations in *FGFR3* were more often observed in low-grade tumors and the papillary urothelial neoplasm of low malignant potential (PUNLMP) + G1 (61.9%) than in high-grade tumors G2 + G3, at 17.2%. It was also observed that *FGFR3* mutations were more frequent in non-invasive tumors' Tis and Ta stages, at 53.4%, than in the invasive stages of T1 and T2, at 12.5%. Mutations correlated with a better survival rate and occurred in a higher level in non-invasive than in advanced diseases, and these values for TaG1, TaG2, TaG3 + T1 and T2 were 67.3%, 43.3%, 20.3% and 6.3% respectively. It was also noticed, but with no statistically significant correlation, that *FGFR3* mutations increase the possibility of disease recurrence [70]. Hosen et al. showed that *FGFR3* mutations have no significant influence on patient survival and that in the Ta, T1, TaG1 and TaG2 diseases, it did not significantly predict the recurrence rate [70].

Knowles et al. also demonstrated that the *FGFR3/HRAS* mutation was often present in the development of urothelial hyperplasia, which can progress to non-invasive papillary tumors with high recurrence rates via the FGFR3/RAS pathway [8].

Van Rhijn [63] conducted a study on a group of 132 patients with primary pT1 bladder cancer. The diagnosis was confirmed after a uropathologist review of the slides. *FGFR3* mutations were identified by a SNaPshot® analysis in 37 of 132 pT1 bladder cancer cases (28%) and an altered P53 expression was determined by standard immunohistochemistry in 71 of them (54%). Both molecular alternations were observed in 8% of patients. In predicting progression, carcinoma in situ and the status of the *FGFR3* mutation were significant but *TP53* was not. It was also mentioned that the presence of *FGFR3* mutations helps to identify patients who have a better disease prognosis because the *FGFR3* mutation occurs with lower grade and altered *TP53* with high-grade pT1 bladder cancer.

Hernández and colleagues [64] analyzed 772 samples from patients with bladder tumors reviewed by expert pathologists. Their results indicated that *FGFR3* mutations were more frequently observed in neoplasms with low malignant potential, at 77%, and in tumors TaG1, at 61%, and TaG2, at 58%, than in tumors TaG3, at 34%, and T1G3, at 17%. They also confirm the association between superficial tumors and a high presence of recurrence. Nevertheless, a significant increase risk was observed only in the group of patients with TaG1 tumors. In this study, another positive correlation of good prognosis and occupancy of FGFR3 was confirmed.

Kompier [71] performed a study on 118 patients with primary and recurrent NMI-BC. They analyzed the *FGFR3* mutation status in the disease process. The analyzed group had 2133 cystoscopies done within the median follow-up of 8.8 years and 414 tumor recurrences developed in 80 patients. *FGFR3* mutations were equally distributed in the recurrences and the primary tumors (63%). Different tumors may have a variety of *FGFR3* mutations types. Mutant or wild-type primary tumors had a similar risk of recurrence but in 81% of recurrences, a mutation was found. In this group, recurrences developed after 10 years and, in comparison with the wild-type primary tumor, occurred in a lower grade and stage.

Therefore, a follow-up surveillance based on the presence of the *FGFR3* mutation analysis with the reduction in the number of cystoscopies may be considered [71].

In another study, Kompier and colleagues [72] confirmed the correlations between a low risk of progression and better disease-specific survival in the primary mutant FGFR3 tumor and worse prognosis in the group of patients with an overexpression of p53.

Williams et al. found that in the selection of patients for the FGFR-targeted therapy, the existence of a fusion protein, which indicates other classes of mutations in a group with a high FGFR3 expression, may be helpful [58].

The study [73] shows that *FGFR3* mutations may influence tumorigenesis by regulating an acute inflammatory response which via the immune cells destroys the tumor cells. Therefore, there may be potential treatment strategy for the early stage of FGFR3-mutated or overexpressed BC based on the synchronal inhibition of FGFR3 and the immune modulators.

Noel [23] conducted a pilot study to assess the *TP53* and *FGFR3* mutations in urine and tumoral tissues samples that had been collected from 103 BC patients. Mutations in *TP53* were detected in 54% of the 103 bladder tumors and the distribution increased with the cellular grade ($p < 0.001$). The *TP53* mutation presented 34% of low- grade (LG) and 62% of high- grade (HG) tumors. The potential prognostic value of *TP53* may indicate a significant difference in the tumor stage ($p = 0.005$). The specificity was 87%, with the positive predictive value (PPV) 76% and with the negative predictive value (NPV) 53%. However, the sensitivity in the urine test was only 34% (Table 1).

In 36% of analyzed tumors, *FRFG3* mutations were identified and their distribution decreased with the cellular grade ($p < 0.001$). They occurred in 62% of LG tumors versus 26% in HG. A negative correlation was also between the *FGFR3* mutations and tumor stage ($p = 0.002$). All predictive capacities were better for the *FGFR3* than for the *TP53* mutations measured in this study, the sensitivity was 43% and the specificity was 98%, with the PPV 94% and the NPV 76% (Table 1) [23].

The results showed that TP53/FGFR3 could be useful as a complementary tool in diagnosis but could not replace urine cytology. The tumor stage and grade are strongly correlated with the *FGFR3* and *TP53* mutations, which are in "mirror distribution" [23].

Kang [24] enrolled 120 patients with primary pT1 BC and examined in this subgroup the utility of expression levels and mutation status of *FGFR3* as a prognostic marker. In this study, 40% of patients had *FGFR3* mutations and those patients also had significantly higher levels of the FGFR3 expression compared with the FGFR3 wild-type BC ($p < 0.001$). The mutation status was not associated with cancer progression, but a low level of FGFR3 correlated with cancer progression and HG tumors ($p = 0.001$ and $p = 0.006$). Therefore, the FGFR3 expression level was, in the multivariate analysis, identified as an independent predictor of cancer progression (Table 1). Significant was also the correlation between the *FGFR3* mutation and a low tumor grade. In tumor recurrence, both the *FGFR3* mutation status and mRNA expression level revealed no significant differences ($p = 0.264$ and $p = 0.856$, respectively).

In conclusion, FGFR3 may be used as a urine-based assay in the detection of primary tumors, recurrences, for prognosis and targeted therapies.

2.5. Tumor-Associated Trypsin Inhibitor (TATI)

TATI is a peptide produced at lower concentrations in many healthy tissues, especially in the gastrointestinal and urogenital tracts but also in the gall bladder, kidney and breast.

It occurs in high concentrations by several tumors such as gynecologic, gastrointestinal, urologic, lung, breast, head and neck cancers [74–79]. An increased level of TATI is also observed in renal failure and in dialysis patients because this peptide is cleared from the circulation by renal excretion. Therefore, a low glomerular filtration rate correlates with an increase in TATI [80].

TATI is connected with tumor aggression because it appears in the co-expression with tumor-associated trypsin, which participates in moderating tumor-associated protease cascades [81].

TATI is produced at high concentrations by mucinous ovarian tumors, and was initially isolated from the urine of a patient with ovarian cancer. The most useful clinical application of this peptide is observed in the detection of ovarian tumors: benign and malignant [82].

TATI occurs in a high level also in other benign and malignant diseases. Pancreatitis and strong acute phase reactions (when serum CRP is clearly increased (>90 mg/L)) such as severe injury or inflammatory diseases trigger a TATI expression. This fact is a limiting factor of the use of TATI as a tumor marker but it does not invalidate this peptide [83]. In cancers, an increased TATI concentration is associated not only with tumor production but also acute phase reactions caused by tissue destruction during cancer invasion [81].

Serum values of TATI have also been used in patients with muscle-invasive and metastatic transitional cell carcinoma, to monitor the response to therapy. In 1996, Pectasides [74] suggested that TATI might be potentially useful in monitoring the efficacy of treatment in transitional cell carcinoma of the bladder. Significantly modified values of TATI were observed in metastatic diseases, in patients with complete or partial remission and non-responders. An important increase in TATI in T2-T4-N0M0 tumors were in the non-responders.

Kelloniemi et al. showed that for the identification group of patients with adverse prognosis in transitional cell carcinoma serum, TATI might be an independent prognostic factor [84].

Shariat [85] indicated that TATI is more specific than NMP22 for the detection of bladder transitional cell carcinoma (TCC). They showed also that higher levels of TATI were in TCC patients and in more invasive stages.

In 2006, Hotakainen [86] reported that a TATI expression was observed in all non-invasive tumors and benign tissues, but the expression was lower in the muscle-invasive tumors. Therefore, they concluded that the TATI expression decreases with the rising stage and grade of the tumor in bladder cancer. Therefore, as for TATI, Shariat [85] showed that higher levels of TATI were associated with more invasive TCC but Hotakainen [86] revealed that the TATI expression decreases with the rising stage. The discrepancy between the results of the studies is most probably related to the different populations of bladder cancer patients. The study by Shariat [85], comprised of 153 consecutive patients who had a history of previous, histologically confirmed bladder cancer, without evidence of muscle invasion (stages Ta, T1 and/or CIS). In the Hotakainen ($n = 28$) group, the individuals were affected with both non-invasive and invasive BC.

Gkialas [27] showed that TATI was significantly more sensitive in stage Ta (80%) than was CYFRA 21-1 (32%), UBC (12%) and cytology (20%). TATI was different also between stages and was more sensitive compared with other tumor markers for stage T1.

Patschan and colleagues [87] confirmed that the TATI level shows a positive correlation with low-stage tumors and the favorable differentiation of bladder cancer. They also showed in univariate analyses, that a decreased level of TATI was associated with high recurrences and cancer-specific mortality.

Liu [26] made a similar conclusion that a decrease in the TATI expression correlated with a more advanced disease. Moreover, in the progression of bladder cancer, the prognostic value of a p53 overexpression can be enhanced by TATI.

Bladder cancer management is one of the most complex and expensive in uro-oncology. An ideal biomarker of the future should be potentially able to detect the disease before its clinical manifestation. The BC mortality rate is another major reason to obtain a similar screening method to that available in other cancers, i.e., prostate and colon.

Currently, flexible cystoscopy remains a mainstay in BC diagnosis and it appears unlikely that available biomarkers would quickly rule out this standard approach in clinical practice. On the other hand, developing markers showing a correlation with cancer aggressiveness and being able to distinguish between aggressive and non-aggressive tumors appears of utmost clinical importance. Hopefully, one of the discussed markers might become helpful in patients' selection for an appropriate treatment plan and personalized cancer medicine. The prospective studies on a larger group of individuals are still needed in order to obtain additional prognostic information that will improve results, reduce adverse effects and in future allow us to individualize bladder cancer treatments.

Author Contributions: All authors made substantial contributions to this work; acquisition and interpretation of data by online search, M.S., M.M.; draft and supervision of the work, M.S.; revision of the work, M.S. All authors have approved the final version and agree to be personally accountable for the author's own contributions.

Funding: This research received no external funding.

Conflicts of Interest: The authors declare no conflict of interest.

Abbreviations

AUC	Area under the curve
BC	Bladder cancer
BCG	Bacille Calmette–Guérin
CIS	Carcinoma in situ
CK	Cytokeratin
CSS	Cancer-specific survival
CYFRA 21.1	Cytokeratin fragment 21.1
DFS	Disease-free survival
ERCC1	Excision repair cross-complementing group 1
HG	High grade
IHC	Immunohistochemistry staining
LG	Low grade
MIBC	Muscle-invasive bladder cancer
NMIBC	Non-muscle invasive bladder cancer
NPV	Negative predictive value
OS	Overall survival
PFS	Progression-free survival
PPV	Positive predictive value
PUNLMP	Papillary urothelial neoplasm of low malignant potential
TURBT	Transurethral resection of bladder tumor
UBC	Urothelial bladder cancer
UC	Urothelial carcinoma

References

1. Siegel, R.L.; Miller, K.D.; Jemal, A. Cancer statistics, 2020. *CA A Cancer J. Clin.* **2020**, *70*, 7–30. [CrossRef]
2. Antoni, S.; Ferlay, J.; Soerjomataram, I.; Znaor, A.; Jemal, A.; Bray, F. Bladder cancer incidence and mortality: A global overview and recent trends. *Eur. Urol.* **2017**, *71*, 96–108. [CrossRef] [PubMed]
3. Sanli, O.; Dobruch, J.; Knowles, M.A.; Burger, M.; Alemozaffar, M.; Nielsen, M.E.; Lotan, Y. Bladder cancer. *Nat. Rev. Dis. Primers* **2017**, *3*, 1–19. [CrossRef] [PubMed]
4. Robertson, A.G.; Kim, J.; Al-Ahmadie, H.; Bellmunt, J.; Guo, G.; Cherniack, A.D.; Hinoue, T.; Laird, P.W.; Hoadley, K.A.; Akbani, R.; et al. Comprehensive molecular characterization of muscle-invasive bladder cancer. *Cell* **2017**, *171*, 540–556. [CrossRef] [PubMed]
5. Humphrey, P.A.; Moch, H.; Cubilla, A.L.; Ulbright, T.M.; Reuter, V.E. The 2016 WHO classification of tumours of the urinary system and male genital organs—Part B: Prostate and bladder tumours. *Eur. Urol.* **2016**, *70*, 106–119. [CrossRef]
6. Czerniak, B.; Dinney, C.; McConkey, D. Origins of bladder cancer. *Annu. Rev. Pathol. Mech. Dis.* **2016**, *11*, 149–174. [CrossRef]
7. Babjuk, M.; Burger, M.; Zigeuner, R.; Shariat, S.F.; van Rhijn, B.W.G.; Compérat, E.; Sylvester, R.J.; Kaasinen, E.; Böhle, A.; Redorta, J.P.; et al. EAU Guidelines on Non–Muscle-invasive urothelial carcinoma of the bladder: Update 2013. *Eur. Urol.* **2013**, *64*, 639–653. [CrossRef]
8. Knowles, M.A.; Hurst, C.D. Molecular biology of bladder cancer: New insights into pathogenesis and clinical diversity. *Nat. Rev. Cancer* **2014**, *15*, 25–41. [CrossRef]
9. Inamura, K. Bladder cancer: New insights into its molecular pathology. *Cancers* **2018**, *10*, 100. [CrossRef]
10. Burger, M.; Catto, J.W.F.; Dalbagni, G.; Grossman, H.B.; Herr, H.; Karakiewicz, P.; Kassouf, W.; Kiemeney, L.A.; Vecchia, C.L.; Shariat, S.; et al. Epidemiology and risk factors of urothelial bladder cancer. *Eur. Urol.* **2013**, *63*, 234–241. [CrossRef]
11. Woldu, S.L.; Bagrodia, A.; Lotan, Y. Guideline of guidelines: Non-muscle-invasive bladder cancer. *BJU Int.* **2017**, *119*, 371–380. [CrossRef] [PubMed]
12. Huang, Y.-L.; Chen, J.; Yan, W.; Zang, D.; Qin, Q.; Deng, A.-M. Diagnostic accuracy of cytokeratin-19 fragment (CYFRA 21–1) for bladder cancer: a systematic review and meta-analysis. *Tumor Biol.* **2015**, *36*, 3137–3145. [CrossRef] [PubMed]

13. Guo, X.-G.; Long, J.-J. Cytokeratin-19 fragment in the diagnosis of bladder carcinoma. *Tumor Biol.* **2016**, *37*, 14329–14330. [CrossRef] [PubMed]

14. Kuang, L.I.; Song, W.J.; Qing, H.M.; Yan, S.; Song, F.L. CYFRA21-1 levels could be a biomarker for bladder cancer: A meta-analysis. *Genet. Mol. Res.* **2015**, *14*, 3921–3931. [CrossRef]

15. Nisman, B.; Barak, V.; Shapiro, A.; Golijanin, D.; Peretz, T.; Pode, D. Evaluation of urine CYFRA 21-1 for the detection of primary and recurrent bladder carcinoma. *Cancer* **2002**, *94*, 2914–2922. [CrossRef]

16. D'Costa, J.J.; Goldsmith, J.C.; Wilson, J.S.; Bryan, R.T.; Ward, D.G. A systematic review of the diagnostic and prognostic value of urinary protein biomarkers in urothelial bladder cancer. *Bladder Cancer* **2016**, *2*, 301–317. [CrossRef]

17. Andreadis, C.; Touloupidis, S.; Galaktidou, G.; Kortsaris, A.H.; Boutis, A.; Mouratidou, D. Serum CYFRA 21–1 in patients with invasive bladder cancer and its relevance as a tumor marker during chemotherapy. *J. Urol.* **2005**, *174*, 1771–1776. [CrossRef]

18. Nisman, B.; Yutkin, V.; Peretz, T.; Shapiro, A.; Barak, V.; Pode, D. The follow-up of patients with non-muscle-invasive bladder cancer by urine cytology, abdominal ultrasound and urine CYFRA 21-1: A pilot study. *Anticancer Res.* **2009**, *29*, 4281–4285.

19. Washino, S.; Hirai, M.; Matsuzaki, A.; Kobayashi, Y. Clinical usefulness of CEA, CA19-9, and CYFRA 21-1 as tumor markers for urothelial bladder carcinoma. *Urol. Int.* **2011**, *87*, 420–428. [CrossRef]

20. Dittadi, R.; Barioli, P.; Gion, M.; Mione, R.; Barichello, M.; Capitanio, G.; Cocco, G.; Cazzolato, G.; De Biasi, F.; Praturlon, S.; et al. Standardization of assay for cytokeratin-related tumor marker CYFRA21.1 in urine samples. *Clin. Chem.* **1996**, *42*, 1634–1638. [CrossRef]

21. Jeong, S.; Park, Y.; Cho, Y.; Kim, Y.R.; Kim, H.-S. Diagnostic values of urine CYFRA21-1, NMP22, UBC, and FDP for the detection of bladder cancer. *Clin. Chim. Acta* **2012**, *414*, 93–100. [CrossRef] [PubMed]

22. Klatte, T.; Seitz, C.; Rink, M.; Rouprêt, M.; Xylinas, E.; Karakiewicz, P.; Susani, M.; Shariat, S.F. ERCC1 as a prognostic and predictive biomarker for urothelial carcinoma of the bladder following radical cystectomy. *J. Urol.* **2015**, *194*, 1456–1462. [CrossRef] [PubMed]

23. Noel, N.; Couteau, J.; Maillet, G.; Gobet, F.; D'Aloisio, F.; Minier, C.; Pfister, C. TP53 and FGFR3 Gene mutation assessment in urine: Pilot study for bladder cancer diagnosis. *Anticancer Res.* **2015**, *35*, 4915–4921. [PubMed]

24. Kang, H.W.; Kim, Y.-H.; Jeong, P.; Park, C.; Kim, W.T.; Ryu, D.H.; Cha, E.-J.; Ha, Y.-S.; Kim, T.-H.; Kwon, T.G.; et al. Expression levels of FGFR3 as a prognostic marker for the progression of primary pT1 bladder cancer and its association with mutation status. *Oncol. Lett.* **2017**, *14*, 3817–3824. [CrossRef] [PubMed]

25. Roperch, J.-P.; Grandchamp, B.; Desgrandchamps, F.; Mongiat-Artus, P.; Ravery, V.; Ouzaid, I.; Roupret, M., Phe, V.; Ciofu, C.; Tubach, F.; et al. Promoter hypermethylation of HS3ST2, SEPTIN9 and SLIT2 combined with FGFR3 mutations as a sensitive/specific urinary assay for diagnosis and surveillance in patients with low or high-risk non-muscle-invasive bladder cancer. *BMC Cancer* **2016**, *16*, 704. [CrossRef]

26. Liu, A.; Xue, Y.; Liu, F.; Tan, H.; Xiong, Q.; Zeng, S.; Zhang, Z.; Gao, X.; Sun, Y.; Xu, C. Prognostic value of the combined expression of tumor-associated trypsin inhibitor (TATI) and p53 in patients with bladder cancer undergoing radical cystectomy. *Cancer Biomark.* **2019**, *26*, 281–289. [CrossRef]

27. Gkialas, I.; Papadopoulos, G.; Iordanidou, L.; Stathouros, G.; Tzavara, C.; Gregorakis, A.; Lykourinas, M. Evaluation of urine tumor-associated trypsin inhibitor, CYFRA 21-1, and urinary bladder cancer antigen for detection of high-grade bladder Carcinoma. *Urology* **2008**, *72*, 1159–1163. [CrossRef]

28. Rabik, C.A.; Dolan, M.E. Molecular mechanisms of resistance and toxicity associated with platinating agents. *Cancer Treat. Rev.* **2007**, *33*, 9–23. [CrossRef]

29. Martin, L.P.; Hamilton, T.C.; Schilder, R.J. Platinum resistance: The role of DNA repair pathways. *Clin. Cancer Res.* **2008**, *14*, 1291–1295. [CrossRef]

30. Metzger, R.; Bollschweiler, E.; Hölscher, A.H.; Warnecke-Eberz, U. ERCC1: Impact in multimodality treatment of upper gastrointestinal cancer. *Future Oncol.* **2010**, *6*, 1735–1749. [CrossRef]

31. Olaussen, K.A.; Dunant, A.; Fouret, P.; Brambilla, E.; André, F.; Haddad, V.; Taranchon, E.; Filipits, M.; Pirker, R.; Popper, H.H.; et al. DNA repair by ERCC1 in Non–Small-Cell Lung Cancer and Cisplatin-Based Adjuvant Chemotherapy. *N. Engl. J. Med.* **2006**, *355*, 983–991. [CrossRef] [PubMed]

32. Simon, G.R.; Sharma, S.; Cantor, A.; Smith, P.; Bepler, G. ERCC1 expression is a predictor of survival in resected patients with non-small cell lung cancer. *Chest* **2005**, *127*, 978–983. [CrossRef] [PubMed]

33. Rosell, R.; Pifarré, A.; Monzó, M.; Astudillo, J.; López-Cabrerizo, M.P.; Calvo, R.; Moreno, I.; Sánchez-Céspedes, M.; Font, A.; Navas-Palacios, J.J. Reduced survival in patients with stage-I non-small-cell lung cancer associated with DNA-replication errors. *Int. J. Cancer* **1997**, *74*, 330–334. [CrossRef]

34. Eldehna, W.M.; Fouda, M.M.; Eteba, S.M.; Abdelrahim, M.; Elashry, M.S. Gene expression of excision repair cross-complementation group 1 enzyme as a novel predictive marker in patients receiving platinum-based chemotherapy in advanced bladder cancer. *Benha Med. J.* **2018**, *35*, 42–48. [CrossRef]

35. Piljić Burazer, M.; Mladinov, S.; Matana, A.; Kuret, S.; Bezić, J.; Glavina Durdov, M. Low ERCC1 expression is a good predictive marker in lung adenocarcinoma patients receiving chemotherapy based on platinum in all TNM stages—A single-center study. *Diagn. Pathol.* **2019**, *14*, 105. [CrossRef]

36. Li, Z.; Qing, Y.; Guan, W.; Li, M.; Peng, Y.; Zhang, S.; Xiong, Y.; Wang, D. Predictive value of APE1, BRCA1, ERCC1 and TUBB3 expression in patients with advanced non-small cell lung cancer (NSCLC) receiving first-line platinum–paclitaxel chemotherapy. *Cancer Chemother. Pharmacol.* **2014**, *74*, 777–786. [CrossRef]

37. Facista, A.; Nguyen, H.; Lewis, C.; Prasad, A.R.; Ramsey, L.; Zaitlin, B.; Nfonsam, V.; Krouse, R.S.; Bernstein, H.; Payne, C.M.; et al. Deficient expression of DNA repair enzymes in early progression to sporadic colon cancer. *Genome Integr.* **2012**, *3*, 3. [CrossRef]

38. Smith, D.H.; Fiehn, A.-M.K.; Fogh, L.; Christensen, I.J.; Hansen, T.P.; Stenvang, J.; Nielsen, H.J.; Nielsen, K.V.; Hasselby, J.P.; Brünner, N.; et al. Measuring ERCC1 protein expression in cancer specimens: Validation of a novel antibody. *Sci. Rep.* **2014**, *4*, 4313. [CrossRef]

39. Sun, J.-M.; Sung, J.-Y.; Park, S.H.; Kwon, G.Y.; Jeong, B.C.; Seo, S.I.; Jeon, S.S.; Lee, H.M.; Jo, J.; Choi, H.Y.; et al. ERCC1 as a biomarker for bladder cancer patients likely to benefit from adjuvant chemotherapy. *BMC Cancer* **2012**, *12*, 187. [CrossRef]

40. Hemdan, T.; Segersten, U.; Malmström, P.-U. 122 ERCC1-negative tumors benefit from neoadjuvant cisplatin-based chemotherapy whereas patients with ERCC1-positive tumors do not—Results from a cystectomy trial database. *Eur. Urol. Suppl.* **2014**, *13*, e122. [CrossRef]

41. Urun, Y.; Leow, J.J.; Fay, A.P.; Albiges, L.; Choueiri, T.K.; Bellmunt, J. ERCC1 as a prognostic factor for survival in patients with advanced urothelial cancer treated with platinum based chemotherapy: A systematic review and meta-analysis. *Crit. Rev. Oncol. Hematol.* **2017**, *120*, 120–126. [CrossRef] [PubMed]

42. Sakano, S.; Ogawa, S.; Yamamoto, Y.; Nishijima, J.; Miyachika, Y.; Matsumoto, H.; Hara, T.; Matsuyama, H. ERCC1 and XRCC1 expression predicts survival in bladder cancer patients receiving combined trimodality therapy. *Mol. Clin. Oncol.* **2013**, *1*, 403–410. [CrossRef] [PubMed]

43. Chen, L.; Liu, Y.; Zhang, Q.; Zhang, M.; Han, X.; Li, Q.; Xie, T.; Wu, Q.; Sui, X. p53/PCDH17/Beclin-1 proteins as prognostic predictors for urinary bladder cancer. *J. Cancer* **2019**, *10*, 6207–6216. [CrossRef] [PubMed]

44. Choundhury, S.; Kolukula, V.; Preet, A.; Albanese, C.; Maria, A. Dissecting the pathways that destabilize mutant p53: The proteasome or autophagy? *Cell Cycle* **2013**, *12*, 1022–1029. [CrossRef]

45. Zhou, G.; Wang, J.; Zhao, M.; Xie, T.-X.; Tanaka, N.; Sano, D.; Patel, A.A.; Ward, A.M.; Sandulache, V.C.; Jasser, S.A.; et al. Gain-of-function mutant p53 promotes cell growth and cancer cell metabolism via inhibition of AMPK activation. *Mol. Cell* **2014**, *54*, 960–974. [CrossRef]

46. Mitra, A.P. Molecular substratification of bladder cancer: Moving towards individualized patient management. *Ther. Adv. Urol.* **2016**, *8*, 215–233. [CrossRef]

47. Ando, K.; Oki, E.; Saeki, H.; Yan, Z.; Tsuda, Y.; Hidaka, G.; Kasagi, Y.; Otsu, H.; Kawano, H.; Kitao, H.; et al. Discrimination of p53 immunohistochemistry-positive tumors by its staining pattern in gastric cancer. *Cancer Medicine* **2014**, *4*, 75–83. [CrossRef]

48. Puzio-Kuter, A.M.; Castillo-Martin, M.; Kinkade, C.W.; Wang, X.; Shen, T.H.; Matos, T.; Shen, M.M.; Cordon-Cardo, C.; Abate-Shen, C. Inactivation of p53 and Pten promotes invasive bladder cancer. *Genes Dev.* **2009**, *23*, 675–680. [CrossRef]

49. Shariat, S.F.; Chade, D.C.; Karakiewicz, P.I.; Ashfaq, R.; Isbarn, H.; Fradet, Y.; Bastian, P.J.; Nielsen, M.E.; Capitanio, U.; Jeldres, C. Combination of multiple molecular markers can improve prognostication in patients with locally advanced and lymph node positive bladder cancer. *J. Urol.* **2010**, *183*, 68–75. [CrossRef]

50. Daizumoto, K.; Yoshimaru, T.; Matsushita, Y.; Fukawa, T.; Uehara, H.; Ono, M.; Komatsu, M.; Kanayama, H.; Katagiri, T. A DDX31/Mutant–p53/EGFR axis promotes multistep progression of muscle-invasive bladder cancer. *Cancer Res.* **2018**, *78*, 2233–2247. [CrossRef]

51. Qamar, S.; Inam, Q.A.; Ashraf, S.; Khan, M.S.; Khokhar, M.A.; Awan, N. Prognostic Value of p53 expression intensity in urothelial cancers. *J. Coll. Physicians Surg. Pak.* **2017**, *27*, 232–236. [PubMed]

52. Ciccarese, C.; Massari, F.; Blanca, A.; Tortora, G.; Montironi, R.; Cheng, L.; Scarpelli, M.; Raspollini, M.R.; Vau, N.; Fonseca, J.; et al. Tp53 and its potential therapeutic role as a target in bladder cancer. *Expert Opin. Ther. Targets* **2017**, *21*, 401–414. [CrossRef] [PubMed]

53. Du, J.; Wang, S.; Yang, Q.; Chen, Q.; Yao, X. p53 status correlates with the risk of progression in stage T1 bladder cancer: A meta-analysis. *World J. Surg. Oncol.* **2016**, *14*, 137. [CrossRef] [PubMed]

54. Shariat, S.F.; Lotan, Y.; Karakiewicz, P.I.; Ashfaq, R.; Isbarn, H.; Fradet, Y.; Bastian, P.J.; Nielsen, M.E.; Capitanio, U.; Jeldres, C.; et al. p53 predictive value for pT1-2 N0 disease at radical cystectomy. *J. Urol.* **2009**, *182*, 907–913. [CrossRef] [PubMed]

55. Moch, H.; Cubilla, A.L.; Humphrey, P.A.; Reuter, V.E.; Ulbright, T.M. The 2016 WHO classification of tumours of the urinary system and male genital organs—Part A: Renal, penile, and testicular tumours. *Eur. Urol.* **2016**, *70*, 93–105. [CrossRef] [PubMed]

56. Sung, J.-Y.; Sun, J.-M.; Chang Jeong, B.; Il Seo, S.; Soo Jeon, S.; Moo Lee, H.; Choi, H.Y.; Kang, S.Y.; Choi, Y.-L.; Young Kwon, G. FGFR3 overexpression is prognostic of adverse outcome for muscle-invasive bladder carcinoma treated with adjuvant chemotherapy11This work was supported by Grant CB-2011-04-01 from Korean Foundation for Cancer Research grant and by a Global Frontier Project Grant (NRF-M1AXA002-2010-0029795) of the National Research Foundation funded by the Ministry of Education, Science and Technology of Korea. *Urol. Oncol. Semin. Orig. Investig.* **2014**, *32*, 49.e23–49.e31. [CrossRef]

57. Akanksha, M.; Sandhya, S. Role of FGFR3 in Urothelial Carcinoma. *Iran. J. Pathol.* **2019**, *14*, 148–155. [CrossRef]

58. Williams, S.V.; Hurst, C.D.; Knowles, M.A. Oncogenic FGFR3 gene fusions in bladder cancer. *Hum. Mol. Genet.* **2012**, *22*, 795–803. [CrossRef]

59. Di Martino, E.; Tomlinson, D.C.; Knowles, M.A. A decade of FGF receptor research in bladder cancer: Past, present, and future challenges. *Adv. Urol.* **2012**, *2012*, 1–10. [CrossRef]

60. Beukers, W.; van der Keur, K.A.; Kandimalla, R.; Vergouwe, Y.; Steyerberg, E.W.; Boormans, J.L.; Jensen, J.B.; Lorente, J.A.; Real, F.X.; Segersten, U.; et al. FGFR3, TERT and OTX1 as a urinary biomarker combination for surveillance of patients with bladder cancer in a large prospective multicenter study. *J. Urol.* **2017**, *197*, 1410–1418. [CrossRef]

61. Hurst, C.D.; Knowles, M.A. Multiomic profiling refines the molecular view. *Nat. Rev. Clin. Oncol.* **2017**, *15*, 203–204. [CrossRef] [PubMed]

62. Van Oers, J.M.M.; Zwarthoff, E.C.; Rehman, I.; Azzouzi, A.-R.; Cussenot, O.; Meuth, M.; Hamdy, F.C.; Catto, J.W.F. FGFR3 mutations indicate better survival in invasive upper urinary tract and bladder tumours. *Eur. Urol.* **2009**, *55*, 650–658. [CrossRef] [PubMed]

63. Van Rhijn, B.W.G.; van der Kwast, T.H.; Liu, L.; Fleshner, N.E.; Bostrom, P.J.; Vis, A.N.; Alkhateeb, S.S.; Bangma, C.H.; Jewett, M.A.S.; Zwarthoff, E.C.; et al. The FGFR3 mutation is related to favorable pT1 bladder cancer. *J. Urol.* **2012**, *187*, 310–314. [CrossRef] [PubMed]

64. Hernandez, S.; Lopez-Knowles, E.; Lloreta, J.; Kogevinas, M.; Amorós, A.; Tardón, A.; Carrato, A.; Serra, C.; Malats, N.; Real, F.X. Prospective study of fgfr3 mutations as a prognostic factor in nonmuscle invasive urothelial bladder carcinomas. *J. Clin. Oncol.* **2006**, *24*, 3664–3671. [CrossRef]

65. Critelli, R.; Fasanelli, F.; Oderda, M.; Polidoro, S.; Assumma, M.B.; Viberti, C.; Preto, M.; Gontero, P.; Cucchiarale, G.; Lurkin, I.; et al. Detection of multiple mutations in urinary exfoliated cells from male bladder cancer patients at diagnosis and during follow-up. *Oncotarget* **2016**, *7*, 67435. [CrossRef]

66. Frantzi, M.; Makridakis, M.; Vlahou, A. Biomarkers for bladder cancer aggressiveness. *Curr. Opin. Urol.* **2012**, *22*, 390–396. [CrossRef]

67. Tomlinson, D.; Baldo, O.; Harnden, P.; Knowles, M. FGFR3 protein expression and its relationship to mutation status and prognostic variables in bladder cancer. *J. Pathol.* **2007**, *213*, 91–98. [CrossRef]

68. Christensen, E.; Birkenkamp-Demtröder, K.; Nordentoft, I.; Høyer, S.; van der Keur, K.; van Kessel, K.; Dyrskjøt, L. Liquid biopsy analysis of FGFR3 and PIK3CA hotspot mutations for disease surveillance in bladder cancer. *Eur. Urol.* **2017**, *71*, 961–969. [CrossRef]

69. Choi, W.; Porten, S.; Kim, S.; Willis, D.; Plimack, E.R.; Hoffman-Censits, J.; McConkey, D.J. Identification of distinct basal and luminal subtypes of muscle-invasive bladder cancer with different sensitivities to frontline chemotherapy. *Cancer Cell* **2014**, *25*, 152–165. [CrossRef]

70. Hosen, I.; Rachakonda, P.S.; Heidenreich, B.; de Verdier, P.J.; Ryk, C.; Steineck, G.; Hemminki, K.; Kumar, R. Mutations inTERTpromoter andFGFR3and telomere length in bladder cancer. *Int. J. Cancer* **2015**, *137*, 1621–1629. [CrossRef]

71. Kompier, L.C.; van der Aa, M.N.; Lurkin, I.; Vermeij, M.; Kirkels, W.J.; Bangma, C.H.; van der Kwast, T.H.; Zwarthoff, E.C. The development of multiple bladder tumour recurrences in relation to the FGFR3mutation status of the primary tumour. *J. Pathol.* **2009**, *218*, 104–112. [CrossRef] [PubMed]

72. Kompier, L.C.; Lurkin, I.; van der Aa, M.N.M.; van Rhijn, B.W.G.; van der Kwast, T.H.; Zwarthoff, E.C. FGFR3, HRAS, KRAS, NRAS and PIK3CA mutations in bladder cancer and their potential as biomarkers for surveillance and therapy. *PLoS ONE* **2010**, *5*, e13821. [CrossRef] [PubMed]

73. Foth, M.; Ismail, N.F.B.; Kung, J.S.C.; Tomlinson, D.; Knowles, M.A.; Eriksson PIwata, T. FGFR3 mutation increases bladder tumourigenesis by suppressing acute inflammation. *J. Pathol.* **2018**, *246*, 331–343. [CrossRef] [PubMed]

74. Pectasides, D.; Bafaloucos, D.; Antoniou, F.; Gogou, L.; Economides, N.; Varthalitis, J.; Athanassiou, A. TPA, TATI, CEA, AFP, β-HCG, PSA, SCC, and CA 19-9 for monitoring transitional cell carcinoma of the bladder. *Am. J. Clin. Oncol.* **1996**, *19*, 271–277. [CrossRef]

75. Järvisalo, J.; Hakama, M.; Knekt, P.; Stenman, U.H.; Leino, A.; Teppo, L.; Maatela, J.; Aromaa, A. Serum tumor markers CEA, CA 50, TATI, and NSE in lung cancer screening. *Lung Cancer* **1993**, *10*, 276. [CrossRef]

76. Sjöström, J.; Alfthan, H.; Joensuu, H.; Stenman, U.; Lundin, J.; Blomqvist, C. Serum tumour markers CA 15-3, TPA, TPS, hCG β and TATI in the monitoring of chemotherapy response in metastatic breast cancer. *Scand. J. Clin. Lab. Investig.* **2001**, *61*, 431–441. [CrossRef]

77. Paavonen, J.; Lehtinen, M.; Lehto, M.; Laine, S.; Aine, R.; Räsänen, L.; Stenman, U.H. Concentrations of tumor-associated trypsin inhibitor and C-reactive protein in serum in acute pelvic inflammatory disease. *Clin. Chem.* **1989**, *35*, 869–871. [CrossRef]

78. Lasson, Å.; Borgström, A.; Ohlsson, K. Elevated pancreatic secretory trypsin inhibitor levels during severe inflammatory disease, renal insufficiency, and after various surgical procedures. *Scand. J. Gastroenterol.* **1986**, *21*, 1275–1280. [CrossRef]

79. Huhtala, M.-L.; Kahanpää, K.; Seppää, M.; Halila, H.; Stenman, U.-H. Excretion of a tumor-associated trypsin inhibitor (TATI) in urine of patients with gynecological malignancy. *Int. J. Cancer* **1983**, *31*, 711–714. [CrossRef]

80. Goumas, P.D.; Mastronikolis, N.S.; Mastorakou, A.N.; Vassilakos, P.J.; Nikiforidis, G.C. Evaluation of TATI and CYFRA 21-1 in patients with head and neck squamous cell carcinoma. *ORL* **1997**, *59*, 106–114. [CrossRef]

81. Tramonti, P.G.; Ferdeghini, M.; Donadio, C.; Annichiarico, C.; Norpoth, M.; Bianchi, R.; Bianchi, C. Serum levels of tumor associated trypsin inhibitor (TATT) and glomerular filtration rate. *Ren. Fail.* **1998**, *20*, 295–302. [CrossRef] [PubMed]

82. Stenman, U.-H.; Koivunen, E.; Itkonen, O. Biology and function of tumor-associated trypsin inhibitor, tati. *Scand. J. Clin. Lab. Investig.* **1991**, *51*, 5–9. [CrossRef] [PubMed]

83. Stenman, U.-H. Tumor-associated trypsin inhibitor. *Clin. Chem.* **2002**, *48*, 1206–1209. [CrossRef] [PubMed]

84. Kelloniemi, E.; Rintala, E.; Finne, P.; Stenman, U.-H. Tumor-associated trypsin inhibitor as a prognostic factor during follow-up of bladder cancer. *Urology* **2003**, *62*, 249–253. [CrossRef]

85. Shariat, S.F.; Herman, M.P.; Casella, R.; Lotan, Y.; Karam, J.A.; Stenman, U.-H. Urinary levels of tumor-associated trypsin inhibitor (TATI) in the detection of transitional cell carcinoma of the urinary bladder. *Eur. Urol.* **2005**, *48*, 424–431. [CrossRef]

86. Hotakainen, K.; Bjartell, A.; Sankila, A.; Järvinen, R.; Paju, A.; Rintala, E.; Haglund, C.; Stenman, U.-H. Differential expression of trypsinogen and tumor-associated trypsin inhibitor (TATI) in bladder cancer. *Int. J. Oncol.* **2006**, *28*, 95–101. [CrossRef]

87. Patschan, O.; Shariat, S.F.; Chade, D.C.; Karakiewicz, P.I.; Ashfaq, R.; Lotan, Y.; Hotakainen, K.; Stenman, U.-H.; Bjartell, A. Association of tumor-associated trypsin inhibitor (TATI) expression with molecular markers, pathologic features and clinical outcomes of urothelial carcinoma of the urinary bladder. *World J. Urol.* **2011**, *30*, 785–794. [CrossRef]

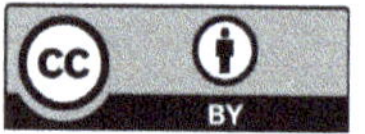

MDPI

St. Alban-Anlage 66

4052 Basel

Switzerland

Tel. +41 61 683 77 34

Fax +41 61 302 89 18

www.mdpi.com

International Journal of Molecular Sciences Editorial Office

E-mail: ijms@mdpi.com

www.mdpi.com/journal/ijms

9 783039 436859